Cardiovascular Disease II

Cardiovascular Disease II

Publisher: iConcept Press Ltd.
Cover design: Pineapple Design Ltd.
Interior design: iConcept Press Ltd.
Typesetting and copy editing: iConcept Press Ltd. and Pineapple Design Ltd.

ISBN: 978-1-922227-577

Printed in the United States of America

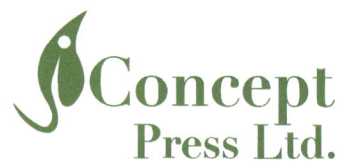

iConcept
Press Ltd.

www.iconceptpress.com

Contents

Preface

Cardiovascular disease is a class of diseases that involve the heart or blood vessels, such as arteries, capillaries and veins. Cardiovascular diseases remain the biggest cause of deaths worldwide, though over the last two decades, cardiovascular mortality rates have declined in many high-income countries. At the same time, cardiovascular deaths and disease have increased at a fast rate in low- and middle-income countries. The causes of cardiovascular disease are diverse but atherosclerosis and/or hypertension are the most common ones.

This book is targeted for researchers, scholars or other health care providers who need a ready reference for cardiovascular disease ranging from causes, signs and symptoms, and diagnosis through treatment and special considerations. There are two volumes. This book is the second volume.

There are totally 13 chapters in this book. Chapter 1 reviews the signs and symptoms of heat stress illnesses, and discusses a formula for heat stress evaluation, discusses guidelines for screening, reviews accommodations for those persons working or playing with physical incapacity and specific illness in hot environments. In addition, it also discusses prevention of heat illness. Chapter 2 shows the effects of different exercises on the cardiovascular system in elderly people. Aerobic exercise is the most known and recommended for prevention, control and treatment of cardiovascular diseases, especially, the hypertension. Yet, the resistance training with low intensity has also present satisfactory results for the hypotensive effect after exercise. Thus, the aerobic and resistance exercises may have a potential protective non-pharmacological effect and also in the associated treatment for diseases such as hypertension. Chapter 3 describes recent evidence of exercise therapy in the prevention of sarcopenia, glucocorticoid caused myopathy and in case of skeletal muscle unloading. The relationships between the muscle contractile and mitochondrial apparatus and the role of oxidative capacity in energy metabolism of skeletal and cardiac muscle, also the extracellular matrix in aging muscle are under the attention. Chapter 4 discusses the spatio-temporal evolution of simultaneously recorded voltage and calcium alternans in the heart. It also discusses whether voltage and calcium alternans can be predicted using slopes of restitution curves.

Chapter 5 deals with the evaluation of the effect of storage under various conditions on the concentrations of diagnostically most important bovine acute phase proteins. These proteins are quantified for diagnostic or monitoring purposes, which demands precise measurement of their concentrations and analytical stability. Chapter 6 reviews the current status of HCM molecular genetics. It addresses the importance of transcriptomics for revealing new diagnostic and therapeutic biomarkers and bioinformatic approaches to improve the translation between the bench and the clinic. Chapter 7 focuses on the role of the immune-system in glaucoma, with special attention on the activation of glial cells from the retina and the increased antigen-presenting activity in macro- and macroglía cells both, in the contralateral (normotensive) and hypertensive eyes of unilateral experimental ocular hypertension. Chapter 8 describes the relationships between severity of hypocholesterolemia, abnormalities of plasma amino acids, severity of hypercatabolism and organ dysfunction, and extreme metabolic disruption in trauma patients with sepsis. It provides further concepts for the interpretation and the practical clinical implications of hypocholesterolemia in human sepsis.

Chapter 9 summarizes recent advances in cyclic nucleotide signaling and its capacity to control abnormal vascular smooth muscle growth in the context of cardiovascular disease. Topics covered include an overview of cyclic AMP and cyclic GMP signals in vascular smooth muscle, the role of newly described activators and stimulators of cyclic nucleotide signaling, and downstream targets of cyclic nucleotide signaling including kinases, growth factors, and matrix-related elements. Chapter 10 describes classifications of endoscopic injuries to the esophagus, the incidence of such burns as well as methods to try to reduce this injury. Chapter 11 proposes the role of autonomic nervous system (ANS), both ANS itself and after the remodeling of it, in atrial fibrillation. A great deal of evidence suggests that ANS plays a very important role in the initiation and maintenance of atrial fibrillation. In Chapter 12, an application of VCG for detection of cardiac ischemia is explained, a synthesized VCG from standard 12-lead ECG signal is constructed, and a new method to convert a VCG to ECG signals by using partial linear transformation is introduced.

Chapter 13 discusses cardiovascular disease in liver cirrhosis. The incidence of cardiovascular diseases in patients with liver cirrhosis is high, and vary according to the underlying cause of liver cirrhosis. Distinctive entities such as cirrhotic cardiomyopathy and a specific cardiovascular pattern limit the compensatory mechanisms to stressful situations. The knowledge of these specificities is fundamental to the cardiovascular approach of patient with liver cirrhosis.

Editing and publishing a book is never an easy task. Each chapter in this book has gone through a peer review, a selection and an editing process so as to guarantee its quality. Without the supports and contributions of the authors and reviewers, this book can never be able to complete. We would like to thank all of the authors in this book and all of the reviewers who participated in the reviewing process: Denis V Abramochkin, Stephen E. Alway, Deepak N. Amarapurkar, Ricardo Y Asano, M. Boerma, Bang V. Bui, Gideon Charach, C. Chelazzi, Kate E. Coldwell, Cihad Dündar, Bülent Elbasan, Cristina O Francisco, Basil O. Ibe, Eugène HJM Jansen, Mehrdad Javadi, Darren Joubert, Dowluru SVGK Kaladhar, Chang-Hyun Kang, Stylianos Karatapanis, Masanori Kawasaki, Shyam S Kothari, Praveen A. S. Kumar, Ismail Laher, Chiara Lazzeri, Xuan Li, Guillermo López-Lluch, William M. Mahoney, Ahmad M Mansour, Gareth D. K. Matthews, Paolo Melillo, Graeme F Nixon, Brian Olshansky, Koh Ono, Alberto Passi, Oscar Pérez-Méndez, Namakkal Soorappan Rajasekaran, David H Rehkopf, Ruth E. Rosenstein, Rasa Ruseckaite, Leonardo Sacconi, Kunihiro Sakuma, Yeon Seok Seo, M Bala Soudarssanane, Fumihiro Tomoda, Kai Wang, Yonghua Wang, Derek S. Wheeler, Jonathon M. Willets, Preecha P Yupapin, Matthew R. Zahner, Juanwen Zhang and Dorota Zysko. We hope that you, the reader, will find this book interesting and useful. Any advices please feel free and are always welcome to tell us.

iConcept Press Ltd
November 2014

Screening for Heat Stress in Workers and Athletes

Lilly Ramphal
Occupational Health Department
Cook Children's Hospital, Fort Worth Texas, USA

1   Introduction

Heat-related illnesses lead to almost 6000 hospital visits per year, or two emergency department visits per 100,000 visits. Heat-related illnesses are most high among men (72%) aged 15 to 19 years and are most often associated with athletic activities (MMWR, July 2011). Two thousand twelve was the warmest year on record in the US since man has begun to record annual temperatures. (National Geographic 2013) Global climate change will continue to have an impact on heat stress in people, on animal survival, and on food availability. The World Health Organization has estimated that over the past 30 years, 150,000 lives have been lost annually due to global heat waves and climate change (Patz *et al.*, 2005). Weather changes have a great impact on athletes and workers by slowing efficiency and decreasing productivity (Basu R) (Costello A & Maslin M). When heat waves occur, overall mortality is also affected among the old and the young, due to their increased risk for dying from respiratory, cerebrovascular, and cardiovascular diseases, such as ischemic heart disease, heart failure, and myocardial infarction (Basu R).

Despite increasing temperatures and environmental levels of carbon dioxide, one third of metropolitan areas do not have heat stress response plans (Bernard S & McGeehin M). Cases of heat stress are handled on a case-by-case basis rather than by being addressed collectively as a public health concern. The National Institute for Occupational Safety and Health initiated heat stress criteria in 1986 and amended them in 2008 regarding worker heat stress safety (MMWR September 1986) (NIOSH 2008). Few people are aware of these criteria, of the risk factors associated with a predisposition to heat stress, or what signs or symptoms to look for that represent risk factors for heat stress. The rules and standards proposed by the Occupational Safety and Health Administration for workplace heat stress are recommendations and still not enforceable (OSHA, 2008).

Screening for heat stress susceptibility in workers and athletes is an issue in need of public health criteria with enforceable rules based on evidence-based research. Screening for heat stress risk factors should consider physical demand level; cardiovascular, pulmonary, and endocrine status; previous history of heat stress; age; diseases; and medications including illegal drug use. Such screening should be part of the recruitment of any person expected to work or play in extremely hot environmental conditions. Older people are at increased risk for cardiovascular and thermoregulatory instability. The aging American workforce, undiagnosed disease, poor hydration while working or playing, and global warming are all factors that contribute to the need to screen workers and athletes for the risk of heat stress (Favata EA & Barnhart S *et.al.*). A summary of the manifestations of heat stress conditions are listed below in chart form.

Several types or workers are at risk for heat stress in the US since they work outdoors for long hours in the sun or are in direct contact with flames or hot equipment (MMWR Sep 1986). These include firefighters, bakery workers, farmers, construction workers, miners, boiler room workers, factory workers, and workers in manufacturing. Athletes at risk for heat stress include football players, runners, soccer players, hockey players, triathlon competitors, marathon runners, weight lifters, swimmers, ice skaters, hurlers, and hunters due to the accelerated cardiovascular state and outdoor nature of these activities.

In addition, certain individuals have higher risks, including those with reduced mental capacity, Alzheimer's disease or dementia, trisomy disorders, dysrhythmias, and congenital heart abnormalities. Persons with reduced mental capacity may not drink fluids on a regular basis, so they should be put on frequent rest cycles and be reminded to drink fluids in hot environments. Aging individuals often have brittle vasoregulatory mechanisms. All these factors can be screened for during physical evaluations.

Type of Heat Illness	Signs and Symptoms	Physiology	First Aid
Heat Stroke	Hot dry skin or profuse sweating Hallucinations Chills Throbbing headache Temperature. 101-105F Confusion/dizziness Slurred speech	Rapid rise in core temperature inability to cool core temperature physical demands exceed cardiac output, cardiovascular challenge, risk for cardiovascular stress and eventual collapse	Call 911 and notify supervisor Move sick person to a cool shaded area Cool worker/athlete using methods such as soaking clothes with water, spraying, sponging, or showering with water, and/or ice immersion
Heat Exhaustion	Heavy sweating Tiredness Weakness/ fatigue Dizziness confusion Clammy moist skin slightly elevated temperature Fast shallow breaths	Body's response to excessive loss of water and salt. Physical challenge exceeds body's ability to thermoregulate	Notify supervisor Move sick person to a cool shaded area Slowly drink water, clear juice, or sports drink If no improvement call 911
Exertional Heat Stroke	Rise in temperature up to 101-104F, Rapid, strong pulse Throbbing headache Dizziness Nausea Confusion Unconsciousness	Rapid rise in core temperature, inability to cool core temperature physical demands exceed cardiac output, cardiovascular challenge, At risk for cardiovascular stress and eventual collapse	Call 911 and notify supervisor Move sick person to a cool shaded area Cool worker/athlete using methods such as soaking clothes with water, spraying, sponging, or showering them with water, an/or ice immersion
Heat Injury	Temperature 104-105, Normal mental status, nausea Often seen in military recruits	Prolonged exposure to heat causes Rise in core temperature which exceeds Thermo-regulating human capacity. At risk for cardiovascular stress and eventual collapse due to organ necrosis	Call 911 and notify supervisor Move sick person to a cool shaded area Cool worker/athlete using methods such as soaking clothes with water, spraying, sponging, or showering them with water, and/or ice immersion
Heat Syncope	Light-headedness Dizziness Fainting	Pooling of fluids due to prolonged standing or sudden rising from sitting, Dehydration is the hallmark or lack of acclimitization	Sit or lie down in a cool place Slowly drink water, clear juice or a sports beverage If no improvement may be Another Heat Illness or condition

Modified and adapted from (OSHA 2011) and NIOSH (2008) Criteria for Heat Stress in Workers

Table 1: Manifestations of Heat Illnesses

This article first reviews the signs and symptoms of heat stress illnesses, then discusses a formula for heat stress evaluation, discusses guidelines for screening, reviews accommodations for those persons working or playing with physical incapacity and specific illness in hot environments and finally discusses prevention of heat illness.

2   Physiology of Temperature Regulation

The human capacity to regulate temperature equilibrium depends on various factors that ultimately impact the body's ability to maintain a steady core temperature (MMWR Sep 1986). Each person's ability to maintain a steady inner core temperature can be influenced by environmental factors, age, gender, cardiovascular health, and even the medications they take (Homer I). The type of clothing barrier that individuals wear influences their ability to cool down core body temperature and adjust to extreme environmental heat as well (Favata E, Buckler G & Gochfield M). Excessive clothing barriers can be extremely important in cases of athletic heat exhaustion and heat stroke mortality.

Substance	Mechanism of action
Legal	
Alcohol	HR decrease, volume depletion
Amphetamine	HR increase, increase in sweating
Anticholinergic	HR lability, abnormal sweating
Antihistamine	HR lability, abnormal sweating
Antihypertensive	HR lability
Benzodiazepine	HR lability, abnormal sweating
Calcium channel blocker	HR lability, venous pooling, abnormal sweating
Diuretic	Volume depletion, decreased vasodilation
Laxative	HR lability, abnormal vasodilation
Neuroleptic	HR lability, abnormal sweating
Phenothiazine	Electrolyte imbalance
Thyroid agonist (improperly controlled)	HR increase, increased sweating
Topiramate	Electrolyte imbalance
Tricyclic antidepressant	Electrolyte imbalance
Illegal	
Cocaine	HR increase, increased sweating
Phencyclidine (PCP)	Abnormal temperature regulation
Lysergic acid diethylamide (LSD)	HR lability, abnormal sweating

Table 2: Legal and illegal medications that impact heat stress susceptibility. Modified from Glazer, 2005, HR indicates heart rate.

Under normal physiological conditions, the human body can maintain a stable core temperature even when stressed by extreme environmental temperatures as long as proper hydration is continuously provided (Maughan RJ& Shirreffs SM *et.al.*)(Bates GP & Schneider J). Skin temperature is several degrees cooler than core temperature. It is regulated by the constriction or dilation of subcutaneous blood vessels, the rate of sweating production, heart rate, and cardiac output. Cardiovascular fitness as well as environmental factors plays an important role in coping with extreme environment. Tolerance to temperature homeostasis via dehydration is more robust when individuals are physically fit and young (Merry T & Ansle P &Cotter J). However, this ability to adapt to heat declines with age, the presence of disease, and a poor level of fitness (Sherwood S & Huber M). Any condition that affects the ability to sweat will also affect a person's ability to maintain a constant body temperature.

Regarding medications, any medication that has the potential to affect the cardiovascular systems, sweating ability, vasodilatation, volume depletion, electrolyte equilibrium, venous pooling, cardiac output, or core temperature via the central nervous system has the potential to affect the risk for heat stress and heat stroke. Most notable among these medications are those listed in Table 2 (Glazer J 2005). The table also reflects the mechanism whereby these medications might impact thermoregulation. Any individual taking these legal or illegal medications is at greater risk for developing heat stress, irrespective of age, weight, or environmental factors. Older individuals are more sensitive to these effects and are also more likely to be on some of these medications due to an increased risk for chronic disease.

3   Formula to Measure Heat Stress Risk

A worthwhile risk assessment model for heat stress that combines both environmental factors and physiological risk factors has been posed in the following simplified formula. The formula incorporates both environmental factors (environmental stress index, or ESI) and personal factors (personal stress index or PSI) as follows:

Environmental Stress Index $= 0.63 T_{ambient} - 0.03$ Relative Humidity $+ 0.002$ Solar Radiation $+ 0.0054 (T_a \times RH) - 0.073 (0.1 + SR)^{-1}$ (Scaled from 0 to 10)

Personal Stress Index $= 5(T_{rectal\text{-}chosen\ endpoint} - T_{rectal\text{-}baseline}) \times (39.5 - T_{rectal\text{-}baseline})^{-1} + 5(HR_{chosen\ enpoint} - HR_{baseline}) \times (180 - HR_0)^{-1}$ (Scaled from 0 to 5)

Variables represent ambient temperature in Celsius degrees (Ta), relative humidity measured in percent (RH), and solar radiation measured by infrared (SR measured in watts/m2). The ESI is the first stress index using direct measurements of infrared solar radiation, heart rate (HR in beats/minute), and rectal temperature (Celsius) measured at baseline (Tre0) and at a chosen endpoint (Tret). Tre0and HR_0 represents the baseline Temperature and heart rate and Tret and HRt are Temperature and heart rate taken at a chosen endpoint in time.

This method considers environmental variations in temperature, humidity, and solar radiation as well as the individual's heart rate and aerobic tolerance and is therefore a good objective measure of risk for heat stress in individuals (Moran D&Pandolf K et.al). For example tachycardia associated with volume depletion, is reflected by the heart rate in this formula. The formula reflects febrile states because it measures rectal temperature. Correlating the PSI and ESI mathematically signals increasing cardiovascular strain and increased need for fluid replacement and work rest cycling thus preventing the risk of heat stress in military recruits.

Limitations of this risk assessment model are that it does not account for certain disease states, such as severe cardiac or respiratory disease. It does not measure stroke volume, cardiac output, central venous pressure, or pulmonary wedge pressures, which are benchmark measurements of cardiovascular and pulmonary compromise in diseased individuals. For this reason, the sensitivity and specificity of this risk assessment formula to screen for heat stressed susceptible persons with severe cardiopulmonary disease is somewhat limited, and other measures suggested later in this article are needed to complement this risk assessment instrument.

4   Recommendations for Screening Workers and Athletes

The medical history intake form is essential when screening for heat stress in individuals. A person's desired level of job activity or athletic activity (physical demand level) is very important to assess as part of the history. Great physical exertion in a hot environment results in more stress on the cardiopulmonary system. Therefore, heat stress screening should be more thorough in individuals who anticipate heavy exertion in hot environments. In such situations, additional objective tests may be needed to improve the sensitivity and specificity of the screening process.

The categories of physical demand of work or play are easy to understand if they are categorized into light (requiring 0 to 19 lb of exertion), medium light (requiring 20 to 30 lb of exertion), medium heavy (requiring 31 to 40 lb of exertion), and heavy (requiring 71 to 100 lb of exertion) physical demand categories. These categories correspond to sedentary administrative type jobs, light cleaning jobs, heavy cleaning jobs, manufacturing jobs with lifting duties, and construction work, respectively. The athletic corollary would be casual walking, light jogging, sprinting, marathon running, and playing football/participating in a triathlon, respectively.

During screening, the medical history should focus on the health and resilience of the cardiovascular and pulmonary systems and the medication history. It is also important to assess whether the individual has had prior episodes of heat stress or heat stroke. Some specific aspects of the screening include obesity, fitness level, cardiac function, and diabetes, as discussed below. *Table 3* summarizes the recommendation for heat stress screening based on physical demand level for individuals who are working or playing in a heat-stressed environment. The three step test is a crude but useful age and gender specific test of cardiovascular resilience (Appendix A).

5   Conditions that lower the heat stress threshold

5.1   Hypertension

High blood pressure is a condition that stresses the cardiovascular system especially if it remains untreated. Labile high blood pressure, systolic or diastolic high blood pressure stresses the cardiovascular tree intermittently during different times of the cardiac pulse cycle. Regardless of when hypertensive stress occurs during the cardiac pulse heat stress will cumulatively damage to the cardiovascular tree. For this reason it is of paramount importance that workers and athletes who are prone to hypertension receive adequate medical management before onging excess heat exposure.

5.2   Obesity

Recent studies indicate that approximately one third of our children and adults fall into the overweight or obese category. A high body mass index (BMI) adds additional burden on the cardiopulmonary system (MMWR Sep 1986) (OSHA Feb 2008)(Wannamethee S& Shaper A. *et.al*).

Thermoregulation of the core temperature can be more challenging if there is increased peripheral insulation. Obesity increases the core temperature and decreases a person's ability to effectively cool down rapidly with the usual cardiovascular thermoregulatory mechanisms. In addition, obesity is an independent risk factor for increased cardiovascular disease (Petrofsky J& Alshahmmari F *et.al*). The association seems to be independent of hormonal factors such as leptin. Therefore, screening for BMI is easy and reasonable to do and should be included as part of the screening protocol for persons who are about to engage in activities that expose them to heat, which will further stress the cardiovascular system. As recommended by the Federal Motor Vehicle Safety Commission (FMCSA) for truck drivers, a BMI >30 kg/m^2 should alert the screening professional that the individual requires health counselling about dietary and exercise goals, assuming there are no cardiac issues that will prevent participation. A BMI >40 kg/m^2 should trigger a need for more frequent rest periods in a heat-stressed environment for various reasons. At this level, FMCSA has data that correlates a high BMI with a risk for labile hypertension, higher mortality from sudden death, and sleep apnea (FMCSA 2009). Such persons can work in the heat for very short periods of time with frequent break sessions for cooling until they decrease their BMI to a safer level.

5.3   Fitness level

Fitness level is an important part of the intake history because a sedentary individual is more likely to succumb to heat stress than an active one. If it is necessary to assess a person's cardiovascular resilience, a simple 3-minute step test and pulse recovery monitoring can easily determine the level of individual fitness. This test must be performed in a standardized manner using a 12-inch step and metronome. The participant steps up and down to a 96-beat-per-minute metronome beat for 3 continuous minutes. Pulse recovery from baseline after 3 minutes of rest is standardized according to the scoring in *Appendix A,* which determines the individual's level of fitness. Fitness levels are not static and can be improved with gradual exercise. If individuals are not fit, their tolerance to heat will be inadequate, and they should not be exposed to long periods in the heat before they improve their fitness and cardiac conditioning.

5.4   Cardiac function

Cardiac screening tests, such as a stress echocardiogram or electrocardiogram, which are considered the gold standard for cost-effective screening (Lee D &Voica F& *et.al*), are recommended only in certain circumstances. If a person is going to be in a medium or heavier physical activity, it is advisable to screen that person for cardiac risk factors with objective tests before he or she is exposed to the stress of a hot environment, in order to mitigate the risk for adverse cardiac events. In addition, at age 35, the cardiopulmonary system of average adults begins a slow aging process that can be mitigated only with exercise and is unpredictably impacted by environmental and genetic factors. For this reason, those older than 35 years should be screened with basic cardiovascular screening tests if they have any cardiovascular risk factors or if they are going to be challenged by physical demands of medium-heavy levels or greater, as indicated in Table 3.

5.5   Diabetes as related to cardiac function

Diabetes is highly associated with ischemic heart disease and cerebrovascular accidents, events that can be provoked by heat stress. For this reason, those exposed to heat should be screened for diabetes, even if they are in a sedentary role. A urinalysis can be used for most screening. (Hayashi T& Kawashima S & *et.al*). For individuals engaging in an activity above a medium physical demand level, the more sensitive serum glucose test is appropriate. A urinalysis positive for glucose also indicates the need for serum glucose testing. A serum glucose level >200 mg/dL indicates the need to stabilize the glucose before the individual is allowed into a heat-stressed environment, as he or she has an increased risk for negative cardiovascular events. Diabetics may have increased thirst if they are hyperglycemic and frequently urinating. For this reason they are also at risk for dehydration which is compounded in a heat stressed environment (FMCSA 2010).

5.6   Congestive Heart Failure and Malignant Arrhythmias

A history of congestive heart failure or the presence of malignant arrhythmias is a marker for underlying cardiovascular fragility. (Pina I) These conditions need close inspection of the present function of the cardiovascular system with measures such as a stress test and evaluation of baseline parameters such as blood pressure, cardiac rhythm under stress and ejection fraction on a periodic basis. Table 2 makes exception for some persons assuming they have normal underlying health. However if that is not the case, and they give a history of congestive heart failure or significant arrhythmias then they should be cleared with a Bruce protocol stress test and normal baseline parameters before being subjected to environmental heat stress. An ejection fraction above 40 is acceptable in the workplace (FMSCA 2010), without the presence of malignant arrhythmias such as ventricular tachycardia, malignant atrial fibrillation, atrial flutter, complete AV block and similar rapid rhythms.

5.7   Advanced Age

Older people may have irregularities in thirst demand-response mechanism. For this reason they can be at greater risk for dehydration and often have to be reminded to drink fluids frequently. Their skin is thinner and does not protect against dehydration and is not as brisk in thermo-regulating against rays from the sun. Age is a greater predictor of cardiovascular fragility and disease as well. Senior citizens are therefore more prone to heat stress (Petrofski J& Alshahmmari F& *et al*). Therefore anyone over 70 years of age deserves greater scrutiny when with regards to heat stress proclivity (OSHA 2011)(NIOSH 2008) (Barrow 1998).

5.8   Dehydration

Loss of intravascular fluid can occur for many reasons many which have been discussed. However many other reasons contribute to dehydration, including excess exposure, psychiatric illnesses such as anorexia nervosa, psychosis, addictive disorders can limit fluid intake due to mental pre-occupation. Geriatric conditions related to chronic neurological disease such as Parkinson's or Alzheimer's disease can contribute to dehydration. Alcoholism can cause intravascular volume depletion for a myriad of reasons including intractable vomiting, gastrointestinal bleeding, intravascular electrolyte abnormalities as well as psychiatric reasons. (Barrow 1998) A dehydrated person is more susceptible to heat illness like a dry pasture is susceptible to fire on hot day. The previously mentioned formula points to the importance of heart rate, baseline temperature as a contributing factor to PSI. If a person starts out with an elevated heart rate or baseline temperature due to dehydration the PSI is already at risk for heat stress.

Weight to be lifted or exertion (lb)	Physical demand level of work or activity	Components of screening needed				
		Medical questionnaire*	BP and BMI	EKG >35 yrs	3-step test	Stress test
0–19	Light	Yes	Yes	No	No	No
20–30	Medium light	Yes	Yes	No	Optional	No
31–40	Medium	Yes	Yes	Yes	Yes	No
41–70	Medium heavy	Yes	Yes	Yes	Yes	Optional
71–100	Heavy	Yes	Yes	Yes	Yes	Yes

*Focused questionnaire to include cardiopulmonary function, fitness level, prior episodes of heat stress, heart disease, and medications.
BP indicates blood pressure; BMI, body mass index; EKG, electrocardiogram

Table 3: Summary recommendations for heat stress screening for workers and athletes. Copyright Ramphal 2011.

6 Accommodation of Heat Stress-susceptible Persons

The American with Disabilities Act Amendment (ADAA) requires employers to accommodate employees who have gone through a disabling disease process that makes them incapable of accomplishing their usual work due to medical disability (ADAA, 2008). The expanding focus of the ADAA places the burden on employers to accommodate workers after clearance from their personal physician. Guidelines from the Federal Motor Carrier Safety Administration (FMCSA), which appear in *Table 4,* specifically address recovery from cardiovascular and pulmonary instability and are applicable to a wide range of situations, including heat stress screening.

Rest/work cycles based on physical demand and temperature, as shown in *Table 5,* also applied. The threshold limit values (TLVs) in this Table are based on the assumption that nearly all acclimatized, fully clothed workers with adequate water and salt intake should be able to function effectively under the given working conditions without exceeding a deep body temperature of 38°C (100.4°F). They are also based on the assumption that the Wet Bulb Globe Temperature (WBGT) of the resting place is the same as or very close to that of the workplace. Where the WBGT of the work area is different from that of the rest area, a time-weighted average should be used (ACGIH 1992-93). In consideration of the ADAA, it is important that if a person is determined to be at greater risk for heat stress then the rest/work cycles should be higher than for a person that does not have a high heat stress risk. Accommodation cycles should be adjusted to account for heat stress risk to 50% outdoor 50% indoor or outdoor work in two to four hour cycles to allow for cooling off periods in people who are at risk. Onsite body temperature monitors and appropriate oral fluid hydration should be made available to prevent heat stress incidents. NIOSH recommendations have been updated to reflect recommendations for employers to prevent heat stressed employees (NIOSH 2008).

Variable	Guideline
High blood pressure	Disqualify if blood pressure exceeds 160/100
Blood glucose	Disqualify if serum glucose ≥200 mg/dL and refer to PCP
Urinanalysis	Defer to serum glucose if dipstick is positive for glucose
Disqualifying medications	Refer to PCP for possible alternative change of medications[†]
Body mass index	Refer for counseling if >40 kg/m^2 Screen for sleep apnea
Cardiac arrhythmias	Disqualify if there is a malignant arrhythmia Clear with benign arrhythmia after medication control and normal baseline stress echo biannually
Myocardial infarction	Wait 2 months then clear with normal baseline stress echo and normal biannual echo; ejection fraction must be >40%
Cardiac stent placement	Wait 1 week then clear with normal baseline stress echo cardiogram; repeat every 2 years
Cardiac bypass	Wait 3 months then clear with normal baseline stress echo; repeat every 2 years; ejection fraction must be >40%

[†]Disqualifying medications are specific for underlying cardiac or pulmonary diseases that may not be capable of substitution. PCP indicates primary care physician.

Table 4: Guidelines for truck driver certification that apply to heat stress screening. Based on 2010 guidelines from the Federal Motor Carrier Safety Administration, available at: http://www.fmcsa.dot.gov/rules-regulations/rules-regulations.htm

Work/rest regimen each hour	Work load		
	Light	Moderate	Heavy
Continuous work	30.0°C (86°F)	26.7°C (80°F)	25.0°C (77°F)
75% work, 25% rest	30.6°C (87°F)	28.0°C (82°F)	25.9°C (78°F)
50% work, 50% rest	31.4°C (89°F)	29.4°C (85°F)	27.9°C (82°F)
25% work, 75% rest	32.2°C (90°F)	31.1°C (88°F)	30.0°C (86°F)

Table 5: Work/rest regimen based on work load and temperature. From American Conference of Governmental Industrial Hygienists 1992-93

7   Prevention of Heat Related Illness

Heat related illnesses and deaths are extremely preventable in medicine in healthy individuals, the young, old, mentally ill, and chronically ill. The air-conditioned environment is the most protective factor against heat-related illness and death. During extremely hot days, people should be encouraged to spend time in activities in air-conditioned places such as shopping malls, public libraries, movie theatres, or local heat relief shelters. Summertime meals should be cool meals, prepared and taken with plenty of fluids, if medical conditions do not preclude fluid intake. Protective clothing should include shade for the head and face with a hat or umbrella. Mid-day exposure during the hottest part of the day should be avoided (CDC 2011) (NIOSH 2008).

Work or athletic practice should include a buddy system to monitor signs and symptoms of excess heat exposure and to assure proper cycling behaviour every 3-4 hours into cool areas for short spans of relief from the heat. The old, young, infirm, and chronically ill are more susceptible to exposure so cycling is especially important in these groups. People who live alone should be checked at least twice a day during extremely hot periods to assure they are not suffering.

The horror of losing an infant in a car seat from heat exposure after just a few minutes emphasizes the importance of never leaving infants or small animals in the back of a car during the summer even if it is just for a few minutes. During athletic events planning ahead to hydrate, cool down, and transport an athlete if necessary requires training and preparation with adequate first aid kits that include mineral water, ice, tubs for immersion, tarps, thermometers and trained staff that knows how to use such equipment (OSHA 2011).

8   Conclusion

In our increasingly warmer global climates, specific screening and first aid treatment is necessary to prevent morbidity and mortality in the workplace and during sports activities. Most people who are screened using these simple tests and guidelines will avoid undesirable outcomes. The recommendations for screening individuals superimposed with existing tools to increase the sensitivity and specificity and identify those at risk for heat stress from those who are less at risk help reduce heat illness and death. These methods also help accommodate individuals who might need to recover from an illness that might temporarily affect cardiovascular fitness. Rarely, there will be those with congenital problems such as Kawasaki's disease, which can cause undetected cardiac complications or the fatal cardiac arrhythmia occurs on a hot summer day on the athletic field or in the workplace. Yet, the goal of primary care providers is to avoid 99.9% of preventable illness. By using the recommended screening tools, they can be better equipped to accomplish this goal.

Acknowledgement

Published with permission from Baylor Proceedings.

Appendix A

	18-25	26-35	36-45	46-55	56-65	65+
Men						
Excellent	50-76	51-76	49-76	56-82	60-77	59-81
Good	79-84	79-85	80-88	87-93	86-94	87-92
Above average	88-93	88-94	92-88	95-101	97-100	94-102
Average	95-100	96-102	100-105	103-111	103-109	104-110
Below average	102-107	104-110	108-113	113-119	111-117	114-118
Poor	111-119	114-121	116-124	121-126	119-128	121-126
Very poor	124-157	126-161	130-163	131-159	131-154	130-151
Women						

Excellent	52-81	58-80	51-84	63-91	60-92	70-92
Good	85-93	85-92	89-96	95-101	97-103	96-101
Above average	96-102	95-101	100-104	104-110	106-111	104-111
Average	104-110	104-110	107-112	113-118	113-118	116-121
Below average	113-120	113-119	115-120	120-124	119-127	123-126
Poor	122-131	122-129	124-132	126-132	129-135	128-133
Very poor	135-169	134-171	137-169	137-171	141-174	135-155

Table 3: Scoring on the 3-Minute Step Test for Men and Women. Scores are the age-adjusted standards based on guidelines published by the YMCA (http://www.exrx.net/Testing/YMCATesting.html). In the test, the participant steps up and down a 12-inch step to a 96-beat-per-minute metronome beat for 3 continuous minutes, and pulse recovery from baseline after 3 minutes of rest is recorded.

References

American Conference of Governmental Industrial Hygienists. (1998). TLV/BEI resources. Available at: http://www.acgih.org/tlv/.

Barrow, M.W. & Clark, K.A. (1998). Heat related Illness.Am Fam Physician. Sep 1;58(3):749-756.

Basu, R. (2009). High ambient temperature and mortality: a review of epidemiologic studies from 2001 to 2008. (2009)Environ Health. Sep 16; 8:40.

Bates, G.P. & Schneider J. (2008). Hydration status and physiological workload of UAE construction workers: A prospective longitudinal observtional study. J Occup Med Toxicol. 3(21).

Bernard, S. & McGeehin, M. (2004). Municipal heat wave response plans. Am J Public Health,;September; 94 (9) 1520-1522.

Costello, A., Maslin, M. & Montgomery, H., Johnson A. & Ekins, P. (2011). Global health and climate change: moving from denial and catastrophic fatalism to positive action. Philos Transact A Math Phys Eng Sci.May 13(369(1942) 1866-82.

Favata, E., Buckler, G. & Gochfield, M. (1990). Heat stress in hazardous waste workers: evaluation and prevention. Occup Med. Jan-Mar(5(1)79-91.

Favata, E.A., Barnhart, S., Bresnitz, E.A., Campbell, V. et al. (1990). Clinical experiences: development of a medical surveillance protocol for hazardous waste workers. Occup Med. Jan- Mar: 5(1):117-25.

Federal Motor Carrier Safety Administration. (2009). Spotlight on sleep apnea. http://www.fmcsa.dot.gov/safety-ecurity/sleep-apnea/sleep-apnea.aspx.

Federal Motor Carrier Safety Administration. Rules and regulations, (2010). Available at http://www.fmcsa.dot.gov/rules-regulations/rules-regulations.htm.

Glazer J. (2005). Information from your family doctor. Heat exhaustion and Heat stroke: what you should know. Am Fam Physician. Jun1 (71(11) 2141-2.

Hayashi, T., Kawashima, S., Nomura, H. et al. (2011). Age, gender, insulin and blood glucose control status alter the risk of ischemic heart disease and stroke among elderly diabetic patients. Cardiovasc Diabetol, Oct6 (10) 86.

Holmer, I.(2010). Climate change and occupational heat stress: methods for Assessment. Glob Health Action. Nov 29(3).

Lee, D., Veroica, F., Husain, M., Al Khdair, D. et al. (2011). Cardiovascular outcomes are predicted by exercise-stress myocardial perfusion imaging: Impact on death, myocardial infarction, and coronary revascularization procedures. Am Heart J. May161 (5) 900-7.

Maughan, R.J., Shirreffs, S.M., Ozgünen, K.T. et al. (2010). Living, training and playing in the heat: challenges to the football player and strategies for coping with environmental extremes. Scand J Med Sci Sports.Oct; 20 Suppl 3:117-24.

Merry, T., Ainsle, P. & Cotter, J. (2010). Effects of aerobic fitness on hypohydration-induced physiological strain and exercise impairment. Acta Physio (Oxf). Feb: 198(2) 179-90.

MMWR, Center for Disease Control. (1986). NIOSH recommendations for occupational safety and health standards. MMWR.Sep26; 35(1 Suppl):1S-33S.

MMWR, Centers for Disease Control and Prevention. (2011). Nonfatal sports and recreation heat illness treated in hospital emergency departments--United States, 2001-2009 MMWR Morbidity Mortal Weekly Rep. July29 (60), 977-80.

Moran, D., Pandolf, K., Heled, Y. & Gonzalez, R. (2003). US Army Research Institute of Environmental Medicine Combined environmental stress and physiological strain indices for physical training guidelines. J Basic Clin Physiol Pharmacol.14(1) 17-30.

National Geographic. (2013). Than K. Accessed at http://news.nationalgeographic.com/news/2013/01/130109-warmest-year-record-2012-global-warming-science-environment-united-states/

NIOSH, National Institute for Occupational Health Safety Criteria. (2008). Accessed at http://www.cdc.gov/niosh/ Occupational Safety and Health Administration (2008);February. Proposed Rules and Standards Related to Heat Stress. Accessed at www.osha.gov/SLTC/heatstress/index.html

Patz, J.A., Campbell-Lendrum, D., Holloway, T. & Foley, J.A. (2005). Impact of regional climate change on human health. Nature. Nov 17,438(7066):310-7.

Petrofsky, J., Alshahmmari, F., Yim, J.E. et al. (2011). The interrelationship between locally applied heat,ageing and skin blood flow on heat transfer into and from the skin. J Med Eng Technol. Jul 35(5):262-74.

Pina, I. (2010) Cardiac rehabilitation in heart failure: a brief review and recommendations. Curr Cardiol Rep. May 12(3) 223-9.

Sherwood, S. & Huber, M. (2010). An adaptability limit to climate change due to heat stress. Proc Natl Acad Sci USA. May 25 107(21) 9552-9555.

The ADA Amendments Act of 2008. (2008). Public Law 110-325. Available At http://www.access-board.gov/about/laws/ada-amendments.htm

Wannamethee, S., Shaper, A., Whincup, P., Lennon, L. & Sattar, N. (2011). Obesity and risk of incident heart failure in older men with and without pre-existing coronary heart disease: does leptin have a role? J Am Coll Cardiol. Oct 25(58(18)1870-7.

Impact of Physical Exercise on the Cardiovascular System in Elderly

Claudio Joaquim Borba-Pinheiro
Instituto Federal do Pará, Brazil
Laboratório de Biociências da Motricidade Humana (LABIMH)
Universidade Federal do Estado do Rio de Janeiro, Brazil

Marco Aurélio Gomes de Oliveira
Grupo Multidisciplinar de Desenvolvimento em Ritmos Biológicos
Universidade de São Paulo, Brazil

André Walsh-Monteiro
Laboratório de Biociências e Comportamento
Instituto Federal do Pará (IFPA), Brazil

Nébia Maria Almeida de Figueiredo
Laboratório de Biociências da Motricidade Humana (LABIMH)
Universidade Federal do Estado do Rio de Janeiro, Brazil

Estélio Henrique Martin Dantas
Laboratório de Biociências da Motricidade Humana (LABIMH)
Universidade Federal do Estado do Rio de Janeiro, Brazil

1   Introduction

The cardiovascular diseases are health problems faced by countries around world. Researches shows that the increased in cardiovascular diseases is associated with different variables such as: body composition, diabetes mellitus, dyslipidemia, poor eating habits, historic family and physical inactivity. All these variables, over the years, to a greater or lesser extent, have contributed to an increase incidence of cardiovascular disease in elderly (Mosca, 2004; Bielemann *et al.*, 2009; National Institute on Aging, 2011; Estruch *et al.*, 2013).

Physical exercises are considered a potential support in the prevention, control and treatment of cardiovascular diseases (National Institute on Aging, 2011; Oliveira *et al.*, 2012). While it is well known that physical inactivity is a major risk factor for cardiovascular disease, there is still a search for the mechanisms by which exercise exerts its positive effect. Skeletal muscle type fibre is affected to some extent by physical exercise. The different fibre types possess anti-inflammatory and glucometabolic properties that can decrease risk in this disease, because skeletal muscle fibre composition may be a mediator of the protective effects of exercise against cardiovascular disease (Andersen *et al.*, 2013).

However, there is a need for a planning and control by a trained professional for appropriate exercise prescription according to patient assessments (Melo *et al.*, 2006; Park *et al.*, 2006).

In this respect, the cardiovascular system plays a fundamental role in facilitating of these responses, including thermoregulation and delivery/removal of nutrients and waste products. Cardiac parasympathetic reactivation following a training session is highly individualized, that has function of a marker of cardiovascular recovery (Stanley *et al.*, 2013).

With this, this chapter aims to present a study on the scientific bases for choice, evaluation and prescription of appropriate exercises, as well as the impacts of these exercises in individuals with cardiovascular diseases and this will be discussed in the following topics:

- Cardiovascular changes in elderly

- Effect of physical exercise on endothelial function

- Acute effect of aerobic and resistance exercise

- Chronic effect of aerobic exercise and resistance exercise

- Aerobic exercise and resistance training for hypertensive elderly

2   Cardiovascular Changes in Elderly

According to the considerations of the World Health Organization (WHO) the world population over 65 years old has rapidly increased in recent decades. For the next five years, the number of individuals aged 65 years old will surpass the number of children under 5 years of age (National Institute on Aging, 2011). This is occurring by rate reduction of births and the increase in life expectancy, due to improvements in health achieved in the 20th century, allowing the reduction of the number of infectious and parasitic diseases in the children, leading to lower rate mortality in this group and the consequent increase in the older population (National Institute on Aging, 2011).

The increase in life expectancy has also brought increased spending on noncommunicable diseases that ascend with age and directly affect economic growth (National Institute on Aging, 2011). According to the considerations of the National Health and Examination Survey, 67% of the U.S.A population with over age 60 was diagnosed with hypertension (Ostchega *et al.*, 2007). Besides of the relationships with lifestyle, this high number is strongly associated with increased life expectancy of the population, which allows greater exposure of the individual to the natural changes that occur in the endothelium over the years, increasing blood pressure levels of population, especially, when associated with genetic predisposition and unhealthy lifestyle habits (Webb & Inscho, 2005; Montalti, 2012).

The endothelium is responsible for the maintenance vascular tonus, creating anticoagulant substances preserving the blood flow, besides maintaining the fluidity of the plasmatic membrane through a single layer of cells organized as a spindle. When the individual reaches the age of 30 years, these cells tend to die and be replaced by others who will not have the same ability to produce vasodilator substances (Bahia *et al.*, 2006). With the passing of years, the endothelium gradually loses the capacity to elasticity as a result of changes in your components. Additionally, these changes cause increased BP, increases oxygen demand in the myocardium, reducing blood flow (Vaitkevicius *et al.*, 1993; Mackey *et al.*, 2002; Behringer *et al.*, 2013; Alssar *et al.*, 2013).

The aging process affects numerous diseases resulting of the physiological changes which may be potentiated by bad living habits. One of these is diabetes mellitus which also is related to hypertension. Over the years, carbohydrate metabolism is altered allowing subjects with genetic predisposition associated with inadequate habits of live can develop type 2 diabetes in the old age (Ferrannini *et al.*, 1996, Muller *et al.*, 1996). Another aspect is the gradual increase of inflammatory cytokines such as TNF and C-reactive protein over the years in patients with type 2 diabetes, which are also associated with the progression of this disease (Del Prato., 2009; Lechleitner *et al.*, 2012).

Insulin resistance arises by genetic predisposition, but also is associated with cultural factors and bad habits of life, preceding type 2 diabetes and has strong contributions to the development of hypertension (Cheung & Li, 2012). These two co-morbidities have a similar pathophysiology, and as a result this, approximately half of all hypertensive patients are insulin resistant. In pathophysiological mechanism of these diseases the elevation of renin – angiotensin - aldosterone system (RAAS), the sympathetic nervous system (SNS), the oxidative stress and vascular dysfunctions are also observed (Cheung & Li, 2012). Figure 1 show the mechanism.

As previously stated, senility has as consequence the occurrence of numerous diseases by the body changes associated with aging. In France, estimates indicate that 8.2% to 14.0% of the population between 65 and 80 years of age are diabetics (Campagha *et al.*, 2005). The Brazilian Society of Diabetes (BSD, 2011) indicates that 18% of elderly Brazilians suffer from this disease, and 50% by type II (BSD, 2011). According to the SBD (2011), the progressive loss of muscular mass with aging causes a decrease in availability of GLUT's (glucose transporters) responsible for the transport of blood glucose into the cells and in consequence, increases blood glucose levels in elderly compared to the young population.

This glycemic elevation and subsequent installation of type II diabetes is associated with endothelial dysfunction and the occurrence of atherosclerosis (Bahia *et al.* 2006). In the elderly, the metabolic syndrome has prevalence ranging from 11% to 43% around the world and is characterized by the presence of diseases such as: obesity, dyslipidemia, hypertension and diabetes, which increase possibilities of a cardiovascular event (Denys, 2009).

In addition, the rate of hypertensive patients with metabolic syndrome is a high number that reaches 85% (Duvnjak *et al.*, 2008). That way, there is a high possibility of the individual developing associated diseases. For this reason, the realization of appropriate physical activity can help control these diseases, even when they are associated (blood pressure, blood glucose, dyslipidemia, etc.).

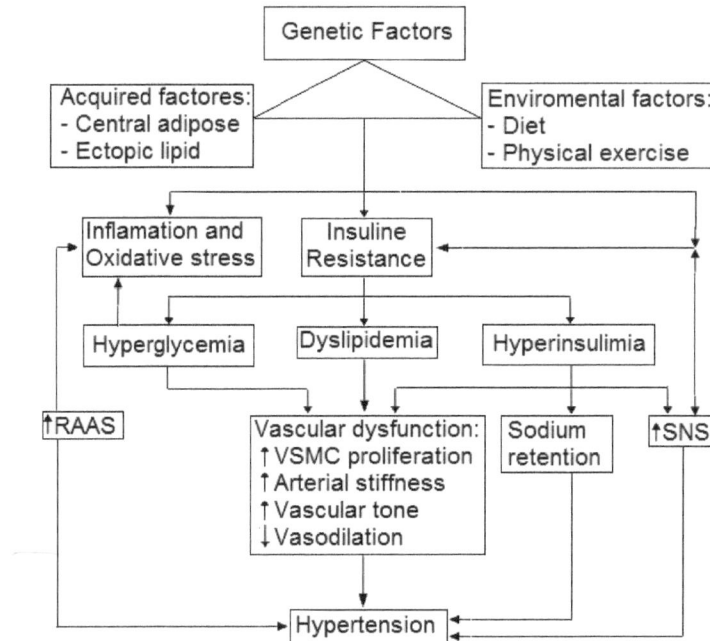

Figure 1: Pathophysiological mechanism between the diabetes and hypertension. VSMC = vascular smooth muscle cell; SNN = sympathetic nervous system; RAAS = renin-angiotensin-aldosterone system (Mugo et al., 2007).

For all above mentioned, the regular physical exercise serves either in preventing as treatment of metabolic syndrome its action affects the hormone levels, the muscular strength, bone metabolism and blood vessels. In the following topics will be presented studies that show acute and chronic effects of physical activity on the cardiovascular system, with emphasis on hypertension, because is a disease that affects millions of people worldwide and it increases with advancing age. We also discussed about the effects and care for prescription of exercise programs.

3   Effect of Physical Exercise on Endothelial Function

The vascular endothelium is represented by cells of the internal layer of all blood vessels and lymphatic system. It is just the small thickness of endothelium at the level of capillaries that allows active and passive molecules exchanges and ions between blood and lymph with the tissues (Cine *et al.*, 1998; Galley & Webster, 2004; Gartner & Hiatt, 2013).

In relation to arterial and venous vessels after the endothelial layer, there are thickness variations of elastic fibers, of smooth musculature and of collagen fibers. The thickness variation of the smooth musculature is directly related to its constriction and dilation capacity by altering the volume, the pressure and flow velocity of blood through in the vessels (Cine *et al.*, 1998; Galley & Webster, 2004; Gartner & Hiatt, 2013).

In physiological system, the vascular endothelium participates in the regulation of events related to blood coagulation, platelet and leukocyte action, besides regulation of vascular tone and inflammatory responses (Marsh & Coombes, 2005). During exercise practices, there is a greater blood pressure in the artery wall which causes the release of vasodilators which together with regulation the autonomic nervous play an important role in improving blood flow (Goto *et al.*, 2003).

The presence of risk factors such as hypertension and dyslipidemia are directly related to the occurrence of endothelial dysfunction that result in the activation of inflammatory and pathological processes that can lead to vascular damage (Singh & Jialal, 2006). These pathological events can be minimized by performing exercises that reduce the occurrence of cardiovascular events (Abramson & Vaccarino, 2002), as will be discussed below.

Nitric Oxide (NO) is one of the endothelial agents most studied having vasodilator effect with important role in maintenance of the endothelial structure integrity. NO is synthesized by the enzyme Nitric Oxide Synthase (NOS) by L-arginine amino acid, yielding NO and L-citrulline. NOS have three isoforms: two constitutive isoforms (eNOS, endothelial, nNOS, neuronal) and one inducible isoform (iNOS), that are associated the cytotoxic inflammatory responses. The NO has variation both in the synthesis as in effects by means in exercises performance (Leung *et al.*, 2008).

Studies have shown that regular physical exercise increases NO production, which increase coronary blood flow, thereby improving cardiac function (Rush *et al.* 2005; Goto *et al.*, 2003). In addition, NO has inhibitory effects on platelet and leukocytes well as induces proliferation of arterial smooth fibers (Ford & Rush, 2007).

These characteristics on vascular tone and antithrombotic reinforce the important role of NO in the preservation of integrity of the blood flow in the individuals, in such a manner that the presence of Reactive Oxygen Species (ROS) can inactivate the NO, which potentializes the formation of atheromatous plaques (Antoniades *et al.*, 2003; Beckman *et al.*, 1990). At the same time, studies show that blockade of NO synthesis causes the promotion of autonomous activity sympathetic, with resulting increased in systemic arterial pressure (Togashi *et al.*, 1992, Souza *et al.*, 2001).

Other studies show that performing aerobic exercise represents an antihypertensive therapy effective in minimizing cardiovascular risk factors (Maiorana *et al.*, 2003; Goldsmith *et al.*, 2000).

The increased NO synthesis appears to be associated with an increase in the bioavailability of its precursor, the amino acid arginine. Oral administration of L-arginine as a supplement increases the vasodilator effect of the lower limbs muscles of individuals that performed resistance exercises increasing the blood perfusion in these muscles as well as maximized the proteins synthesis involved in muscle contraction process (Schaefer *et al.*, 2002). Thus, arginine also contributes to the synthesis of NO that seems to have role potentialized function in transition of the muscle fibers in resistance overloads (Smith *et al.*, 2002).

Besides the NO, studies also show that aerobic exercises, practiced in childhood cause stimulation of some biological modulators that produce beneficial effects in decreasing the incidence of diabetes, hypertension and dyslipidemias also causing inhibition of other pro-inflammatory modulators (Barbeau *et al.*, 2002; Cooper *et al.*, 2004).

The antithrombotic effect of aerobic exercise has been identified by the reduction serum levels of important inflammatory modulators, such as C-Reactive Protein (CRP), Interleukin-6 (IL-6) and Tumor Necrosis Factor-α (TNF-α), which has been associated with the presence and progression of chronic diseases (Petersen & Pedersen, 2005; Greenberg & Obin, 2006; Visser *et al.*, 2001; Barbeau *et al.*, 2002; Brazil *et al.*, 2007). One of the benefits of aerobic exercise on blood vessels is associated with the response to post-exercise hypotension. Even though many components are involved in this response, the reduction in peripheral vascular resistance is certainly the one who has the most noticeable effects on the endothelium.

Once again NO have an important role vasodilator associated with a reduction in sympathetic autonomic response (Chen & Bonham, 2010). Added to this process, endothelial function tends to improve with regular exercise practice with induction angiogenic in the most active muscle groups of the exercises, increasing capillarity action and improving blood flow (Porter *et al.*, 2002; Prior *et al.*, 2003).

Another angiogenic effect caused by exercise is related to Endothelial Progenitor Cells (EPC) (Asahara *et al.*, 1997). Studies show that exercise training increases the migration of EPC into the peripheral circulation and these cells secrete angiogenic modulators, such as: Endothelial Growth Factor (EGF) and granulocyte colony-stimulating factor (G-CSF) (Adams *et al.*, 2008; Bonsignore *et al.*, 2010). This migration of EPC can cause both neovascularization as vascular repair (Hill *et al.*, 2003). In addition, the exercise at moderate intensities shows strong positive correlation between EPC and NO (Yang *et al.*, 2007).

4   Acute Effect of Aerobic and Resistance Exercises

According to scientific literature, the controlled physical exercises has contributed for maintenance blood pressure because after executing the exercise, the blood pressure is reduced to values lower than those presented in the beginning of the exercise (Taylor-Tolbert *et al.*, 2000; Melo *et al.*, 2006; Park *et al.*, 2006).

This acute effect is known as post exercise hypotension (PEH) and can last a few minutes or even a few hours, it is observed both in hypertensive individuals (Taylor-Tolbert *et al.*, 2000; Hagberg *et al.*, 1987; Melo *et al.*, 2006), in borderline hypertensive individuals (Headley *et al.*, 1998; Park *et al.*, 2006) as well as in normotensive individuals (Forjaz *et al.*, 2000; Wallace *et al.*, 1999). Particularly for hypertensive patients PEH has significant clinical value.

The first report of PEH occurred in 1897 by Leonard Hill when he observed the process in an individual who ran 400 yards and 90 minutes after the proof revealed a PEH (Hill, 1897). Decades later (Schneider & Truesdell, 1922) also observed this same process in a test sit and rise from a chair five times every 15 seconds. However, investigations on the effects of PEH in the organism, the type of exercise, the population that this effect is more evident and the mechanism by which occurs, gained more evidence from the end of year 1970.

In this period, Fitzgerald (1981) after not present significant response to drugs, he decided to abandon the pharmacological treatment and began a running training allied to food reeducation. Between the years 1976 and 1979 he began to monitor your blood pressure three times / day, it went on to note that after the routine run approximately 25 min, their blood pressure reduced to levels lower than baseline.

PEH has been reported both in normotensive as in hypertensive individuals, in its turn, these latter have lower reduction of blood pressure when compared to normotensive groups (Forjaz *et al.*, 2000; Oliveira *et al.*, 2012). One possible explanation for this may be that in normotensive, the baroreflex mechanism prevents the occurrence of PEH as a form of not affect orthostatic tolerance (McDonald, 2002).

Already in the systemic form, two explanations can help understand the pressure reduction after exercise: the first is the cardiac output reduction caused by decreased systolic volume and second explication by reducing peripheral vascular resistance (PVR) (Rezk *et al.*, 2006; Rueckert *et al.*, 1996).

Currently there are two types of physical exercises that are most studied by researchers to assess the PEH phenomenon, which are: aerobic and resistance exercises. Resistance exercise began to be discussed recently, having still controversial results due to the use of different training protocols involving: number of sets and sessions, number of repetitions, rest intervals, number of exercises and intensity of effort as well as level of fitness physical, age and profile pressure of the individual (Annunciation & Polito, 2011; Oliveira *et al.*, 2012).

The effect mechanism PEH by resistance exercise realized in the intensity of 40% 1RM (one repetition maximum test) is promoted by reduced cardiac output and maintenance of PVR, while in intensity of 80% 1RM the cardiac output decreased continues, however, with the increase in PVR (peripheral vascular resistance). In this way, resistance exercise with lower intensity promotes PEH both Systolic Blood Pressure (SBP) as Diastolic Blood Pressure (DBP), in turn the highest intensity allows only reduction in SBP (Rezk *et al.*, 2006).

In the aerobic exercise, Rueckert *et al.* (1996) observed the two hypotensive mechanisms at different times of the recovery after training, primarily by decreasing PVR and posterior decrease in cardiac output. Studies have shown the existence of acute hypotensive effect in hypertensive patients after the first training session with aerobic exercise (Taylor-Tolbert *et al.*, 2000; Kokkinos & Papademetriou, 2000).

Behind all this, there is an adaptation of the autonomic nervous system to the new body physiological condition after physical activity, occurring inhibition of sympathetic nerve activity that favors the reduction in blood pressure as a consequence of the reduction in PVR (Floras *et al.*, 1989; Halliwill *et al.*, 1996).

In resistance exercise, the study of Melo *et al.* (2006) showed a greater reduction in blood pressure after low-intensity exercise in hypertensive women that used angiotensin-converting enzyme (ACE). In the same study PEH remained by 10pm below the levels shown in the pressure control session.

It is observed that both SBP and DBP remained at low levels (p <0.05), compared with the control session for up to 10h after the final of the resistance training session. The experimental session was performed with six exercises, three sets of 20 repetitions at an intensity of 40% 1RM (Melo *et al.*, 2006).

The intensity used by Melo *et al.* (2006) corroborates the results encountered by Koltybn & Focht (1999) after verifying reductions in SBP and maintenance DBP in individuals who performed resistance exercise at 40% of 1RM, whereas increased SBP and DBP maintenance when performing training with 80% of 1 RM, suggesting that low-intensity resistance exercise has hypotensive effect greater than that realized at high intensity.

Recently, (Keese *et al.*, 2011) investigated the hypotensive response in 4 different sessions: control, aerobic exercise, resistance exercise and concurrent exercise (aerobic and resistance exercises together in the same session). During the recovery period of this study, after 120 minutes the concurrent exercise session presented greater hypotensive effect compared to the other two exercise groups and the control session (Keese *et al.*, 2011). It is noteworthy that studies using this methodology are recent and should be conducted in populations with different age groups as well as different pressure profiles.

The PEH through aerobic exercise was observed in cycle ergometer or treadmill ergometer at intensities ranging from 40% - 100% of heart rate reserve and VO2max or maximum predicted heart rate (Casonatto & Polito, 2009). But, there is still no consensus in the scientific literature of the ideal intensity to obtain PEH (Polito & Casonatto, 2009) because both the low (Forjaz *et al.*, 1998) as of high intensities (Macdonald *et al.*, 2001) showed capacity to provoke PEH in hypertensive patients. However, studies with greater intensity are able to cause greater duration and magnitude (Piepoli *et al.*, 1994; Forjaz *et al.*, 2004).

Regarding the duration of exercise, numerous studies advocate the hypothesis when higher the realization of aerobic activity, the greater the effects on the duration and magnitude of PEH (March *et al.*, 2005; Forjaz *et al.*, 1998; Jones *et al.*, 2007).

The study of March *et al.* (2005) submitting 9 volunteers pre-hypertensive at 4 sessions of aerobic exercise with the same intensity, around 75% of heart rate reserve and different durations of training, varying in 10, 20, 40 and 80 min. It was noted that the PEH had greatest magnitude and duration when applied for longer training protocol. Stanley *et al.* (2013) demonstrate that the time required for complete cardiac autonomic recovery after an aerobic training session is up to 24h following low-intensity exercise, 24–48 h following threshold-intensity exercise and at least 48h following high-intensity exercise.

The mechanism through which the PEH occurs after the realization of aerobic exercise still needs further study for effective prescription of training with greater hypotensive effect as well as population profile that best responds to exercise.

The responses to resistance exercise are similar to aerobic, reducing cardiac output and PVR. It is known that the reduction of PVR is associated with the release of vasodilator substances in the endothelium, such as NO, and adenosine prostaglandins. However, the PEH persist even with the blocking release of these substances. Another component that is directly involved in PVR is the reduction of sympathetic nerve activity, which also allows the occurrence of PEH (Annunciation & Polito, 2011).

In resistance exercise, the probably action hypotensive occurs through different pathways, that are depend on the intensity of the effort employed by the exercise. At low intensities with 40% of 1RM in resistance exercise hypotension is presented by reduction of CO and maintenance of PVR, since at high intensities as 80% of 1RM, the PEH is reduced by reduction of the CO, but with a slight increase in the PVR (Rezk *et al.*, 2006).

The aerobic exercise mechanism PEH is associated only to the PVR, possibly due to vasodilation in smaller vessels as a result of arterial stiffness which also can be caused by increasing age (Hagberg, *et al.* 1987; Rueckert *et al.* 1996; Brandes *et al.* 2005).

The mechanism PEH after aerobic and resistance exercises, the training prescription that shows greater hypotensive effect and population profile that best responds to the type of exercise, are still poorly known. However, the studies identified in the scientific literature present different hypotheses to explain the phenomenon of PEH for resistance exercise and for the aerobic, but both have action with the two responsible for the mediation of blood pressure, which are: cardiac output (CO) and peripheral vascular resistance (PVR).

Finally, the blood pressure reduction was noted in the end of century XIX and gained visibility in the end of century XX. The experiments, with aerobic and resistance exercises presented positive effect even utilizing different protocols. However, although there are studies showing that resistance exercise performed at low intensity promotes hypotension for up to 10h, these should be viewed with caution because the study population was exclusively hypertensive individuals. For this reason, it is necessary to compare groups of different profile, as well as verification of the volume and intensity that fits best for patient profile evaluated.

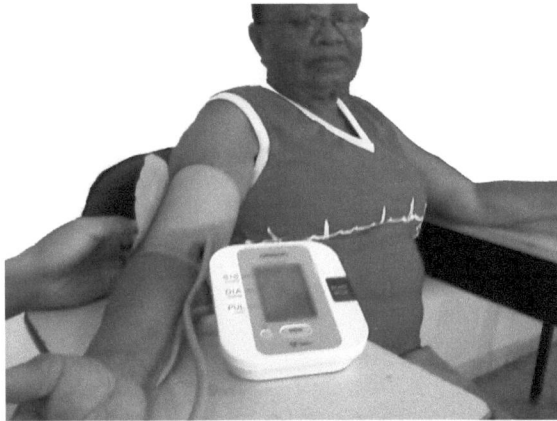

Figure 2: Blood pressure assessment first and after resistance training program. Photography courtesy of Oliveira, M.C. Resistance Training program of the Laboratory of State University of Pará – Brazil.

5   Chronic Effect of Aerobic and Resistance Exercises

The regular practice of appropriate physical activity may represent a reduction of government public spending with pathologies associated to cardiovascular diseases, and in addition, heavily contribute to the improvement in the health and quality of life for people in all ages (Bielemann *et al.*, 2009). The physical activity is associated with numerous systemic changes that result in adaptations of the organism seeking the homeostasis after performing a training session with physical exercise.

In this way, chronic exercise is associated with changes in body composition, in the lipid and glycemic index, muscle strength and blood pressure (Volaklis *et al.*, 2013). All these factors act directly or indirectly on the endothelium, consequently, the regular exercise is a potential agent to improve and maintain the integrity of the vascular tissue (Volaklis *et al.*, 2013).

These adaptations take place mainly at the molecular level, dividing into neurohumoral and autonomic effects which cause reduced sympathetic tone and increased of the sympathetic vascular changes due to increased vasodilation endothelial and NO synthesis, as well as cardiac adaptations as physiological hypertrophy, prevention of calcification, besides, non-cardiac adaptations musculoskeletal improvement, increased aerobic capacity and reduced blood viscosity. However, in certain areas such as in the venous system and microcirculation, studies are preliminary and warrant further attention by the scientific community (Gielen *et al.*, 2010).

In the last decade, numerous studies have demonstrated that endothelial progenitor cells are stimulated with the realization of physical activity. These cells are produced by the bone marrow and are able to migrate to a region of lesioned endothelium, passing to differentiate into mature cells, and thus perform an important role in the regeneration process of the endothelium (Volaklis *et al.*, 2013). However, the changes brought about by physical exercise are not limited to the endothelium. It was found that blood pressure reductions in around 3 mmHg can mean reduced risk of suffering encephalic vascular accident in up to 14%, as well as 5-9% reduced risk in cardiovascular morbidity in trained individuals (Meka *et al.*, 2008).

In a study of animal model for hypertension was observed decreased of sensitivity in the baroreceptors activity; however this situation is reversed with the low intensity training (Andersen & Yang,

1989). In human's low-intensity aerobic exercise also promoted chronic reducing of blood pressure, this being conducted among 40% to 60% VO_{2max} with high volume weekly or related to the daily session (Alvez & Forjaz, 2007). For Whelton *et al.* (2002) in a meta-analysis that evaluated 54 controlled trials of aerobic training, it was found a mean reduction in systolic of 3.7 mmHg and 2.6 mmHg diastolic blood pressure.

In another meta-analysis study that investigated the chronic effects of resistance exercise on blood pressure, it was found reduced blood pressure between 3.2 and 3.5mmHg (Cornelissen & Fagard, 2005a). Even though seem little, as previously mentioned, the progressive reduction of the blood pressure through the physical activity significantly reduces the risk of death from cardiovascular disease (Meka *et al.*, 2008). One factor for this are little work which aim to assess the chronic effects of resistance exercise in the cardiovascular system, another problem, as previously mentioned, is the profile and criteria for sample selection because trained volunteers, sedentary, normotensive, hypertensive users of antihypertensive medications, can present similar and/or different responses, but by different mechanisms which influence the results and consequently the conclusions. What can also be seen in meta-analysis study by Cornelissen & Fagard (2005b) evaluated 75 studies with healthy adults: normotensive and hypertensive patients for a minimum of four week intervention, this study observed reduction of - 6.9mmHg in hypertensive groups, while normotensive obtained - 2.4mmHg of reduction in blood pressure.

Given the above, one should consider the small number of investigations which aim to assess the characteristics of physical exercise in the process of chronic reduction in blood pressure. However, comparing resistance exercise with aerobic, there is a disparity in the number of studies in favor of aerobic exercise. Given this, there is a need for more studies to be verified a better way to prescribe resistance exercise with the objective of reducing chronic blood pressure. For Andersen *et al.* (2013) in an investigation in skeletal muscle morphology with risk of cardiovascular events in a sample of 466 71 years-old men without cardiovascular disease, of which 295 were physically active (strenuous physical activity at least 3 h / week) was concluded that higher skeletal muscle proportion of type-I fibres was associated with lower risk of cardiovascular events and a higher proportion of type-II fibres was associated with higher risk of cardiovascular events. These relations were only observed in physically active men. Skeletal muscle fibre composition may be a mediator of the protective effects of exercise against cardiovascular disease, which can justify the need for maintenance of resistance training at moderate and low intensities (aerobic and resistance exercises) for an appropriate hypotensive effect.

In turn, both exercises triggers physiological mechanisms endothelial that allow blood pressure control in the medium and long term, and the reduction of public spending on cardiovascular events coming from the hypertension can justify the use of training programs with these exercises for normotensive and hypertensive populations with greater professional care for hypertensive patients.

6   Aerobic and Resistance Exercises for Hypertensive Elderly

The American College of Sport Medicine (ACSM) recommends performing aerobic and resistance exercise to control blood pressure in hypertensive individuals, provided they are not suffering from cardiovascular or renal complications arising from these diseases (Pescatello *et al.*, 2004). The physical exercise, especially aerobic should be associated to pharmacological treatment, as well as the change in lifestyle of hypertensive patients are, especially, recommended for the maintenance and control of blood pressure (Pescatello *et al.*, 2004).

However, there is a major risk for hypertensive patients of increase in blood pressure while performing any physical activity. This increase occurs by activation of the sympathetic nervous system with the objective of optimize and redistribute blood flow in the recruited muscles during exercise, and for that reason can cause problems such as: cerebral aneurysm or myocardial ischemia (Vongpatanasin *et al.*, 2011). But interestingly, as blood flow is directed to the left ventricle during cardiac diastole, the high elevation of diastolic pressure during exercise seems to cause a protective effect against cardiac ischemia, although it is the perilous increase of systolic pressure at this moment. This was observed by Vongpatanasin *et al.* (2011) with 469 elderly patients after exercise on a cycle ergometer.

The use pharmacologic therapy show also protective effect in the elevation process of blood pressure during exercise. Was what showed Gomides *et al.* (2010) submitting to a group of 10 hypertensive patients to a protocol with execution of a leg extension exercise to muscular failure in series of 100%, 80% and 40% of 1RM in two phases: initially with using the Atenolol (β-adrenergic blockade) and other group with placebo. The training series conducted with the drug therapy showed lower pressure values than those performed with placebo (Gomides *et al.*, 2010).

For Haykowsky *et al.* (1996) The association of physical activity and increased blood pressure, especially when associated with the valsalva maneuver, cause pressure rises with higher values 480/350mmHg during exercise, which can lead to intracranial aneurysms. However, no study that shows caused death of individuals, but is prudent to consider this increase in blood pressure during exercise caused by maneuver valsalsa (Haykowsky *et al.*, 1996).

The valsalva maneuver is a hemodynamic process characterized by forced expiration against a closed glottis, increasing intrathoracic pressure and systemic circulation, leading the individual to dizziness, syncope and to brain injuries (Zhang *et al.*, 2012). However, this is inevitable when the exercise intensity is equal or greater than 80% 1RM, and as a consequence can increase abruptly the pressure 58±28 mmHg. Already with higher loads, intrathoracic pressure exceeds 100 mmHg, which corresponds to increases about 60%, that is, more than the voluntary valsalva maneuver (Maccartney *et al.*, 1999).

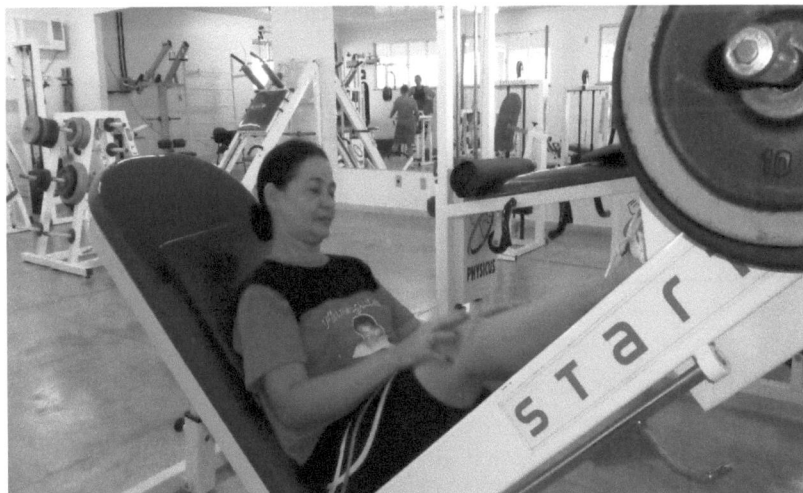

Figure 3: Resistance training for the treatment of hypertension patients. Photography courtesy of Oliveira, M.C. Resistance training program of the Laboratory of State University of Pará – Brazil.

Clinical trials have shown that aerobic exercise combining resistance exercise promotes the prevention and control of hypertension, and both when combined in the training program, provide best results for hypertension (Fletcher *et al.*, 2001; Keese *et al.*, 2011). The frequency of the training program should be 5 times / week, beginning with progressively lighter activity and subsequently moderate activity, for this, the intensity can be evaluated by a treadmill and strength tests in order to establish the maximum heart rate and also maximum strength (Brazilian Society of Hypertension, 2010; Sorace *et al.*, 2012).

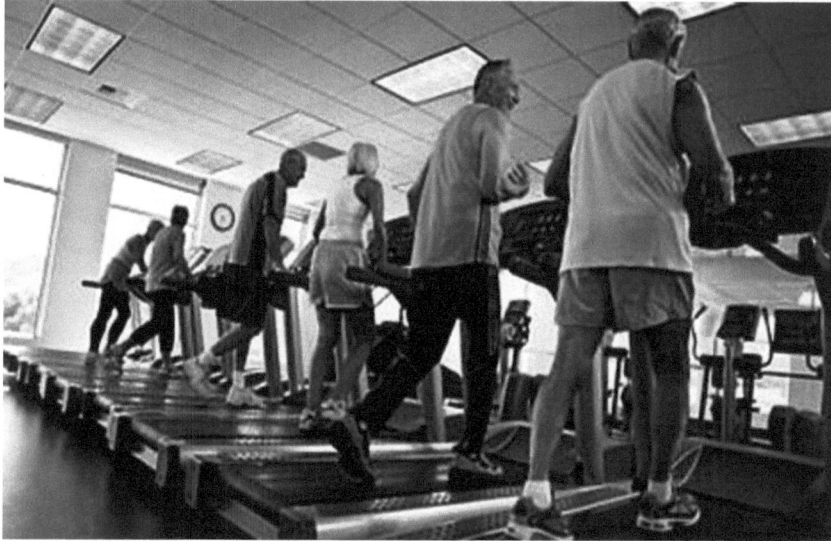

Figure 4: Aerobic training for treatment of hypertension. Figure Google image without restrictions on its use.

In the impossibility of realize the aerobic test, the calculation HR_{max} = 220-age can be used, except for individuals who use β-blockers and/or calcium inhibitor drugs channel (Brazilian Society of Hypertension, 2010). The benefits of resistance training are already known in the skeletal and muscular systems, but only in recent years its effect on the vascular system has be studied with greater frequency. In the case of hypertension, it must be realized as a complement to aerobic training between two and three times/week with 1 to 3 sets of 8 to 15 repetitions until concentric failure (Brazilian Society of Hypertension, 2010). But aerobic exercise can be done every day of the week in intensity between 40% and 60% of reserve VO_2 in activities such as walking, running and cycling that has duration longer than 30 min, continuous or accumulated through the day (Pescatello *et al.*, 2004). Table 1 presents the types of exercises, physical modality, as well as intensity and frequency based on systematic studies on this topic.

It is worth emphasizing, that although exercises are indicated for hypertension, it should be prevented if the individual has blood pressure above 160 mmHg and 105 mmHg for systolic and diastolic, respectively, because these pressure levels can cause cardiac ischemia or intracranial aneurysms (Brazilian Society of Hypertension, 2010).

It is also recommended that the patient be evaluated by a cardiologist before commencing physical activity, as well as the activity is accompanied by a physical education professional, qualified to prescribe and evaluate the training.

Exercises	Time	Intensity	Volume
Aerobic Training - Walking - Run - Bicycling	>30 minutes	Between 40-60% VO_{2max} or 50-70% HR_{max}	3 times/week
Resistance Training	*	Between 40-55% of 1RM	Among 1-3 sets of 12 to 20 reps; 6-8 exercises per training. With intervals of 1 minute rest between sets and repetitions to allow the reduction of BP before a new stimulus.

* The duration of resistance exercise will depend on the amount present in the training exercises, well as the rest interval during the sessions and repetitions numbers.

Table 1: Recommended Physical Activities for hypertensive population.

7   Final Considerations

Recent advances on the understanding of the influence of physical activity as non-pharmacological treatment in the prevention and control of cardiovascular disease, in particular to hypertension are evident in scientific literature. With that, monitoring by adequately trained health professionals in a multidisciplinary and interdisciplinary relationship with a physical education professional, cardiologist, nutritionist, among others, allows the elderly has better quality of life through the exercises programs. Thus, physical exercise, especially, the aerobic exercise being complemented by low-intensity resistance training is a good recommendation because they presented real gains in reducing blood pressure in hypertensive patients, particularly when combined with pharmacological treatment.

It is worth noting also, that the cultural habits of a population, ease of access, as well as costs related to the practice of physical exercise can be determinant to motivate the elderly to practice this or that type of training. Given all that was addressed, and also considering the recommendations of the official health organs such as the World Health Organization, American College of Sport Medicine and National Institute on Aging, the controlled exercises can benefit the people with hypertension.

References

Abramson JL, Vaccarino V. (2002) *Relationship between physical activity and inflammation among apparently healthy middle-aged and older US adults. Arch Intern Med. 162 (11): 1286-92.*

Adams V, Linke A, Breuckmann F, Leineweber K, Erbs S, Krankel N, et al. (2008) *Circulating progenitor cells decrease immediately after marathon race in advanced-age marathon runners. Eur J Cardiovasc Prev Rehabil.15(5):602-7.*

Alves LL, Forjaz C. (2007) *influência da intensidade e do volume do treinamento aeróbico na redução da pressão arterial de hipertensos [in Portuguese]. R. bras. Ci e Mov. 15(3): 115-122.*

Andresen M.C, Yang M. (1989) *Arterial baroreceptor resetting: contributions of chronic and acute processes. Clin. Exp. Pharmacol. Physiol. 15 (2):19–30.*

Andersen K., Lind L., Ingelsson E., Ärnlöv J., Byberg L., Michaëlsson K et al. (2013). Skeletal muscle morphology and risk of cardiovascular disease in elderly men. European J Preventive Cardiology. Online Published in October 3, doi:10.1177/2047487313506828.

Antoniades C, Tousoulis D, Tentolouris C, Toutouzas P, Stefanadis C. (2003) Oxidative stress, antioxidant vitamins, and atherosclerosis. Herz. 28 (7):628-38.

Anunciação PG, Polito MD. (2011) A review on post-exercise hypotension in hypertensive individuals. Arq Bras Cardiol. 96(5):100-109.

Asahara T, Murohara T, Sullivan A, Silver M, van der Zee R, Li T et al. (1997) Isolation of putative progenitor endothelial cells for angiogenesis. Science. 275(5302):964-7.

Bahia L, Aguiar L, Villela NR, Bottino D, Bouskela E. (2006) The endothelium in the metabolic syndrome.Arq Bras Endocrinol Metab. 50(2):291-303.

Barbeau P, Litaker MS, Woods KF, Lemmon CR, Humphries MC, Owens S et al. (2002) Hemostatic and inflammatory markers in obese youths: effects of exercise and adiposity. J Pediatr. 141:415-20.

Behringer EJ, Shaw RL, Westcott EB, Socha MJ, Segal SS. (2013) Aging impairs electrical conduction along endothelium of resistance arteries through enhanced Ca2+-activated K+ channel activation. Arterioscler Thromb Vasc Biol. 33(8):1892-901.

Beckman J, Beckman TW, Chen J, Marshall PA, Freeman BA. (1990) Apparent hydroxyl radical production by peroxynitrite: implications for endothelial injury from nitric oxide and superoxide. Proc Natl Acad Sci USA. 87(4):1620-4.

Bielemann R, Knuth A, Hallal. (2010) Physical activity and cost savings for chronic diseases to the Health System. Rev. Bras de Ativ física & Saude.15(1); 9-14.

Bonsignore MR, Morici G, Riccioni R, Huertas A, Petrucci E, Veca M, et al. (2010) Hemopoietic and angiogenetic progenitors in healthy athletes: different responses to endurance and maximal exercise. J Appl Physiol. 109(1):60-7.

Brandes RP, Fleming I, Busse R. (2005) Endothelial aging. Cardiovasc Res. 2005; 66 (2): 286-94.

Brasil AR, Norton RC, Rossetti MB, Leão E, Mendes RP. (2007) C-reactive protein as an indicator of low intensity inflammation in children and adolescents with and without obesity. J Pediatr. (Rio Janeiro);83:477-80.

Campagna A, Bourdel-Marchasson I, Simon D. (2005) Burden of diabetes in an aging population: prevalence, incidence, mortality, characteristics and quality of care. Diabetes Metab. 31(2):535-552.

Casonatto J, Polito M. (2009) Post-exercise hypotension: a systematic review [in Portuguese]. Rev Bras Med Esporte. 15(2):151-157.

Chen CY, Bonham AC. (2010) Post-exercise hypotension: central mechanisms. Exerc Sport Sci Rev; 38(3):122-127.

Cheung BM, Li C. (2012) Diabetes and hypertension: is there a common metabolic pathway? Curr Atheroscler Rep. 14(2):160-6.

Cines DB, Pollak ES, Buck CA, Loscalzo J, Zimmerman GA, McEver RP, et al. Endothelial cells in physiology and in the pathophysiology of vascular disorders.Blood. 1998 15;91(10):3527-61.

Cooper DM, Nemet D, Galassetti P. (2004) Exercise, stress, and inflammation in the growing child: from the bench to the playground. Curr Opin Pediatr.16:286-92.

Cornelissen VA, Fagard RH. (2005a) Effects of endurance training on blood pressure, blood pressure-regulating mechanisms, and cardiovascular risk factors. Hypertension. 46(4):667-675.

Cornelissen VA, Fagard RH. (2005b) Effect of resistance training on resting blood pressure: a meta-analysis of randomized controlled trials. J Hypertens. 23(2):251-925.

Del Prato S. (2009) Role of glucotoxicity and lipotoxicity in the pathophysiology of Type 2 diabetes mellitus and emerging treatment strategies. Diabet Med. 26:1185-1192.

Denys K. (2009) Metabolic syndrome in the elderly: an overview of the evidence. Acta Clin Belg. 64(1):23-34.

Duvnjak L, Bulum T, Metelko Z. (2008) Hypertension and the metabolic syndrome. Diabetol Croat. 37(4):83-89.

El Assar M, Angulo J, Rodríguez-Mañas L. (2013) Oxidative stress and vascular inflammation in aging. Free Radic Biol Med. 10(65C):380-401.

Estruch R, Ros E, Salas-Salvadó J, Covas MI, Corella D, Arós F et al. (2013) Primary Prevention of Cardiovascular Disease with a Mediterranean Diet. N Engl J Med. 368(14):1279-90.

Ferrannini E, Vichi S, Beck-Nielsen H, et al. (1996) Insulin action and age. European Group for the Study of Insulin Resistance. Diabetes. 45;947-953.

Fitzgerald W. (1981) Labile hypertension and jogging: new diagnostic tool or spurious discovery? Br Med J (Clin Res Ed); 282: 542–544.

Fletcher GF, Balady GJ, Amsterdam EA, Chaitman B, Eckel R, Fleg J. et al. (2001) Exercise standards for testing and training: a statement for healthcare professionals from the American Heart Association. Circulation;104(14):1694-740.

Floras JS, Sinkey CA, Aylward PE, Seals DR, Thoren PN, Mark AL. (1989) Post-exercise hypotension and sympathoinhibition in borderline hypertensive men. Hypertension. 14(1):28-35.

Focht, BC, Koltyn KF. (1999) Influence of resistance exercise of different intensities on 15 state anxiety and blood pressure. Med Sci Sports Exerc. 31:456-463.

Forjaz CL, Santaella DF, Rezende LO, Barretto AC, Negrão CE. (1998) Effect of exercise duration on the magnitude and duration of post-exercise hypotension [in Portuguese]. Arq Bras Cardiol. 70(2):99-104.

Forjaz CL, Tinucci T, Ortega KC, Santaella DF, Mion D Jr, Negrão CE. (2000) Factors affecting post-exercise hypotension in normotensive and hypertensive humans. Blood Press Monit. 5(5-6):255-262.

Forjaz CL, Cardoso CG Jr, Rezk CC, Santaella DF, Tinucci T. et al. (2004) Post-exercise hypotension and hemodynamics: the role of exercise intensity. J Sports Med Phys Fitness. 44(1):54-62.

Fukai T, Siegfried MR, Ushio-Fukai M, Cheng Y, Kojda G, Harrison DG. (2000) Regulation of the vascular extracellular superoxide dismutase by nitric oxide and exercise training. J Clin Invest. 105:1631-9.

Galley HF, Webster NR. (2004) Physiology of the endothelium. Br J Anaesth. Jul;93(1):105-13.

Gartner LP, Hiatt JL. (2013) Color atlas and text of histology. Edition:6, Lippincott. Wiliams & Wilkins Ed, Baltimore, SA.

Gielen S, Schuler G, Adams V. (2010) Cardiovascular Effects of Exercise Training : Molecular Mechanisms.Circulation. 122:1221-1238.

Goldsmith RL, Bloomfield DM, Rosenwinkel ET. (2000) Exercise and autonomic function. Coron Artery Dis. 11:129-35.

Gomides RS, Costa LA, Souza DR, Queiroz AC, Fernandes JR, Ortega KC et al. (2010) Atenolol blunts blood pressure increase during dynamic resistance exercise in hypertensives. Br J Clin Pharmacol.70(5):664-673.

Goto C, Higashi Y, Kimura M, Noma K, Hara K, Nakagawa K et al. (2003) Effect of different intensities of exercise on endothelium-dependent vasodilatation in humans: role of endothelium-dependent nitric oxide and oxidative stress. Circulation. 108(5):530-5.

Greenberg AS, Obin MS. (2006) Obesity and the role of adipose tissue in inflammation and metabolism. Am J Clin Nutr. 83:461S-465S.

Hagberg JM, Montain SJ, Martin WH. (1987) Blood pressure and hemodynamic responses after exercise in older hypertensives. J Appl Physiol. 63(1):270-276.

Halliwill JR, Taylor JA, Eckberg DL. (1996) Impaired sympathetic vascular regulation in humans after acute dynamic exercise. J Physiol. 495(1):279-288.

Haykowsky MJ, Findlay JM, Ignaszewski AP. (1996) Aneurysmal subarachnoid hemorrhage associated with weight training: three case reports. Clin J Sport Med. 6(1):52-55.

Headley SA, Keenan TG, Manos TM, Phillips K, Lachowetz T, Keenan HA. et al. (1998) Renin and hemodynamic responses to exercise in borderline hypertensives. Ethn Dis. 8(3):312-318.

Hilberg T. (2008) Physical activity in the prevention of cardiovascular diseases: epidemiology and mechanisms. Hamostaseologie. 28 (1): 9-15.

Hill JM, Zalos G, Halcox JP, Schenke WH, Waclawiw MA, Quyyumi AA, et al. (2003) Circulating endothelial progenitor cells, vascular function, and cardiovascular risk. N Engl J Med. 348(7):593-600.

Hill L. (1987) Arterial pressure in man while sleeping, resting, working and bathing. J Physiol. (Lond). 22:26-29.

Jones H, George K, Edwards B, Atkinson G. (2007) Is the magnitude of acute post-exercise hypotension mediated by exercise intensity or total work done? Eur J Appl Physiol. 102(1):33-40.

Keese F, Farinatti P, Pescatello L, Monteiro W. (2011) A comparison of the immediate effects of resistance, aerobic, and concurrent exercise on postexercise hypotension. J Strength Cond Res. 25(5):1429-1436.

Kokkinos PF, Papademetriou V. (2000) Exercise and hypertension. Coron Artery Dis. 11:99-102.

Leung FP, Yung LM, Laher I, Yao X, Chen ZY, Huang Y. (2008) Exercise, vascular wall and cardiovascular diseases: an uptade (part1). Sports Med. 38(12):1009-24.

Lechleitner M, Herold M, Dzien-Bischinger C, Hoppichler F, Dzien A.Tumour necrosis factor-alpha plasma levels in elderly patients with Type 2 diabetes mellitus-observations over 2 years. Diabet Med. 2002;19(11):949-53.

MacDonald JR, Hogben CD, Tarnopolsky MA, MacDougall JD. (2001) Post exercise hypotension is sustained during subsequent bouts of mild exercise and simulated activities of daily living. J Hum Hypertens. 15(8):567-71.

MacDonald JR. (2002) Potential causes, mechanisms, and implications of post exercise hypotension. J Hum Hypertens. 16(4):225-36.

Mach C, Foster C, Brice G, Mikat RP, Porcari JP. (2005) Effect of exercise duration on postexercise hypotension. J Cardiopulm Rehabil. 25(6):366-369.

Mackey RH, Sutton-Tyrrell K, Vaitkevicius PV, Sakkinen PA, Lyles MF, Spurgeon HA et al. (2002) Correlates of aortic stiffness in elderly individuals: a subgroup of the Cardiovascular Health Study. Am J Hypertens. 15(1):16–23.

Maiorana A, O'Driscoll G, Taylor R, Green D. (2003) Exercise and the nitric oxide vasodilator system. Sports Med. 33:1013-35.

Marsh SA, Coombes JS. (2005) Exercise and the endothelial cell. Int J Cardiol. 99(2):165-9.

McCartney N. (1999) Acute responses to resistance training and safety. Med Sci Sports Exerc. 31(1):31-37.

Meka N, Katragadda S, Cherian B, Arora RR. (2008) Endurance exercise and resistance training in cardiovascular disease. Ther Adv Cardiovasc Dis. 2(2):115–121.

Melo CM, Alencar Filho AC, Tinucci T, Mion D Jr, Forjaz CL. (2006) Post-exercise hypotension induced by low-intensity resistance exercise in hypertensive women receiving captopril.Blood Press Monit. 11(4):183-189.

Montalti M, Bargiani M, Montalti B, Mucci N, Cupelli V, Arcangeli G.Risk assessment of arterial hypertension in a working population. G Ital Med Lav Ergon. 2012;34(3):199-201.

Mosca L. Heart Disease Prevention in Women. Circulation. 2004; 109 (1): 158-160.

Mugo MN, Stump CS, Rao PG et al. (2007) Hypertension and diabetes mellitus. In: Black HR, Elliott WJ, editors. Hypertension: A Companion to Braunwald's Heart Disease. Elsevier. p. 409.

Muller DC, Elahi D, Tobin JD, Andres R. (1996) The effect of age on insulin resistance and secretion: A review. Semin Nephrol. 16:289-298.

National Institute on Aging. Global Health and Aging. (2011) World Health Organization. 11(7737):1-28.

Oliveira MA, Borba-Pinheiro CJ, Rocha-Junior OR, Reis TET, Monteiro-Santos R, Souza AC, Walsh-Monteiro A. (2012) Efecto hipotensor después de ejercicio de resistencia en mujeres mayores con hipertensión [in Spanish]. Rev Motricidad Humana; Edición 13 (1).

Ostchega Y, Dillon CF, Hughes JP, Carroll M, Yoon S. (2007) Trends in hypertension prevalence, awareness, treatment, and control in older U.S. adults: data from the National Health and Nutrition Examination Survey 1988 to 2004. J Am Geriatr Soc. 55:1056–1065.

Park S, Rink LD, Wallace JP. (2006) Accumulation of physical activity leads to a greater blood pressure reduction than a single continuous session, in prehypertension. J Hypertens. 24(9):1761-170.

Pescatello, LS, Franklin BA, Fagard R, Farquhar WB, Kelley GA, Ray CA et al. (2004) American College of Sports Medicine position stand. Exercise and hypertension. Med Sci Sports Exerc. 36:533-553.

Petersen AM, Pedersen BK. (2005) The anti-inflammatory effect of exercise. J Appl Physiol. 98:1154-62.

Piepoli M, Isea JE, Pannarale G, Adamopoulos S, Sleight P, Coats AJ. (1994) Load dependence of changes in forearm and peripheral vascular resistance after acute leg exercise in man. J Physiol. 478(2):357-62.

Porter M M et al. (2002) Capillary supply of the tibialis anterior muscle in young, healthy, and moderately active men and women. J Appl Physiol, 92(4):1451-1457.

Prior BM et al. (2003) Exercise-induced vascular remodeling. Exerc Sport Sci Rev; 31(1):26-33.

Rezk CC, Marrache RC, Tinucci T, Mion D Jr, Forjaz CL. (2006) Post-resistance exercise hypotension, hemodynamics, and heart rate variability: influence of exercise intensity. Eur J Appl Physiol. 98:105-112.

Rueckert PA, Slane PR, Lillis DL, Hanson P. (1996) Hemodynamic patterns and duration of post-dynamic exercise hypotension in hypertensive humans. Med Sci Sports Exerc. 28(1):24-32.

Rush JWE, Denniss SG, Graham DA. (2005) Vascular nitric oxide and oxidative stress: determinants of endothelial adaptations to cardiovascular disease and to physical activity. Can J Appl Physiol. 30(4):442-74.

Rush JWE, Ford RJ. (2007) Nitric oxide, oxidative stress and vascular endothelium in health and hypertension. Clin Hemorh Microc. 37(1-2):185-92.

Sociedade Brasileira de Diabetes (Brazilian Diabetes Society). Diabetes in the elderly. From in: http://www.diabetes.org.br/colunistas-da-sbd/diabetes-em-pacientes-especiais/1826. Accessed in 29 May of 2013.

Sociedade Brasileira de Hipertensão (Brazilian Diabetes Society). (2010) VI Diretrizes brasileiras de hipertensão [in Portuguese]. Rev Bras Hipertens. 17(1):25-30.

Schaefer A, Piquard F, Geny B, Doutreleau S, Lampert E, Mettauer B, et al. (2002) Arginine reduces exercise-induced increase in plasma lactate and ammonia. Int J Sports Med. 403-7.

Schneider EC, Truesdell D. (1922) A statistical study of the pulse rate and the arterial blood pressures in recumbence, standing, and after a standard exercise. Am J Physiol.61:29-74.

Singh U, Jialal I. (2006) Oxidative stress and atherosclerosis. Pathophysiology. 13 (3):129-42.

Smith LW, Smith JD, Criswell DS. (2002) Involvement of nitric oxide synthase in skeletal muscle adaptation to chronic overload. J Appl Physiol. 92(5):2005-11.

Sorace P, Churilla JR, Magyari PM. (2012) Resistance Training for Hypertension. ACSM's Health & Fitness Journal. 16(1):13-17.

Souza HCD, Ballejo G, Salgado MCO, Silva VJD, Salgado HC. (2001) Cardiac sympathetic overactivity and decreased baroreflex sensitivity in L-NAME hypertensive rats. Am J Physiol - Heart Circ Physiol. 280: 844-50.

Stanley J, Peake JM, Buchheit M. (2013) Cardiac Parasympathetic Reactivation Following Exercise: Implications for Training Prescription [In press]. Sport Med. 10.1007/s40279-013-0083-4

Taylor-Tolbert NS, Dengel DR, Brown MD, McCole SD, Pratley RE, Ferrell RE. (2000) Ambulatory blood pressure after acute exercise in older men with essential hypertension. Am J Hypertens. 13(1):44-51.

Togashi H, Sakuma I, Yoshioka M, Kobayashi T, Yasuda H, Kitabatake A et al. (1992) A central nervous system action of nitric oxide in blood pressure regulation. J Pharmacol Exp Ther. 262: 343-7.

Vaitkevicius PV, Fleg JL, Engel JH, O'Connor FC, Wright JG, Lakatta LE. et al. (1993) Effects of age and aerobic capacity on arterial stiffness in healthy adults. Circulation. 88:1456–1462.

Visser M, Bouter LM, McQuillan GM, Wener MH, Harris TB. (2001) Low-grade systemic inflammation in overweight children. Pediatrics. 107:E13.

Volaklis K, Takmakidis S Halle M. (2013) Acute and chronic effects of exercise on circulating endothelial progenitor cells in healthy and diseased patients. Clin Res Cardiol. 102:249–257.

Vongpatanasin W, Wang Z, Arbique D, Arbique G, Adams-Huet B, Mitchell JH. (2011) Functional sympatholysis is impaired in hypertensive humans. The Journal of Physiology, 589(5):1209-1220.

Wallace JP, Bogle PG, King BA, Krasnoff JB, Jastremski CA. (1999) The magnitude and duration of ambulatory blood pressure reduction following acute exercise. J Hum Hypertens. 13(6):361-366.

Webb C, Inscho EW. (2005) Age-related changes in the cardiovascular system. In Prisant LM (ed). Hypertension in the Elderly. Totowa: Elsevier. 11-21.

Whelton SP, Chin A, Xin X, He J. (2002) Effect of aerobic exercise on blood pressure: A meta-analysis of randomized, controlled trials. Ann Intern Med. 136:493-503.

Yang Z, Wang JM, Chen L, Luo CF, Tang AL, Tao J. (2007) Acute exercise-induced nitric oxide production contributes to upregulation of circulating endothelial progenitor cells in healthy subjects. J Hum Hypertens. 21(6):452-60).

Zhang XY, Cao TS, Yuan LJ. (2012) The Mechanics of Left Ventricular Filling During the Strain Phase of the Valsalva Maneuver in Healthy Subjects. Am J Med Sci. 1(1)1-3.

Exercise in Rehabilitation of Sarcopenic and Myopathic Muscle: Effect on Intra- and Extracellular Compartments

Teet Seene

Department of Functional morphology, Institute of Exercise Biology
University of Tartu, Estonia

Priit Kaasik

Department of Functional morphology, Institute of Exercise Biology
University of Tartu, Estonia

1   Introduction

Aging and inactivity or disuse is associated with a decline in muscle mass, structure, strength and endurance (Evans, 2010; Seene *et al.*, 2012). A sedentary lifestyle, bed rest, spaceflight and hindlimb suspension lead the skeletal muscle to microcirculatory disturbances, atrophy, protein loss, changes in contractile properties and fiber type switching (Trappe, 2009; Evans, 2010). In both young and aged skeletal muscle, oxidative stress increases in response to unloading (Siu *et al.*, 2008) and may have an important role in mediating muscle atrophy. Unloading results in a decrease in the number of myonuclei and an increase in the number of apoptotic myonuclei in skeletal muscle (Leeuwenburg *et al.*, 2005).Heat-shock protein 70 (HSP 70) inhibits caspase-dependent and caspase-independent apoptotic pathways and may function in the regulation of muscle size via the inhibition of necrotic muscle fiber distribution and apoptosis in aged muscle (Ogata *et al.*, 2009). The decline in muscle mass primarily results from type II fiber atrophy and loss in the number of muscle fibers. Increased variability in fiber size, accumulation of non-grouping, scattered and angulated fibers and the expansion of extracellular space are characteristic to muscle atrophy (Buford *et al.*, 2010). Beyond the loss of muscle size due to reduced fiber number and myofibrillar proteins that underlie muscle weakness in the elderly (Clark & Manini, 2008), impairments in neural activation have been found, as well as potential alterations in other muscular properties that may reduce contractile quality defined as reduction in involuntary force production per unit muscle size (Gonzales *et al.*, 2000; Stackhouse *et al.*, 2001). The functional and structural decline of the neuromuscular system is a recognized cause of decreased strength, endurance what lead to the impaired performance of daily activities, and loss of independence in the elderly (Manini & Clark, 2012). Loss of muscle strength in older adults is weakly associated with the loss of lean body mass (Gandevia, 2001). It means that muscle weakness in older adults is more related to impairments in neural activation and/or reductions in the intrinsic force-generating capacity of skeletal muscle (Manini & Clark, 2012).

The number and magnitude of associations for low physical performance or disability are greater for low muscle strength than low muscle mass (Gandevia, 2001), and higher aerobic capacity is related to an increase in the abilities of cardiovascular factors in the elderly (Sagiv *et al.*, 2010; Seppet *et al.*, 2013). But it is still unclear whether aerobic exercise training is superior to resistance training or other exercise models in altering effect on the elderly (Netz, 2009). However, it is clear that purposeful life-long physical activity has proven to have a positive effect on health via many disease-specific mechanisms and seems to provide the highest health benefits (Kujala, 2011).

Aging skeletal muscle becomes less powerful, fat is redistributed from the depot to muscle (Toth & Tchernof, 2000), and altered collagen synthesis and post-translational changes in the structure of collagen reduce the elasticity of ligaments (Kjaer *et al.*, 2006).The properties of muscle strength and stiffness that control balance between the ability of muscle fibers to resist stretching come from having a critical degree of cross-linking of collagen molecules to form fibers. With age, the number of cross-links increases and makes the collagen fibers too stiff for optimal function (Freemont & Hoyland, 2007).Skeletal muscle reloading after unloading has been shown to increase the recovery of motor activity, which is as fast as the recovery of muscle strength, but mechanical properties depend on the metabolism and regeneration of the muscle structures from disuse atrophy (Seene *et al.*, 2012). The qualitative remodeling of contractile proteins plays a certain role in impaired locomotion and general weakness in aging. Thus, when atrophic muscle become active again, muscle mass increases in a relatively short period of time but the recovery of muscle strength takes much longer(Pottle & Gosselin, 2000).

Dexamethasone treatment increased aged muscle wasting much more than in the young (Seene *et al.*, 2003) and the main reason is the loss of myofibrillar proteins from muscle (Evans, 1997; Attaix *et al.*, 2005). The catabolic action of glucocorticoids on skeletal muscle was found to depend on the functional activity of muscle (Goldberg & Goodman, 1969; Seene & Viru, 1982). Exercise with simultaneous glucocorticoid treatment is an effective measure in retarding skeletal muscle atrophy (Hickson & Davis, 1981; Hickson *et al.*, 1986) and provides protection against one of the major effects of glucocorticoid-muscle wasting (Czerwinski-Helms & Hickson, 1987). The search for possibilities to rehabilitate the loss of physical function by exercise therapy in the elderly to prevent diseases is one of the challenges nowadays caused by the increase in the number of aging people in the society (Seene & Kaasik, 2012a;2012b). The capacity to evoke structural and functional rearrangements in aging skeletal muscle depends on the oxidative potential of the fibers (Seene *et al.*, 2009). The integral indicator of muscle protein metabolism, the turnover rate, provides a mechanism by which exercise can change the renewal of contractile proteins in accordance with the needs of muscle contractile apparatus (Seene *et al.*, 2012). As oxidative capacity of skeletal muscle decreases in the elderly, endurance exercise seems to be effective in its restoration as it stimulates mitochondrial biogenesis and improves their functional parameters (Hood, 2009; Ljubicic *et al.*, 2010; Seppet *et al.*, 2013). Comparison of high oxidative capacity (cardiac muscle) and relatively low oxidative capacity (skeletal muscle) changes in elderly energy metabolism show that adaptation capacity is higher in cardiac muscle (Seppet *et al.*, 2013)

The purpose of this review is to discuss recent evidence of exercise therapy in the prevention of sarcopenia, glucocorticoid caused myopathy and in case of skeletal muscle unloading, what is characteristic in aging population. The relationships between the muscle contractile and mitochondrial apparatus and the role of oxidative capacity in energy metabolism of skeletal and cardiac muscle, also the extracellular matrix (ECM) in aging muscle are under the attention.

2   Reasons of Muscle Weakness in the Elderly

Aging leads to changes in skeletal muscle quantity and quality and these changes are a major cause for increased prevalence of disability of the aging population (Evans *et al.*, 2010; Seene *et al.*, 2012). In addition to sarcopenia, osteopenia and organopenia are characteristic to increasing age and may contribute to the development of disability(Manini, 2009).

Sarcopenia was already defined as the age-related loss of muscle mass (Janssen, 2010). It is know that muscle mass and strength are causally linked and changes in mass are responsible for changes in strength. It was shown that muscle strength does not solely depend on muscle mass (Moritani & deVires, 1979). In elderly people, the decline in muscle strength is more rapid than the concomitant loss of muscle mass (Delmonico *et al.*, 2009; Frontera *et al.*, 2000) and loss of muscle mass during disuse is associated with loss of strength only in the range of 10% (Clark *et al.*, 2006). This standpoint is also supported by the experiments, where muscle mass is gained but the age-related decline in muscle strength is not prevented (Delmonico *et al.*, 2009). The fact that the loss of muscle strength in elderly people is weakly associated with the loss of lean body mass, demonstrates that the loss of strength is more related to impairments in the neural activation of muscle (Gandevia, 2001).

Aging is a physiological process that includes a gradual decrease in skeletal muscle mass, strength and endurance coupled with an ineffective response to tissue damage (Figure 1).

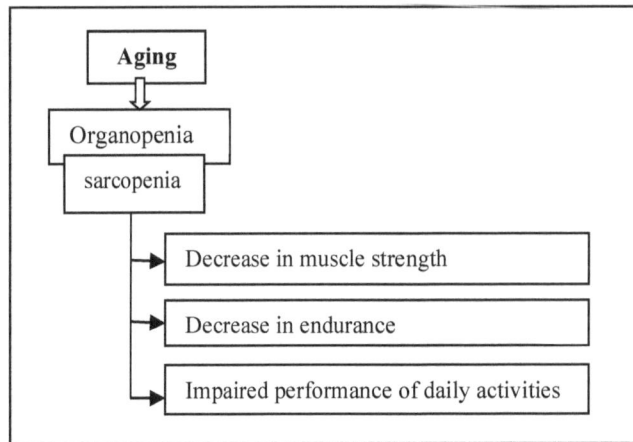

Figure 1: Reasons of the decline in physiological capacities in elderly.

Aging and a reduced physical level are mainly responsible for the progressive decline in several physiological capacities in the elderly (Kadi & Ponsot, 2010). Decrease in the protein synthesis rate is affected by the translational process occurring in older human skeletal muscle, whereas the transcriptional process appears to be unaltered when compared with those in younger men (Roberts *et al.*, 2010). Skeletal muscle fibers have a remarkable capacity to regenerate (Bassaglia & Gautron, 1995) and this depends on the number of satellite cells under the basal lamina of fibers and their oxidative capacity (Shultz & Darr, 1990). Autografting of gastrocnemius muscle in old rats shows that regeneration proceeds at a significantly slower rate in comparison with young animals (Kaasik *et al.*, 2007). A decrease in the number of satellite cells has been shown in fast-twitch (FT) muscle fibers of elderly subjects (Verney *et al.*, 2008). In sarcopenic muscle, the decrease in the satellite cell pool and the length of telomeres might explain the higher prevalence of muscle injuries and delayed muscle regeneration (Kadi & Ponsot, 2010). Functionally heterogeneous satellite cells with different properties may be recruited for different tasks, for example muscle regeneration (Ono *et al.*, 2010; Tatsumi, 2010).

After severe damage, muscles in old rodents did not regenerate as well as muscles in adults (Kaasik *et al.*, 2012). It has been shown that the decreased regeneration capacity of muscles is due to extrinsic causes, but it is likely a combination of both extrinsic and intrinsic factors that contribute to reduce muscle regeneration, than an intrinsic limitation of muscles (Carlson *et al.*, 2001; Conboy *et al.*, 2005). A contraction-induced muscle injury to weight-bearing muscles in old rodents causes deficits in muscle mass and force (Rader & Faulkner, 2006). It has been shown that the degradation rate of contractile proteins in rat skeletal muscle during aging increased about two times and muscle strength and motor activity decreased at the same time (Kaasik *et al.*, 2007). Aging-induced sarcopenia is a result of decreased synthesis and increased degradation of myofibrillar proteins, which leads to the slower turnover rate of muscle proteins, particularly contractile proteins and this, in turn, leads to the decrease in muscle strength (Figure 2). Increasing dietary protein intake in combination with the use of anabolic agents attenuates the muscle loss (Evans, 2010). In essence, sarcopenia is an imbalance between protein synthesis and degradation rate.

Aging skeletal muscle

> Decreased synthesis rate of muscle proteins

> Increased degradation rate of muscle proteins

> Slow turnover rate of muscle proteins
> Muscle atrophy

> Impaired neural activation

> Reduced contractile quality

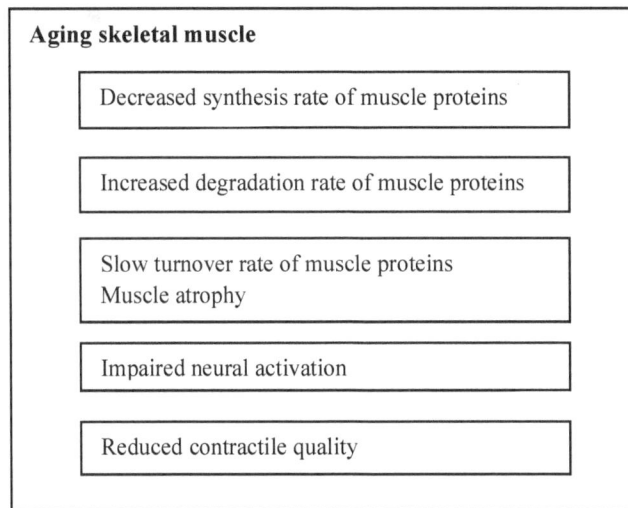

Figure 2: Changes in skeletal muscle what are leading to the loss of independence in the elderly.

As muscle size is not the sole contributor to loss in physical activity in the elderly, it is important to evaluate all aspects in the etiology of disability. In the literature, there are many descriptions for the identification of risk factors for loss in physical activity among the elderly (Clark & Manini, 2010). The decline in muscle strength is a result of a combination of neurologic and muscular factors (Figure 2), such as the impairment of neural activation due to a reduction in descending excitatory drive from supraspinal centers, suboptimal motor unit recruitment and neuromuscular transmission failure (Stackhouse *et al.*, 2001; Weisleder *et al.*, 2006). Muscle atrophy, reduced contractile quality due to changes in the myofibrillar machinery and infiltration of adipocytes into muscle fibers are also reasons for the decrease of muscle strength and physical activity (Delmonico *et al.*, 2009; Seene *et al.*, 2012). Decrease in skeletal muscle strength contractile proteins synthesis rate and increase in muscle protein degradation rate demonstrate that the contractile machinery in elderly is potentially structurally and functionally damaged (Figure2). Such an integral indicator of contractile protein metabolism as their turnover rate shows that in senescent rats, myosin heavy chain (MyHC) turned over about 35% and actin about 10% more slowly than in young elderly (Seene *et al.*, 2003; Kaasik *et al.*, 2007). Functional rearrangements in the contractile apparatus of senescent rats also show a decrease in MyHC fastest isoforms relative content in skeletal muscle (Pehme *et al.*, 2004). Changes in MyHC isoforms' composition in skeletal muscle may be related to slower ATP splitting in the elderly because of decrease in muscle mitochondrial ATP production (Abate & Chandalia, 2003). It has been demonstrated that skeletal muscle mitochondrial dysfunction occurs with age (Rooyackers *et al.*, 1996). The reason is a decrease in mitochondrial DNA copy numbers, decreased mRNA in genes encoding muscle mitochondrial proteins (Barazzoni *et al.*, 2000), reduced oxidative enzyme activity and a decreased mitochondrial protein synthesis rate (Short *etal.*, 2003). Neuronal or chemical meditators may also play a role in signaling hypothalamus from the periphery to stimulate the center of sympathetic nerves signaling the paraventricular nucleus of the hypothalamic center (Nair, 2005). It is generally known that skeletal muscle protein synthesis in humans decreases with age (Yarasheki *et al.*, 2002; Short *et al.*, 2004). Studies have shown that the synthesis rate of MyHC and mitochondrial proteins decreases, but others like sarcoplasmic proteins have a relatively high synthesis rate in the elderly (Nair, 2005). It has been shown that the age-related decrease in muscle protein is not a global effect on all proteins, but is selective for certain proteins (Nair, 2005). Proteins that have a faster turnover rate contribute more to the skeletal muscle synthesis rate despite their small amount. Proteins which constitute a major part of muscle proteins but have a slow turnover rate play a smaller role in the synthesis rate of skeletal muscle proteins (Nair, 2005).

3   Effect of Unloading on Muscle Function

The gradual development of functional limitations over an extended period of time is affected by a natural age-related decline in physical and biological properties, which already starts in midlife and increases the risk for a decline in physical functioning in later life (von Bonsdorff & Rantanen, 2011).During aging, the physical system suffers to a different extent and rate in diverse parts of the body. This result in reduced functional reserve, a decrease in vital capacity, deterioration of the capillary blood supply and a decrease in muscle mass (Mechling & Netz, 2009).One of the reasons for the development of muscle weakness in the elderly is decreased physical activity (Powers *et al.*, 2007). Inactivity and aging cause a marked relative increase in the endo- and perimysial connective tissue, which results in changes in the mechanical properties of skeletal muscle (Figure 3).

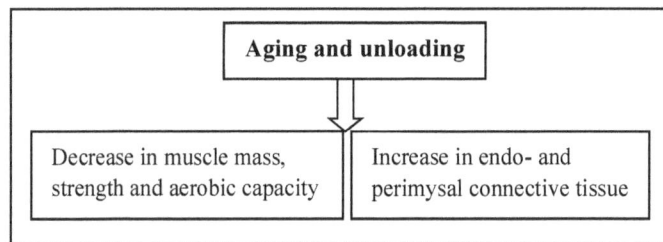

Figure 3: Effect of aging and inactivity on skeletal muscle mechanical properties.

Myofibrillar basal lamina becomes thicker and more rigid with age and increased cross-linking of collagen molecules make fibrils more resistant to degradation by collagenase (Goldspink *et al.*, 1994). The muscle tissue response to unloading seems to more express than connective tissue response (Kjaer *et al.*, 2006; Mackey *et al.*, 2008). The connective structures are protected from rapid changes in tissue mass while muscle, which is known to act as a protein store of the organism, is subject to substantial and fast changes in tissue mass. Despite the small changes in connective tissue mass, important changes occur in the tissue structures during unloading and aging (Seene *et al.*, 2012; Seene & Kaasik, 2012a;2012b).

Unloading has shown to decrease protein synthesis rate in skeletal muscle by 46% (Ferrando *etal.*, 1996). The decreased muscle mass, reduction in strength and aerobic capacity are the typical changes in elderly during bedrest (Evans, 2010). Increase of dietary protein intake attenuates the protein degradation rate during bedrest (Stuart *et al.*, 1990) and in combination with anabolic agents prevents the muscle loss (Katsanos *et al.*, 2008; Symons *et al.*, 2009).

Due to the differences in plasticity of young and old skeletal muscle, young muscle mass increases faster than old after reloading (Suetta *et al.*, 2009), but the recovery of muscle strength both in young and old takes more time than gain of muscle mass (Pottle &Gosselin, 2000). Regain of muscle strength after unloading takes longer in old than in young (Suetta *et al.*, 2009). The recovery of locomotory activity after hindlimb suspension is as fast as the recovery of muscle strength and related to the regeneration of the muscle structures from disuse atrophy (Itai *et al.*, 2004). Muscle metabolism can be restored faster than full recovery of muscle function as cross-sectional area and myonuclear domain size require more time for restoration of neural and mechanical properties of muscle (Desaphy *et al.*, 2005; Ohira, 2006).It has also been proposed that aging militates against the loss of collagen stability due to mechanical over-extension (Willett *et al.*, 2010) but the growth hormone is more important in strengthening the matrix tissue than forming muscle fiber hypertrophy in aged musculotendinous tissue (Doessing *et al.*, 2010). After severe damage, muscle in old rodents does not regenerate as well as muscle in adults (Conboy *et al.*, 2005). A contraction-induced muscle injury to weight-bearing muscles in old age cause deficits in muscle mass and force (Rader & Faulkner, 2006).The fact that an increase in muscular strength lags behind that in muscular mass shows that an increase in muscular mass contains functionally immature muscle fibers during the recovery process following disuse atrophy (Seene *et al.*, 2012).

4   Effect of Glucocorticoid Caused Myopathy on Intracellular and Extra-cellular Compartments

The anti-inflammatory effect of glucocorticoids is the reason for their wide exploitation in various clinical scenarios. A side effect of glucocorticoids is muscle atrophy.Glucocorticoid caused myopathy as well as Cushing's disease lead to a marked reduction in muscle mass, wasting of muscle, loss of strength and selective atrophy of FT muscle fibers (Seene, 1994).

Aging caused sarcopenia is associated with muscle weakness and impaired locomotion. Glucocorticoids treatment significantly decreases muscle strength and motor activity of laboratory animals and humans (Seene *et al.*, 2003; Attaix *et al.*, 2005). The reduced muscle mass in aging and dexamethasone treatment reflect a loss of myofibrillar proteins (Seene *et al.*, 2012;Seene & Kaasik, 2012b). In both laboratory animals and humans, the synthesis rate of myofibrillar but not of sarcoplasmatic proteins decreases with age (Attaix, 2005; Kaasik *et al.*, 2012). The treatment of adult and aged laboratory animals with glucocorticoids leads to muscle wasting but this effect was much more rapid in aged animals (Dardavet *et al.*, 1995). One of the reasons for this is that glucocorticoids decrease the stimulatory effect of insulin and insulin-like growth factor-1(IGF-1) in the skeletal muscle of old rats twice as much as in adults (Dardavet *et al.*, 1998) and increase the expression of myostatin, a negative regulator of skeletal muscle (Artaza *et al.*, 2002). In FT muscle fibers, an excess of glucocorticoids causes a break-down of thick and thin myofilaments and disintegration of individual myofibrils (Figure 4).

One of the important consequences of aging is impaired locomotion and general weakness (Attaix *et al.*, 2005). Daily motor activity of old rats has a tendency to decrease in comparison with young rats. Glucocorticoids treatment significantly reduced daily motor activityand muscle strengthin atrophic muscle in both young and old age groups (Short & Nair, 2000; Kaasik *et al.*, 2007). The qualitative remodeling of contractile proteins probably plays a certain role in this. Glucocorticoids treatment decreased hindlimb grip strength in both age groups but significantly more in the old than in the young group (Seene *et al.*, 2003; Kaasik *et al.*, 2007). In the everyday life of senescent rats, a decrease in muscle strength plays a more important role than daily motor activity.

```
┌─────────────────────────────────────────────────────┐
│  Myopathic muscle                                     │
│                                                       │
│   ┌─────────────────────────────────────────────┐   │
│   │ Disintegration and atrophy of myofibrils      │   │
│   └─────────────────────────────────────────────┘   │
│                                                       │
│   ┌─────────────────────────────────────────────┐   │
│   │ Break-down of thick and thin myofilaments      │   │
│   └─────────────────────────────────────────────┘   │
│                                                       │
│   ┌─────────────────────────────────────────────┐   │
│   │ Loss of myofibrillar protein                  │   │
│   └─────────────────────────────────────────────┘   │
│                                                       │
│   ┌─────────────────────────────────────────────┐   │
│   │ Slow turnover rate of contractile proteins     │   │
│   └─────────────────────────────────────────────┘   │
│                                                       │
│   ┌─────────────────────────────────────────────┐   │
│   │ Muscle wasting and impaired locomotion         │   │
│   └─────────────────────────────────────────────┘   │
│                                                       │
└─────────────────────────────────────────────────────┘
```

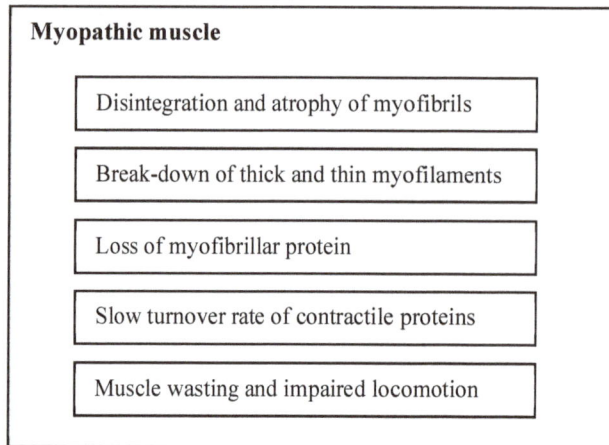

Figure 4: Reasons of muscle wasting in glucocorticoid caused myopathic skeletal muscle.

An excess of glucocorticoids has some similarities in its effect on the intracellular and extracellular compartments of skeletal muscle, *e.g.*, the decreased synthesis of proteins (Seene, 1994; Ahtikoski *et al.*, 2004). The downregulation of collagen synthesis during glucocorticoids administration shows that ECM components decrease. As shown previously (Seene *et al.*, 1988), MyHC synthesis rate only decreased in FT muscles, while the expression of collagen I, III, and IV mRNA decreased in both FT and slow-twitch (ST) muscles. It seems that glucocortioids treatment similarly influences fibril- and network-forming collagen expression in ST and FT muscles but differs at this point from contractile protein myosin synthesis, which was depressed only in FT muscles (Riso *et al.*, 2008).The second principal difference between contractile proteins and ECM during an excess of glucocorticoids is' the degradation rate of proteins. Glucocorticoids increased the degradation of contractile proteins in skeletal muscle about two times but the expression of matrix metalloproteinase-2 (MMP-2) mRNA did not simultaneously significantly change although the degradation of collagens occurs mainly through MMP activity (Everts *et al.*, 1996). This is surprising as it was shown earlier that ST muscles contain significantly more collagen than FT muscles (Kovanen *et al.*, 1984b).

The concentration of endomysial collagen is higher around FT fibers (Kovanen *et al.*, 1984a), but as the downregulation of synthesis and unchanged degradation of type IV collagen are very similar to fibrillar collagen, and this shows that mechanical stability in skeletal muscle fibers, which is ensured by collagen IV, does not differ between ST and FT fibers. The effect of glucocorticoids on muscle weakness is applied through damaged contractile machinery of FT muscle fibers' intracellular compartment (Seene *et al.*, 2003; Riso *et al.*, 2008).

5   Regeneration Capacity of Myopathic Muscle

The intensity of regeneration depends on the number of satellite cells under the basal lamina of muscle fibers, the size of the muscle, the type of injury and the twitch characteristics of the muscle (Järva *et al.*, 1997b; Seene *et al.*, 2008; Seene *et al.*, 2009). Autografting of gastrocnemius muscle in old animals shows that regeneration proceeds significantly more slowly in comparison with young animals. Glucocorticoids treatment decreased regeneration capacity both in young and old animals. Slower regeneration in old animals and after glucocorticoids treatment in young and old groups is in good correlation with the decreased number of satellite cells (Kaasik *et al.*, 2007). Previous work has shown that glucocorticoids treatment caused destructive changes in satellite cells on the ultrastructural level, which are similar to mother cell damage (Seene *et al.*, 1988). MyHC composition during regeneration shifts from fast to slower type and this process is regulated by the cycle of denervation and reinnervation in regenerating skeletal muscle fibers (Järva *et al.*, 1997a).

Glucocorticoids treatment led to quite similar results both in the young and the old but these changes are more significant in the aging group. Both aging and glucocorticoids induced sarcopenic muscles have diminished regenerative capacity (Kaasik *et al.*, 2007).

It has been shown that the turnover rate of contractile proteins in aging animals and in young adults after the infusion of glucocorticoids decreases (Seene *et al.*, 2003; Pehme *et al.*, 2004) and precursor cells required for muscle regrowth are morphologically and functionally damaged (Seene *et al.*, 1988). These changes together may be one of the reasons for sarcopenia. The mechanisms responsible for sarcopenia in aged skeletal muscle are largely unknown, but muscle satellite cells required for the repair of fibers certainly exhibit impaired activation (Barani *et al.*, 2003) and proliferation (Machida & Booth, 2004) compared to young muscle.

Autografting of skeletal muscle has been used as a model of muscle regeneration. Higher oxidative capacity of muscle tends to ensure its faster regeneration (Carlson, 1986; White & Devor, 1993). It has been shown that the synthesis rate of contractile proteins depends on muscle oxidative potential (Seene *et al.*, 2004). In aging rats, the MyHC and actin synthesis rates decrease by about 30% and 23%, respectively (Kaasik *et al.*, 2007). It is known that aging is related to a dramatically reduced MyHC synthesis rate (Balagopal *et al.*, 1997) without any change in MyHC on the transcriptional level (Welle *et al.*, 1996). Muscle wasting is also associated with increased protein degradation, particularly that of contractile proteins. Accumulation of abnormal proteins during aging is believed to result from defects in protein breakdown but very few experimental data support this hypothesis (Attaix *et al.*, 2005). Results show that the degradation rate of contractile proteins in skeletal muscle during aging increased about two times, and glucocorticoids treatment significantly increased the degradation rate in both age groups (Kaasik *et al.*, 2007). Previous works have shown that dexamethasone associated degradation starts from the periphery of myofibrils in muscle fibers with low oxidative potential (Seene *et al.*, 1988). This destruction process starts from myosin filaments and thereafter spreads all over the myofibrillar apparatus (Seene *et al.*, 1988). It has been shown that contractile proteins turned over slowly in old animals and subjects as well as in young rodents after dexamethasone treatment (Seene, 1994).

6 Exercise Therapy in Prevention and Management of Sarcopenia and Myopathy

Exercise therapy is a wide and systematic approach to the regular use of specific movements to improve different body functions, mobility and fitness (Figure 5). Exercise therapy is a useful tool for the prevention and management of different injuries and diseases. On many occasions, specific exercise programs are tailored for rehabilitation needs. For example, in case of glucocorticoid caused myophaty, both endurance and strength exercise training has been shown to play a preventive role in the development of muscle atrophy, but a combination of both with different frequency, intensity and duration seems to be also promising (Seene & Kaasik, 2012b).

More than four decades ago, the preventive role of exercise in the development of muscle atrophy during glucocorticoid administration was shown (Goldberg & Goodman, 1969). From the historical viewpoint, endurance exercise has been found to be an effective measure in retarding skeletal muscle atrophy associated with the administration of glucocorticoids (Seene & Viru, 1982; Hickson *et al.*, 1984; Czerwinski-Helms & Hickson, 1987). From the contraction nature, four model systems have given the desired effect: endurance exercise, strength exercise, muscle functional overload, and in vitro cell culture stimulation (Czerwinski & Hickson, 1990). Later intensive short-lasting exercise training has shown to have an anticatabolic effect on the contractile apparatus and the ECM of skeletal muscle (Riso *et al.*, 2010). Glucocorticoids increased myofibrillar protein degradation in FT muscles, while fibril- and network-forming collagen specific mRNA levels decreased at the same time in FT and ST muscles (Riso *et al.*, 2008). Both the myofibrillar apparatus and the ECM play a crucial role in changes of muscle strength during glucocorticoid administration and following muscle loading (Riso *et al.*, 2010).

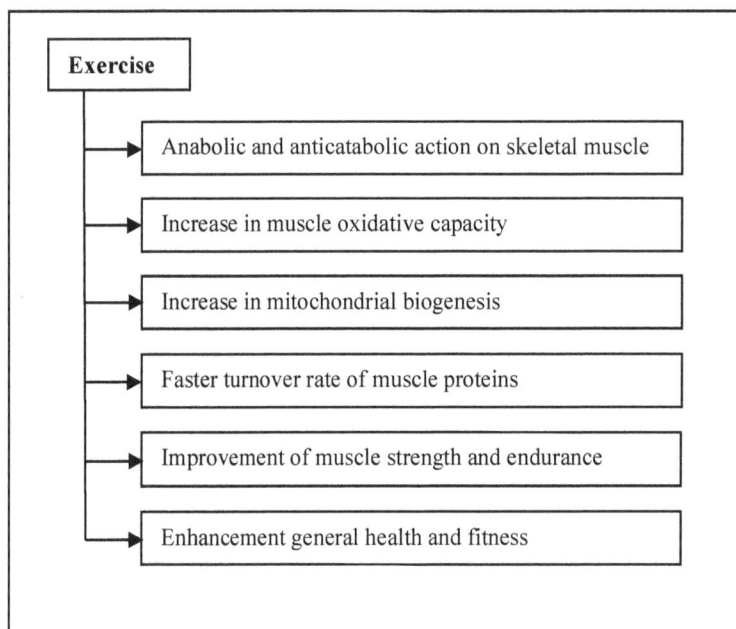

Figure 5: Effect of exercise rehabilitation of sarcopenia and myopathic muscle

6.1   Effect of Resistance Exercise

Muscle atrophy contributes to but does not completely explain the decrease in force in the elderly. The age-related decrease in muscle mass and strength is a consequence of the complete loss of fibers associated with the decrease in the number of motor units and fiber atrophy (Rader & Faulkner, 2006). In recent years, resistance exercise has become one of the fastest growing forms of physical activity for different purposes: improving athletic performance, enhancing general health and fitness, rehabilitation after surgery or an injury, or just for the pleasure of exercise (Fry, 2004). Resistance exercise has shown to be an effective measure in the elderly, improving glucose intolerance, including improvements in insulin signaling defects, reduction in tumor necrosis factor-α, increases in adiponectin and IGF-1 concentrations, and reductions in total and abdominal visceral fat (Flack *et al.*, 2011). Resistance exercise improves skeletal muscle metabolism and through it muscle function in the elderly and their life quality (Figure 5).Resistance exercise enhances the synthesis rate of myofibrillar proteins but not that of sarcoplasmic proteins (Moore *et al.*, 2009) and this is related to mammalian target of rapamycin by activating proteins within the nitrogen – activated proteinkinase signaling (Moore *et al.*, 2011). A significant difference was observed between previously trained young and old participants in recovery from resistance training (McLester, *et al.*, 2003). These results suggest a more rapid recovery in the young group. It seems that recovery from more damaging resistance exercise is slower as a result of age, whereas there are no age-related differences in recovery from less damaging metabolic fatigue (Fell & Williams, 2008).

It has been shown that resistance training, during which the power of exercise increased less than 5% per session, caused hypertrophy of both FT and ST muscle fibers, an increase of myonuclear number via fusion of satellite cells with damaged fibers or the formation of new muscle fibers as a result of myoblasts' fusion in order to maintain myonuclear domain size (Seene *et al.*, 2010).

Aging, unloading and glucocorticoids are related to a decreased protein synthesis rate in skeletal muscle, particularly that of myofibrillar proteins (Pehme *et al.*, 2004; Seene *et al.*, 2012). It has been found that the relative content of MyHC I and IId isoform increased and MyHC IIb decreased with age. Heavy resistance training decreased the relative content of MyHC IId isoform in old rats' muscle (Pehme *et al.*, 2004). Compensatory hypertrophy of the plantaris muscle by tenotomy of the gastrocnemius muscle decreased the relative content of MyHC IIb and IIa isoforms in old rats. Simultaneous compensatory hypertrophy and heavy-resistance training increased the proportion of MyHC IIb and decreased MyHC IId isoforms in old animals' muscle. Heavy resistance training also prevented the age-related decrease in the relative content of MyHC IIb isoform in rat plantaris muscle (Pehme *et al.*, 2004).

As training status of participants in studies examining aging and muscle function is different, there are difficulties in comparing indices of muscle recovery in old and inactive subjects after severe lengthening contractions with the recovery from training-induced fatigue in older humans(Fell & Williams, 2008). Contractile proteins turned over faster in type I and IIA fibers than in IIB fibers and the turnover rate of skeletal muscle proteins in skeletal muscle depends on the functional activity of the muscle (Seene *et al.*, 2009). The turnover rate of myofibrillar proteins in aging skeletal muscle is related to the changes in MyHC isoforms' composition (Seene *et al.*, 2012). The effect of resistance training on the increase of the turnover rate of skeletal muscle contractile proteins in old age is relatively small (Seene *et al.*, 2012). Adaptational changes first appeared in newly formed or regenerating fibers and these changes lead to the remodeling of the contractile apparatus and an increase in the strength generating capability of muscle. These changes are more visible in muscle fibers with higher oxidative capacity. When unloaded, muscle becomes active again, muscle mass increases in a relatively short period of time but the recovery of muscle strength takes longer (Pottle & Gosselin, 2000; Seene *et al.*, 2012). The recovery of locomotory activity after unloading is as fast as the recovery of muscle strength. It is related to the regeneration of muscle structure form disuse atrophy (Itai *et al*, 2004). This fact suggests the presence of functionally immature muscle fibers during the recovery process following disuse atrophy (Itai *et al*, 2004). So, the recovery of skeletal muscle mechanical properties depends on the structural and metabolic peculiarities of the skeletal muscle (Seene *et al.*, 2009). As a complex of factors contributes to the development of muscle wasting and weakness in the elderly, skeletal muscle unloading and glucocorticoid caused myopathy, it is complicated to find one certain measure for rehabilitation. As lack of strength is one of the central reasons for muscle weakness, it seems to be most realistic to use resistance training for this purpose in the elderly. Resistance training is a strong stimulus for muscle metabolism in the elderly, particularly for the contractile machinery of muscle (Figure 5).

6.2   Effect of Endurance Exercise

As oxidative capacity of skeletal muscle decreases in the elderly, endurance training is effective in stimulating mitochondrial biogenesis and improving their functional parameters (Hood, 2009; Ljubicic *et al.*, 2010). In combination with resistance training, the oxidative capacity and subsequently the turnover rate of contractile proteins in elderly skeletal muscle increases. This increase of the turnover rate of muscle proteins leads to the increase in skeletal muscle plasticity. It has recently been shown that the plasticity of individual development in the elderly makes it possible to modify the age-associated decline even in maximal physical performance (Suominen, 2011). Another positive influence of endurance training in the elderly is related to an increase in the ability of cardiovascular factors and to a lesser extent, to an increase in muscle mitochondrial concentration and capacity (Sagiv *et al.*, 2010). The increase in muscle oxidative capacity and contractile property is an effective measure for enhancing life quality in the elderly by improving skeletal muscle functional capacity and plasticity (Figure 5). Regular aerobic exercise provides a foundation for an increase in muscle oxidative capacity in the elderly; it means that adequate physical performance is an essential element of a healthy and productive life among the elderly. With older age managing everyday activities becomes less self-evident although there are gender differences in physical functioning (Kuh *et al.*, 2005). Functional limitation is an objective measure of the consequences of disease and impairment (Guralnik & Ferrucci, 2003).

It seems that the turnover rate of contractile proteins provides a mechanism by which the effect of exercise causes changes in accordance with the needs of the contractile apparatus. As the contractile protein turnover rate depends on the oxidative capacity of muscle and muscle oxidative capacity decreases in the elderly, it is obvious that enduarnce exercise stimulates an increase in the oxidative capacity of skeletal muscle by an increase in mitochondrial biogeneses and supports faster protein turnover during resistance training in order to increase muscle function (Figure 5). It has been shown that the aging-associated reduction in AMP- activated protein kinase (AMPK) activity may be a factor in reduced mitochondrial function (Reznick *et al.*, 2007). In response to contractile activity, AMPK activation was registered only in aging FT muscles (Thomson *et al.*, 2009). It is known that AMPK is activated in response to endurance exercise (Winder & Hardie, 1996)] and related to the metabolic adaptation of skeletal muscle. Later it has been shown that $\alpha 1$ isoform of AMPK is the regulator of skeletal muscle growth, but not of metabolic adaptation (McGee *et al.*, 2008). As factors such as health, physical function and independence constitute components of quality of life in the elderly, physiological functioning of skeletal muscle in the elderly has significance in determining the ability to maintain independence and an active interaction with the environment (Spirduso & Cronin, 2001; Seene *et al.*, 2012). Successful aging is guaranteed when elderly people use widespread participation exercise for further improving their fitness and reducing the risk of disability(Kramer & Erickson, 2007).

6.2.1   Effect of Endurance Exercise on Skeletal and Cardiac Muscle Energetics

In contrast to cardiac muscle (high oxidative capacity), hypertrophy of skeletal muscle (relatively low oxidative capacity) is not developed during endurance type of exercise training. Skeletal muscles respond to exercise by increasing the fiber composition towards increased proportion ofoxidative fibres at the expense of proportion ofglycolytic fibres(Green *et al.*,1983). This change do not give rise to overall muscle size as oxidative fibres CSA is less than glycolytic ones (van Wessel *et al.*, 2010). The proteasome-, lysosome- and Ca^{2+}-mediated protein degradation occurs at higher ratesin oxidative than glycolytic fibres (van der Vusse *et al.*, 1992).The mechanisms stimulating either oxidative mechanisms or hypertrophy seem to exclude each other (van Wessel *et al.*, 2010). Increased mitochondrial biogenesis via AMPK may be accompanied by suppression of the myofibrillar protein synthesis through pathways mediated by mitogen activated protein kinase (MAPK) and nuclear factor kappa B (van Wessel *et al.*, 2010). Further support for that assumption comes from the finding that exercise, though increasing oxidative metabolism, yet suppresses myofibre growth in myostatin knock-out mice (Matsakas *et al.*, 2012). These facts imply that cardiac and skeletal muscles possess distinctmechanisms for regulation of the balance between the capacities of oxidative potential and hypertrophy in response to endurance type of exercise training. These muscle type specific differences in adaptation to endurance type of exercise training can be revealed also at the level of ATP consumption. In cardiac muscle endurance exercise training results in enhanced myosin ATPase activity along with increased contractility (Pierce et al., 1989). This change based on the myosin isoenzyme shift towards increased fast V1 (α) isoform (Rupp, 1981; Jin *et al.*, 2000) and alterations in regulation of myosin ATPase. Endurance type of exercise training results in increased myofilament sensitivity to Ca^{2+}(Wisloff *et al.*, 2001), and probably due to augmented expression of atrial myosin light chain-1 isoform (Diffee *et al.*, 2003)that increases the capacity to consume ATP by myofibrils. Endurance exercise training also promotes the expression of sarcoplasmatic reticulum (SR) Ca^{2+}ATPase (SERCA2) together with increased Ca^{2+} transport into SR (Tate *et al.*, 1996). In addition, Ca^{2+} removal through trans sarcolemmal route is facilitated due to activation of Ca^{2+}-ATPase localized in sarcolemma (Pierce *et al.*, 1989). Exercise increases the capacity of ATP consumption in cardiac cells, but not in skeletal muscles, which respond to exercise training by shifting the myofibre profile towards increased proportion of oxidative fibres characterized with markedly lower ATPase activity (Bottinelli, 2001; Nuhr *et al.*, 2003). This change is beneficial as it increases the economy of ATP utilization for cross-bridge cycling (Baldwin & Haddad, 2001). Endurance type of exercisetraining stimulates also the Na^+-K^+-ATPase activity in skeletal muscle(Mohr *et al.*, 2007) but not in myocardium (Pierce *et al.*, 1989).

Endurance training stimulates mitochondrial biogenesis (Figure 5) and improves the functional capacity of mitochondria in producing ATP in skeletal muscles (Hood, 2001; Menshikova *et al.*, 2006; Ljubicic *et al.*, 2010). Upregulated mitochondrial biogenesis manifests as increases in mitochondrial content per gram of tissue (Hollozy, 1967), mitochondrial volume relative to fibre area (Tyler *et al.*, 1998), and tissue activity of mitochondrial enzymes (Silva *et al.*, 2009). These changes occur simultaneously in oxidative and glycolytic muscle fibres (Hollozy, 1967; Baldwin *et al.*, 1972). Increased mitochondrial contribution to energy metabolism is associated with transition from carbohydrate utilization to fat utilization and this is the reason of improvement of the endurance capacity (Spina *et al.*,1996).

Responses of mitochondria to endurance exercise in cardiac cells are ambiguous. Endueance exercise has resulted in increased tissue activities of mitochondrial enzymes, suggesting enhanced oxidative capacity in heart of mammals (Stuewe *et al.*, 2000; Sun *et al.*, 2008).Endurance exercise is also known not to induce alterations in mitochondrial enzymes and yield in cardiac muscle (Kemi *et al.*, 2007). Endurance training has shown decreased the oxidation rate of palmitoylcarnitine/malate without changes in pyruvate, 2-oxoglutarate and succinate oxidation (Terblanche *et al.*, 2001). The controversies regard also to morphometric studies.For example increased mitochondria-to-myofibril ratio (Bozner &Meessen,1969) or no change in this parameter (Anversa *et al.*, 1982). Endurance training, though resulting inhypertrophy and increased oxidative capacity ofheart, did not increase the volume density of mitochondria (Kayar *et al.*, 1986), mitochondrial volume, despite increased weight and size of the heart

(Paniagua *et al.*, 1977).The nature of conflicting data on mitochondrial biogenesis are not clear. Many reasons like training intensity,training volume, time for recovery,gender and age differences lead to contraversial results (Noble *et al.*,1999).Ttraining-induced changes in oxidative capacity and size of the striated muscle fibres tend to mutually exclude each other through altered balance between the biosynthesis of contractile proteins and mitochondria (van Wessel *et al.*, 2010).It is clear that the mechanisms of mitochondrial biogenesis differ from those that underlie muscle hypertrophy. Myocytes follow specific and powerful mechanisms capable to preferentially promote the biosynthesis of mitochondria in response to increased workload.

Most of these mechanisms converge at peroxisome proliferator-activated receptor gamma coacivator-1alpha (PGC-1α), a regulator of oxidative metabolism and mitochondrial content in muscle cells. PGC-1α binds to DNA-binding transcription factors, such as the nuclear respiratory factors NRF-1 and NFR-2, and trans-activates genes involved in the control over electron transport chain, mitochondrial protein import, and transcription factors Tfam, TFB1M, and TFB2M (Gleyzer *et al.*,2005).Endurance training increases the activity and expression of PGC-1α in muscle cells through multiple mechanisms. Glucocorticoids activate PGC-1α through genomic and non-genomic effects (Scheller &Sekeris, 2003). Exercise training activates the p38 MAPK (Akimoto *et al.*,2005) which phosphorylates the PGC-1α repressor protein p160^{MBP} that relieves the inhibitory effect of repressor on PGC-1α, thereby permitting PGC-1α to interact with target proteins (Fan *et al.*,2004).p38 MAPK also increases the transcriptional activity of PGC-1α through phosphorylation (Puigserver *et al.*,2001).AMP produced in exercising muscle cells stimulates AMPK that in turn upregulates the expression of PGC-1α(Lee *et al.*,2006;Narkar *et al.*,2008). PGC-1αactivated by reversible deacetylation carried out by class III histone deacylase SIRT1 (Menzies&Hood,2012).SIRT1 upregulates the expression of PGC-1α through formation of the SIRT1-MyoD-PGC-1α complex on PGC-1α promoter (Amat *et al.*,2009).Endurance exercise upregulation of SIRT1 occurs rapidly, as its mRNA level increases together with mRNAs for PGC-1α, cytochrome c, and citrate synthase in muscle tissue after intensive cycling (Dumke *et al.*,2009). A relevant mechanism appears to be mediated by stimulation of AMPK, as SIRT2 activates the liver kinase B1, a serine-threonine kinase that impels AMPK (Pillai *et al.*,2010). In heart and skeletal muscleSIRT3 is localized exclusively within mitochondria andthe muscle SIRT3 protein content increases in parallel to elevations in citrate synthase activity and PGC-1α content among distinct muscle types(Palacios *et al.*, 2009; Gurd *et al.*,2011).Electrical stimulation resulted in increases in SIRT3 protein and PGC-1α proteins in an AMPK-independent manner (Gurd *et al.*,2011).These data are in accordance with observations that endurance exercise training increases SIRT3 and mitochondrial content in skeletal muscle (Hokary *et al.*,2010). SIRT3 activates also mitochondrial enzymes, such as succinate dehydrogenase, isocitrate dehydrogenase, glutamate dehydrogenase, NDUFA9 subunit of complex I of the respiratory chain, and acetyl-coenzyme A synthase, the targeted activation of SIRT3 may provide a means for shifting metabolism towards use of fatty acids thereby protecting failing heart (Pillai *et al.*,2010).

Endurance exercise training stimulates PGC-1α through activation of cyclic-nucleotide regulatory binding protein (CREB), in association with upregulation of mitochondrial proteins in heart and skeletal muscle (Wu *et al.*,2006). The CREB-mediated mechanism is specifically targeted by catecholamines.It has been shown thatp53, a tumour suppressor protein,involve in mitochondrial biogenesis. p53 increases the expression of synthesis of cytochrome c oxidase 2 (SCO2), an important protein for assambling the cytochrome c oxidase complex what is controlling the rate of mitochondrial respiration (Matoba *et al.*,2006).p53 translocate into mitochondria for interaction with and activation of the mitochondrial DNA polymerase γ (Achanta *et al.*,2005).p53 also interacts with Tfam (Park *et al.*,2009).The importance of p53 in regulation of mitochondrial biogenesis wasconfirmed (Saleem *et al.*,2009).

7 Summary

Aging is a physiological process that includes a gradual decrease in skeletal muscle mass, strength and endurance coupled with an ineffective response to tissue damage. Aging and a reduced physical level are mainly responsible for the progressive decline in several physiological capacities in the elderly.Changes in skeletal muscle mass and function with advancing age are the reasons of the disability of aging population. Glucocorticoid treatment and skeletal muscle unloading are leading to the atrophy of muscle, loss of myofibrillar protein, changes in ECM and decrease of muscle strength and motor activity. As a complex of factors supporting development of skeletal muscle wasting and weakness in the elderly in case of muscle unloading and glucocorticoid caused myopathy it is complicated to find one certain facility for rehabilitation. As oxidative capacity of skeletal muscle decreases in elderly and endurance training is known as effective tool in stimulation of mitochondrial biogenesis and improves their functional parameters, it seems that combination with resistance exercise training the oxidative capacity and subsequently the turnover rate of muscle contractile proteins in elderly skeletal muscle increase and leads to the increase of muscle plasticity. Physiological functioning of skeletal muscle in elderly has significance in determining the ability to maintain independence and an active interaction with the environment.

As aging associated reductions in AMPK activity may be the factor in the reduced mitochondrial function and in response to endurance exercise AMPK is activating, explain the use of endurance exercise training in prevention of disability and diseases.

In contrast to cardiac muscle, hypertrophy of skeletal muscle is not developed during endurance type of exercise training. Skeletal muscles respond to exercise by increasing the fiber composition towards increased proportion of oxidative fibres at the expense of proportion of glycolytic fibres.This change doesnot give rise to overall muscle size as oxidative fibres CSA is less than glycolytic ones. The proteasome-, lysosome- and Ca^{2+}-mediated protein degradation occurs at higher rates in oxidative than glycolytic fibres.The mechanisms stimulating either oxidative mechanisms or hypertrophy seem to exclude each other. Increased mitochondrial biogenesis via AMPK may be accompanied by suppression of the myofibrillar protein synthesis through pathways mediated by MAPK and nuclear factor kappa B. Exercise increases the capacity of ATP consumption in cardiac cells, but not in skeletal muscles, which respond to exercise training by shifting the myofibre profile towards increased proportion of oxidative fibres characterized with markedly lower ATPase activity. This change is beneficial as it increases the economy of ATP utilization for cross-bridge cycling. Endurance type of exercisetraining stimulates also the Na^{+}-K^{+}-ATPase activity in skeletal musclebut not in myocardium.

Acknowledgements

This study was supported by the funds of the Ministry of Education and Research of Estonia, research project number TKKSB1787.

References

Abate, N. & Chandalia, M. (2003). The impact of ethnicity on type 2 diabetes. Journal of Diabetes and its Complications, 17, 39–58.

Achanta, G., Sasaki, R., Feng, L., Carew, J.S., Lu, W., Pelicano, H., Keating, M.J. & Huang, P. (2005). Novel role of p53 in maintaining mitochondrial genetic stability through interaction with DNA Pol gamma. The EMBO Journal, 24, 3482–3492.

Ahtikoski, A.M., Riso, E.-M., Koskinen, S.O. Risteli, J., & Takala, T.E. (2004). Regulation of type IV collagen gene expression and degradation in fast and slow muscles during dexamethasone treatment and exercise.Pflügers Archiv: European Journal of Physiology,448, 123–130.

Akimoto, T., Pohnert, S.C., Li, P., Zhang, M., Gumbs, C., Rosenberg, P.B., Williams, R.S. & Yan, Z. (2005). Exercise stimulates PGC-1a transcription in skeletal muscle through activation of the p38 MAPK pathway.The Journal of Biological Chemistry, 280, 19587–19593.

Amat, R., Planavila, A., Chen, S.L., Iglesias, R., Giralt, M. & Villarroya, F. (2009). SIRT1 controls the transcription of the peroxisome proliferator-activated receptor-gamma Co-activator-1alpha (PGC-1alpha) gene in skeletal muscle through the PGC-1alpha autoregulatory loop and interaction with MyoD. The Journal of Biological Chemistry, 284, 21872–21880.

Anversa, P., Beghi, C., Levicky, V., McDonald, S.L. & Kikkawa, Y. (1982). Morphometry of right ventricular hypertrophy induced by strenuous exercise in rat. The American Journal of Physiology, 243, 856–861.

Artaza, J.N., Bhasin, S., Mallidis, C., Taylor, W., Ma, K. & Gonzales-Gadavid, N.F. (2002). Endogenous expression and localization of myostatin and its relation to myosin heavy chain distribution in C2C12 skeletal muscle cells. Journal of Cell Physiology, 190, 170–179.

Attaix, D., Mosoni, L., Dardevet, D., Combaret, L., Mirand, P.P. & Grizard J. (2005). Altered responses in skeletal muscle protein turnover during aging in anabolic and catabolic periods. The International Journal of Biochemistry & Cell Biology, 37, 1962–1973.

Balagopal, P., Rooyackers O.E., Adey, D.B., Ades, P.A. & Nair, K.S. (1997). Effect of aging on in vivo synthesis of skeletal muscle myosin heavy-chain and sarcoplasmic protein in humans. American Journal of Physiology. Endocrinology and Metabolism, 273, E790-E800.

Baldwin, K.M. & Haddad, F. (2001). Effects of different activity and inactivity paradigms on myosin heavy chain gene expression in striated muscle. Journal of Applied Physiology, 90, 345–357.

Baldwin, K.M., Klinkerfuss, G.H., Terjung, R.L., Mole, P.A. & Holloszy, J.O. (1972). Respiratory capacity of white, red, and intermediate muscle: adaptative response to exercise. American Journal of Physiology, 222, 373–378.

Barani, A.E., Durieux, A.C., Sabido, O. & Freyssenet, D.F. (2003). Age-realted changes in the mitotic and metabolic characteristics of muscle-derived cells.Journal of Applied Physiology,95, 2089–2098.

Barazzoni, R., Short, K.R. & Nair, K.S. (2000). Effects of aging on mitochondrial DNA copy number and cytochrome c oxidase gene expression in rat skeletal muscle, liver, and heart. The Journal of Biological Chemistry, 275, 3343–3347.

Bassaglia, Y., & Gautron, J. (1995). Fast and slow rat muscles degenerate and regenerate differently after cruch injury. Journal of Muscle Research and Cell Motility, 16, 420–429.

Bottinelli, R. (2001). Functional heterogeneity of mammalian single muscle fibres: do myosin isoforms tell the whole story? Pflügers Archiv: European Journal of Applied Physiology, 443, 6–17.

Bozner, A. & Meessen, H. (1969). The ultrastructure of the myocardium of the rat after single and repeated swim exercises. Virchows Archiv. B: Cell Pathology, 3, 248–269.

Buford, T.W., Anton, S.D., Judge, A.R., Marzetti, E., Wohlgemuth, S.E., Carter, C.S., Leeuwenburgh, C., Pahor, M. & Manini, T.M. (2010). Models of accelerated sarcopenia: Critical pieces for solving the puzzle of age-related muscle atrophy. Ageing Research Reviews, 9, 369–383.

Carlson, B.M. (1986). Regeneration of entire skeletal muscles.Federation Proceedings, 45, 1456–1460.

Carlson, B.M., Dedkov, E.I., Borisov, A.B. & Faulkner, J.A. (2001). Skeletal muscle regeneration in very old rats. The Journals of Gerontology. Series A, Biological Sciiences and Medical Sciences, 56, B224–B233.

Clark, B.C. & Manini, T.M. (2010). Functional concequences of sacropenia and dynapenia in the elderly. Current Opinion in Clinical Nutrition and Metabolic Care, 13, 271–276.

Clark, B.C. & Manini, T.M. (2008). Sarcopenia =/= dynapenia. The Journals of Gerontology. Series A, Biological Sciences and Medical Sciences, 63, 829–834.

Clark, B.C., Manini, T.M., Bolanowski, S.J. & Ploutz-Snyder, L.L. (2006). Adaptations in human neuromuscular function following prolonged unweighting: IINeurological properties and motor imagery efficacy. Journal of Applied Physiology, 101, 264–272.

Conboy, I.M., Conboy, M.J., Wagers, A.J., Girma, E.R., Weissman, I.L. & Rando, T.A. (2005). Rejuvenation of aged progenitor cells by exposure to a young systemic environment. Nature, 433, 760–764.

Czerwinski, S.M., & Hickson, R.C. (1990). Glucocorticoid receptor activation during exercise in muscle. Journal of Applied Physiology, 68, 1615–1620.

Czerwinski-Helms, S.M., & Hickson, R.C. (1987). Specificity of activated glucocorticoid receptor expression in heart and skeletal muscle types. Biochemical and Biophysical Research Communications, 142, 322–328.

Dardevet, D., Sornet, C., Savary, I., Debras, E., Patureau-Mirand, P.,& Grizard, J. (1998). Glucocorticoid effects of insulin IGF-1 regulated muscle protein metabolism during aging. The Journal of Endocrinology, 156, 83–89.

Dardevet, D., Sornet, C., Taillandier, D., Savary,I., Attaix, D. & Grizard, J. (1995).Sensitivity and protein turnover response to glucocorticoids are different in skeletal muscle from adult and old rats. Lack of regulation of the ubiquitin-proteasome proteolytic pathway in aging. The Journal of Clinical Investication,96, 2113–2119.

Delmonico, M.J., Harris, T.B., Visser, M., Park, S.W., Conroy, M.B., Valasquez-Mieyer, P., Boudreau, R., Manini, T.M., Nevitt, M., Newman, A.B. & Goodpaster, B.H. (2009). Longitudinal study of muscle strength, quality, and adipose tissue infiltration. The AmericanJournal of Clinical Nutrition, 90, 1579–1585.

Desaphy, J.F., Pierno, S., Liantonio, A., De Luca, A., Didonna, M.P., Frigeri, A., Nicchia, G.P., Svelto, M., Camerino, C., Zallone, A. & Camerino, D.C. (2005). Recovery of the soleus muscle after short-and long-term disuse induced by hindlimb unloading: effects on the electrical properties and myosin heavy chain profile. Neurobiology of Disease, 18, 356–365.

Diffee, G.M., Seversen, E.A., Stein, T.D. & Johnson, J.A. (2003). Microarray expression analysis of effects of exercise training: increase in atrial MLC-1 in rat ventricles. American Journal of Physiology. Heart and Circulatory Physiology, 284, 830-837.

Doessing, S., Heinemeier, K.M., Holm, L., Mackey, A.L., Schjerling, P., Rennie, M., Smith, K.,Reitelseder, S., Kappelgaard, A.M., Rasmussen, M.H., Flyvbjerg, A. &Kjaer, M. (2010).Growth hormone stimulates the collagen synthesis in human tendon and skeletal muscle without affecting myofibrillar protein synthesis. The Journal of Physiology, 588, 341–351.

Dumke, C.L., Davis, J.M., Murphy, E.A. Nieman, D.C., Carmichael, M.D., Quindry, J.C., Travis Triplett, N., Utter, A.C., Gross Gowin, S.J., Henson, D.A., McAnulty, S.R. & McAnulty L.S. (2009). Successive bouts of cycling stimulates genes associated with mitocondrial biogenesis. European Journal of Applied Physiology, 107, 419–427.

Evans, W. (1997). Functional and metabolic consequences of sarcopenia. The Journal of Nutrition, 127,998S–1003S.

Evans, W.E. (2010). Skeletal muscle loss: cachexia, sarcopenia, and inactivity. The American Journal of Clinical Nutrition, 91(suppl), 1123S–1127S.

Everts, V., van der Zee, E., Creemers, L. & Beertsen, W. (1996).Phagocytosis nad intracellular digestion of collagen, its role in turnover and remodeling. The Histochemical Journal, 28, 229–245.

Fan, M., Rhee, J., St-Pierre, J., Handschin, C., Puigserver, P., Lin, J., Jäeger, S., Erdjument-Bromage, H., Tempst, P. & Spiegelman, B.M. (2004). Suppression of mitochondrial respiration through recruitment of p160 myb binding protein to PGC-1: modulation by p38 MAPK. Genes & Development, 18, 278–289.

Fell, J.W., & Williams, A.D. (2008). The effect of aging on skeletal muscle recovery from exercise: possible implications for the aging athlete. Journal of Aging and Physical Activity,16,97–115.

Ferrando, A.A., Lane, H.W., Stuart, C.A., Davis-Street, J., & Wolfe, R.R. (1996). Prolonged bed rest decreases skeletal muscle and whole body protein synthesis. The American Journal of Physiology, 270, E627–E633.

Flack, K.D., Davy, K.P., Hulver, M.W., Winett, R.A., Frisard, M.I. & Davy, B.M. (2011). Aging, resistance training, and diabetes prevention. Journal of Aging Research, doi:10.4061/2011/127315

Freemont, A.J., & Hoyland, J.A. (2007). Morphology, mechanisms and pathology of musculoskeletal ageing. Journal of Pathology, 211, 252–259.

Frontera, W.R., Suh, D., Krivickas, L.S., Huges, V.A., Goldstein, R. & Rubenoff, R. (2000). Skeletal muscle fiber quality in older men and women. The American Journal of Physiology - Cell Physiology, 279, C611–C618.

Fry, A.C. (2004). The role of resistance exercise intensity on muscle fibre adaptations. Sports Medicine, 34, 663–679.

Gandevia, S.C. (2001). Spinal and supraspinal factors in human muscle fatigue. Physiological Reviews, 81,1725–1789.

Gleyzer, N., Vercauteren, K. & Scarpulla, R.C. (2005). Control of mitochondrial transcription specificity factors (TFB1M and TFB2M) by nuclear respiratory factors (NRF-1 and NFR-2) and PGC-1 family coactivators. Molecular and Cell Biology, 25, 1354–1366.

Goldberg, A.L., & Goodman,H.M. (1969). Relationship between cortisone and muscle work in determining muscle size. The Journal of Physiology, 200, 667–675.

Goldspink, G., Fernandes, K., Williams, P.E. & Wells, D.J. (1994). Age-related changes in collagen gene expression in the muscles of mdx dystrophic and normal mice. Neuromuscular Disorders, 4, 183–191.

Gonzales, E., Messi, M.L. & Delbono, O. (2000). The specific force of single intact extensor digitorum longus and soleus mouse muscle fibers declines with aging. The Journal of Membrane Biology, 178, 175–183.

Green, H.J., Reichmann, H. & Pette, D. (1983). Fibre type specific transformations in the enzyme activity pattern of rat vastus lateralis muscle by prolonged endurance training. Pflügers Archiv: European Journal of Physiology, 399, 216-222.

Guralnik, J.M., & Ferrucci, L. (2003). Assessing the building blocks of function: utilizing measures of functional limitation. American Journal of Preventive Medicine, 25, 112–121.

Gurd, B.J., Holloway, G.P., Yoshida, Y. & Bonen, A. (2011). In mammalian muscle, SIRT3 is present in mitochondria and not in the nucleus; and SIRT3 is upregulated by chronic muscle contraction in an adenosine monophosphate-activated protein kinase-independent manner. Metabolism, 9, 1–9.

Hickson, R.C. & Davis, J.R.(1981). Partial prevention of glucocorticoid –induced muscle atrophy by endurance training. American Journal of Physiology, 241, E226–E232.

Hickson, R.C., Galassi, T.M., Capaccio, J.A. & Chatterton, R.T. (1986). Limited resistance of hypertrophied skeletal muscle to glucocorticoids. Journal of Steroid Biochemistry, 24, 1179–1183.

Hickson, R.C., Kurowski, T.T., Capaccio, J.A. & Chatterton, R.T.(1984). Androgen cytosol binding in exercise-induced sparing of muscle atrophy. The American Journal of Physiology,247, E597–E603.

Hokary, F., Kawasaki, E., Sakai, A. Koshinaka, K., Sakuma, K. & Kawanaka, K. (2010). Muscle contractile activity regulates Sirt3 protein expression in rat skeletal muscles. Journal of Applied Physiology, 109, 332–340.

Holloszy, J.O. (1967). Biochemical adaptations in muscle. Effects of exercise on mitochondrial oxygen uptake and respiratory enzyme activity in skeletal muscle. The Journal of Biological Chemistry, 242, 2278–2282.

Hood, D.A. (2001). Invited review: contractile activity-induced mitochondrial biogenesis in skeletal muscle. Journal of Applied Physiology, 90, 1137–1157.

Hood, D.A. (2009). Mechanisms of exercise-induced mitochondrial biogenesis in skeletal muscle. Applied Physiology, Nutrition, and Metabolism, 34, 465–472.

Itai, Y., Kariya, Y., Hoshino, Y. (2004). Morphological changes in rat hindlimb muscle fibres during recovery from disuse atrophy. Acta Physiologica Scandinavica, 181, 217–224.

Janssen, I. (2010). Evolution of sarcopenia research. Applied Physiology, Nutrition, and Metabolism, 35, 707–712.

Järva, J., Alev, K. & Seene, T. (1997a). Myosin heavy chain composition in regenerating skeletal muscle grafts. Basic and Applied Myology, 7, 137–141.

Järva, J., Alev, K. & Seene, T. (1997b). The effect of autografting on the myosin composition in skeletal muscle fibers. Muscle & Nerve, 20, 718–727.

Jin, H., Yang, R., Li, W., Lu, H., Ryan, A.M., Ogasawara, A.K., Van Peborgh, J. & Paoni, N.F. (2000). Effects of exercise on cardiac function, gene expression and apoptosis in rats. American Journal of Physiology. Heart and Circulatory Physiology, 279, 2994–3002.

Kaasik, P., Umnova, M., Alev, K., Selart, A. & Seene, T. (2012).Fine architectonics and protein turnoverrate in myofibrils of glucocorticoid caused myopathic rats. Journal of Interdisciplinary Histopathology,doi: 10.5455/jihp.20120606081246

Kaasik, P., Umnova, M., Pehme, A., Alev, K., Aru, M., Selart, A. & Seene, T. (2007). Ageing and dexamethasone associated sarcopenia: Peculiarities of regeneration. The Journal of Steroid Biochemistry and Molecular Biology, 105, 85–90.

Kadi, F. & Ponsot, E. (2010). The biology of satellite cells and telomeres in human skeletal muscle: effects of aging and physical activity. Scandinavian Journal of Medicine & Science inSports, 20, 39–48.

Katsanos, C.S., Chinkes, D.L., Paddon-Jones, D., Zhang, X., Aarsland, A. & Wolfe, R.R. (2008). Whey protein ingestion in elderly results in greater muscle protein accural than ingestion of its constituent essential amino acid content. Nutrition Research, 28, 651–658.

Kayar, S.R., Conley, K.E., Claassen, H. & Hoppeler, H. (1986). Capillarity and mitochondrial distribution in rat myocardium following exercise training. The Journal of Experimental Biology, 120, 189–199.

Kemi, O.J., Høydal, M.A., Haram, P.M. Garnier, A., Fortin, D., Ventura-Clapier, R. & Ellingsen, O. (2007). Exercise training restores aerobic capacity and energy transfer systems in heart failure treated with losartan. Cardiovascular Research, 76, 91–99.

Kjaer, M., Magnusson, P., Krogsgaard, M., Moller, J.B., Olesen, J., Heinemeier, K., Hansen, M., Haraldsson, B., Koskinen, S., Esmarck, B. & Langberg, H. (2006). Extracellular matrix adaptation of tendon and skeletal muscle to exercise. Journal of Anatomy, 208:445–450

Kovanen, V.,Suominen, E. & Heikkinen, E. (1984a.) Collagen of slow twitch and fast twitch muscle fibres in different types of rat skeletal muscle. European Journal of Applied Physiology and Occupational Physiology, 52, 235–242.

Kovanen, V., Suominen, E. & Heikkinen, E. (1984b). Mechanical properties of fast and slow skeletal muscle with special reference to collagen and endurance training.Journal of Biomechanics, 17, 725–735.

Kramer, F. & Erickson, K.I. (2007). Capitalizing on cortical plasticity: influence of physical activity on cognition and brain function. Trends in Gognitive Scienceş, 11, 342–348.

Kuh, D., Bassey, E.J., Butterworth, S., Hardy, R.. & Wadsworth, M.E.J. (2005). Grip strength, postural control, and functional leg power in a representative cohort of British men and women: associations with physical activity, health status, and socioeconomic conditions.The Journals of Gerontology. Series A, Biological Sciences and Medical Sciences, 60, 224–231.

Kujala, U.M. (2011). Physical activity, genes, and lifetime predisposition to chronic disease. European Review of Aging and Physical Activity, 8, 31–36.

Lee, W.J., Kim, M., Park, H.S., Kim, H.S., Jeon, M.J., Oh, K.S., Koh, E.H., Won, J.C., Kim, M.S., Oh, G.T., Yoon, M., Lee, K.U. & Park, J.Y. (2006). AMPK activation increases fatty acid oxidation in skeletal muscle by activating PPAR alpha and PGC-1. Biochemical and Biophysical Research Communications, 340, 291–295.

Leeuwenburgh, C., Gurley, C.M., Strotman, B.A. & Dupont-Versteegden, E.E. (2005). Age-realted differences in apoptosis with disuse atrophy in soleus muscle. American Journal of Applied Physiology Regulatory, Integrative and Comparative Physiology, 288, R1288–R1296.

Ljubicic, V., Joseph, A.M., Saleem, A., Uquccioni, G., Collu-Marchese, M., Lai, R.Y., Nguyen, L.M. & Hood, D.A. (2010). Transcriptional and post-transcriptional regulation of mitochondrial biogenesis in skeletal muscle: effects of exercise and aging. Biochimica et Biophysica Acta, 1800, 223–234.

Machida, S. & Booth, F.W. (2004). Increased nuclear proteins in muscle satellite cells in aged animals as compared to young growing animals. Experimental Gerontology, 39, 1521–1525.

Mackey, A.L., Heinemeier, K.M., Koskinen, S.O.A. & Kjaer, M. (2008). Dynamic adaptation of tendon and muscle connective tissue to mechanical loading. Connective Tissue Research, 49, 165–168.

Manini, T.M. (2009). Organ-o-penia. Journal of Applied Physiology, 106, 1759–1760.

Manini, T.M. & Clark, B.C. (2012). Dynapenia and aging: an uptate. The Journals of Gerontology. Series A, Biological Sciences and Medical Sciences, 67, 28–40.

Matoba, S., Kang, J.G., Patino, W.D., Wragg, A., Boehm, M., Gavrilova, O., Hurley, P.J., Bunz, F. & Hwang, P.M. (2006). P53 regulates mitochondrial respiration. Scince, 312, 1650–1653.

Matsakas, A., Macharia, R., Otto, A., Elashry, M.I., Mouisel, E., Romanello, V., Sartori, R., Amthor, H., Sandri, M., Narkar, V. & Patel, K. (2012). Exercise training attenuates the hypermuscular phenotype and restores skeletal muscle function in the myostatin null mouse. Experimental Physiology, 97, 125-140.

McGee, S.L., Mustard, K.J., Hardic, D.G. & Baar, K. (2008). Normal hypertrophy accompanied by phosphorylation and activation of AMP-activated protein kinase a1 following overload in LKB1 knockout mice. Journal of Physiology, 586, 1731–1741.

McLester, J.R., Bishop, P.A., Smith, J., Wyers, L., Dale, B., Kozusko, J., Richardson, M., Nevett, M.E. & Lomax,R. (2003). A series of studies – a practical protocol for testing muscular endurance recovery. Journal of Strength and Conditioning Research,17,259–273.

Mechling, H. & Netz, Y. (2009). Aging and inactivity-capitalizing on the protective effect of planned physical activity in old age. European Review of Aging and Physical Activity, 6, 89–97.

Menshikova, E.V., Ritov, V.B., Fairfull, L., Ferrell, R.E., David E. Kelley, D.E. & Goodpasteret B.H. (2006). Effects of exercise on mitochondrial content and function in aging human skeletal muscle. The Journal of Gerontology. Series A, Biological Sciences and Medical Sciences,61, 534–540.

Menzies, K.J. & Hood, D.A. (2012). The role of SirT1 in muscle mitochondrial turnover. Mitochondrion, 12, 5–13.

Mohr, M., Krustrup, P., Nielsen, J.J., Nybo, L., Rasmussen, M.K., Juel, C. & Bangsbo, J. (2007). Effect of two different intense training regimes on skeletal muscle ion transport proteins and fatigue development. American Journal of Physiology. Regulatory, Integrative and Comparative Physiology, 292, 1594–1602.

Moore, D.R., Atherton, P. J., Rennie, M.J., Tarnopolski, M.A. & Phillips, S.M. (2011). Resistance exercise enhances mTOR and MAPK signalling in human muscle over that seen at rest after bolus protein ingestion. Acta Physiologica, 201, 365–372.

Moore, D.R., Tang, J.E., Burd, N.A., Rerecich, T., Tarnopolski, M.A. & Phillips, S.M. (2009). Differential stimulation of myofibrillar and sarcoplasmic protein synthesis with protein ingestion at rest and after resistance exercise. Journal of Physiology, 587, 897–904.

Moritani, T. & deVries, H.A. (1979). Neural factors versus hypertrophy in the time course of muscle strength gain. American Journal of Physical Medicine, 58, 115–130.

Nair, K.S. (2005). Aging muscle. The American Journal of Clinical Nutrition, 81, 953–963.

Narkar, V.A., Downes, M., Yu, R.T., Embler, E., Wang, Y.X., Banayo, E., Mihaylova, M.M., Nelson, M.C., Zou, Y., Juguilon, H., Kang, H., Shaw, R.J. & Evans, R.M. (2008). AMPK and PPAR delta agonists are exercise mimetics. Cell, 134, 1–11.

Netz, Y. (2009). Type of activity and fitness benefits as moderators of the effect of physical activity on affect in advanced age: a review. European Review of Aging and Physical Activity, 6, 19–27.

Noble, E.G., Moraska, A., Mazzeo, R.S., Roth, D.A., Olsson, M.C., Moore, R.L. & Fleshner, M.(1999). Differential expression of stress proteins in rat myocardium after free wheel or treadmill run training. Journal of Applied Physiology, 86, 1696–1701.

Nuhr, M., Crevenna, R., Gohlsch, B., Bittner, C., Pleiner, J., Wiesinger, G., Fialka-Moser, V., Quittan, M. & Pette, D. (2003). Functional and biochemical properties of chronically stimulated human skeletal muscle. European Journal of Applied Physiology, 89, 202–208.

Ogata, T., Machida, S., Oishi, Y., Higuchi, M. & Muraoka, I. (2009). Differential cell death regulation between adult-unloaded and aged rat soleus muscle. Mechanisms of Ageing and Development, 130, 328–336.

Ohira, Y., Yoshinaga, T., Ohara, M., Kawano, F., Wang, X.D., Higo, Y., Terada, M., Matsuko, Y., Roy, R.R., Edgerton, V.R. (2006). The role of neural and mechanical influences in maintaining normal fast and slow muscle properties. Cells, Tissues, Organs, 182, 129–142.

Ono, Y., Boldrin, L., Knopp, P., Morgan, J.E. & Zammit, P.S. (2010). Muscle satellite cells are a functionally heterogeneous population in both somite-derived and branchiomeric muscles. Developmental Biology, 337, 29–41.

Palacios, O.M., Carmona, J.J., Michan, S., Chen, K.Y., Manabe, Y., Ward, J.L.3rd, Goodyear, L.J. & Tong, Q. (2009). Diet and exercise signals regulate SIRT3 and activate AMPK and PGC-1alpha in skeletal muscle. Aging, 1, 771–783.

Paniagua, R., Vázques, J.J. & López-Moratalla, N. (1977). Effects of physical training on rat myocardium. An enzymatic and ultrastructural morphometric study. Revista Española de Fisiologia, 33, 273–281.

Park, J.-Y., Wang, P.-Y., Matsumoto, T. Sung, H.J., Ma, W., Choi, J.W., Anderson, S.A., Leary, S.C., Balaban, R.S., Kang, J.G. & Hwang, P.M. (2009). P53 improves aerobic exercise capacity and augments skeletal muscle mitochondrial DNA content. Circulation Research, 105, 705–712.

Pehme, A., Alev, K., Kaasik, P. & Seene, T. (2004). Age related changes in skeletal musclemyosin heavy-chain composition: effect of mechanical loading. Journal of Aging and Physical Activity, 12, 29–44.

Pierce, G.N., Sekhon, P.S. & Meng, H.P., Maddaford, T.G. (1989). Effects of chronic swimming training on cardiac sarcolemmal function and composition. Journal of Applied Physiology, 66, 1715–1721.

Pillai, V.B., Sundaresan, N.R., Jeevanandam, V. & Gupta, M.P. (2010). Mitochondrial SIRT3 and heart disease. Cardiovascular Research, 88, 250–256.

Pottle, D. & Gosselin, L.E. (2000). Impact of mechanical load on functional recovery after muscle reloading. Medicine and Science in Sports and Exercise, 32, 2012–2017.

Powers, S.K., Kavazis, A.N. & McClung, J.M. (2007). Oxidative stress and disuse muscle atrophy. Journal of Applied Physiology, 102, 2389–2397.

Puigserver, P., Rhee, J., Lin, J.Wu, Z., Yoon, J.C., Zhang, C.Y., Krauss, S., Mootha, V.K., Lowell, B.B. & Spiegelman, B.M. (2001). Cytokine stimulation of enenrgy expenditure through p38 MAP kinase activation of PPAR gamma coactivator-1. Molecular Cell, 8, 971–982.

Rader, E.P. & Faulkner, J.A. (2006). Recovery from contraction-induced injury is impaired in weight-bearing muscles of old male mice. Journal of Applied Physiology, 100, 656–661.

Reznick, R.M., Zong, H., Li, J., Morino, K., Moore, K.J., Yu, H.J., Liu, Z.-X., Dong, J., Mustard, K.J., Hawley, S.A., Befroy, D., Pypaert, M., Hardie, D.G., Young, L.H. & Shulman, G.I. (2007). Aging-associated reductions in AMP-activated protein kinase activity and mitochondrial biogenesis. Cell Metabolism, 5, 151–156.

Riso, E.-M., Ahtikoski, A., Alev, K., Kaasik, P., Pehme, A. & Seene, T. (2008). *Relationship between extracellular matrix, contractile apparatus, muscle mass and strength in case of glucocorticoid myopathy. The Journal of Steroid Biochemistry and Molecular Biology, 108, 117–120.*

Riso, E.-M., Ahtikoski, A.M., Takala, T.E.S. & Seene, T. (2010). *The effect of unloading and reloading on the extracellular matrix in skeletalmuscle: changes in muscle strength and motor activity. Biology of Sport, 27, 89–94.*

Roberts, M.D., Kerksick, C.M., Dalbo, V.J., Hassell, S.E., Tucker, P.S. & Brown, R. (2010). *Molecular attributes of human skeletal muscle at rest and after unaccustomed exercise: an age comparison. Journal of Strength and Conditioning Research, 24, 1161–1168.*

Rooyackers, O.E., Adey, D.B., Ades, P.A. & Nair, K.S. (1996). *Effect of age in vivo rates of mitochondrial protein synthesis in human skeletal muscle. Proceedings of the National Academy of Sciences of the United States of America, 93, 15364–15369.*

Rupp, H. (1981). *The adaptive changes in the isoenzyme pattern of myosin from hypertrophied rat myocardium as a result of pressure overload and physical training. Basic Research in Cardiology, 76, 79–88.*

Russ, D.W., Grandy, J.S., Toma, K. & Ward, C.W. (2011). *Ageing, but not yet senescent, rats exhibit reduced muscle quality and sarcoplasmic reticulum function. Acta Physiologica, 201, 391–403.*

Sagiv, M., Goldhammer, E., Ben-Sira, D. & Amir, R. (2010). *Factors defining oxygen uptake at peak exercise in aged people. European Review of Aging and Physical Activity, 7, 1–2.*

Saleem, A., Adhietty, P.J. & Hood, D.A. (2009). *Role of p53 in mitochondrial biogenesis and apoptosis in skeletal muscles. Physiological Genomics, 37, 58–66.*

Scheller, K. & Sekeris, C.E. (2003).*The effects of steroid hormones on the transcription of genes encoding enzymes of oxidative phosphorylation. Experimental Physiology, 88, 129–140.*

Seene, T. (1994). *Turnover of Skeletal Muscle Contractile Proteins in Clucocorticoid Myopathy. The Journal of Steroid Biochemistry and Molecular Biology, 50, 1–4.*

Seene, T. & Kaasik, P. (2012a). *Muscle weakness in the elderly: role of sarcopenia, dynapenia, and possibilities for rehabilitation. European Review of Aging and Physical Activity, 9, 109–117.*

Seene ,T. & Kaasik, P. (2012b). *Role of exercise therapy in prevention of decline in aging muscle function: glucocorticoid myopathy and unloading. Journal of Aging Research, Doi: 10.1155/2012/172492*

Seene, T., Kaasik, P., Alev, K., Pehme, A. & Riso, E.-M. (2004). *Composition and turnover of contractile proteins in volume-overtrained skeletal muscle. International Journal of Sports Medicine, 25, 438–445.*

Seene, T., Kaasik, P., Pehme, A., Alev, K. & Riso, E.-M.(2003). *The effect of glucocorticoids on the myosin heavy chain isoforms' turnover in skeletal muscle. The Journal of Steroid Biochemistry and Molecular Biology, 86, 201–206.*

Seene, T.,Kaasik, P. &. Riso, E.-M. (2012). *Review on aging, unloading and reloading: changes in skeletal muscle quantity and quality. Archives of Gerontology and Geriatrics, 54, 374–380.*

Seene, T., Kaasik, P. & Umnova, M., (2009). *Structural rearrangements in contractile apparatus and resulting skeletal muscle remodelling: effect of exercise training. The Journal of Sports Medicine and Physical Fitness, 49, 410-423.*

Seene, T., Pehme, A., Alev, K., Kaasik, P., Umnova, M. & Aru, M. (2010). *Effects of resistance training on fast- and slow-twitch muscles in rats.Biology of Sport,27, 221–229.*

Seene, T., Umnova, M., Alev, K. & Pehme, A. (1988). *Effect of glucocorticoids on contractile apparatus of rat skeletal muscle. Journal of Steroid Biochemistry, 29, 313–317.*

Seene, T., Umnova, M., Kaasik, P., Alev, K. & Pehme, A. (2008). *Overtraining injuries in athletic population. In: Tiidus P. (Ed.), Skeletal Muscle Damage and Repair.Champaign (IL): Human Kinetics, pp. 173–184 & 305–307.*

Seene, T. & Viru, A. (1982). *The catabolic effect of glucocorticoids on different types of skeletal muscle fibres and its dependence upon muscle activity and interaction with anabolic steroids. The Journal of Steroid Biochemistry and Molecular Biology, 16, 349–352.*

Seppet, E., Orlova, E., Seene, T. & Gellerich F.N. (2013). Adaptation of cardiac and skeletal muscle mitochondria to endurance training: implications for cardiac protection. In: Ostadal, B. & Dhalla NS (Eds), Cardiac Adaptations. NY: Springer, vol 4, pp. 375-402.

Short, K.R. & Nair,K.S. (2000). The effect of age on protein metabolism. Current Opinion in Clinical Nutrition and Metabolic Care, 3, 39–44.

Short, K.R., Vittone, J.L., Bigelow, M.L., Proctor, D.N. & Nair, K.S. (2004). Age and aerobic exercise training effects on whole body and muscle protein metabolism. American Journal of Physiology. Endocrinology and Metabolism, 286, E92–E101.

Short, K.R., Vittone, J.L., Bigelow, M.L., Proctor, D.N., Rizza. R.A., Coenen-Schimke, J.M. & Nair, K.S. (2003). Impact of aerobic exercise training on age-related changes in insulin sensitivity and muscle oxidative capacity. Diabetes, 52, 1888–1896.

Shultz, E. & Darr, K. (1990). The role of satellite cells in adaptive or induced fiber transformations. In: Pette, D. (Ed.), The dynamic state of muscle fibers. Berlin: W.de Gruyter, pp 667–681.

Silva, L.A., Pinho, C.A., Scarabelot, K.S., Fraga, D.B., Volpato, A.M., Boeck, C.R., De Souza, C.T., Streck, E.L. & Pinho, R.A. (2009). Physical exercise increases mitochondrial function and reduces oxidative damage in skeletal muscle. European Journal of Applied Physiology, 105, 861–867.

Siu, P.M., Pistilli, E.E. & Alway, S.E. (2008). Age-dependent increase in oxidative stress in gastrocnemius muscle with unloading. Journal of Applied Physiology, 105, 1695–1705.

Spina, R.J., Chi, M.M., Hopkins, M.G., Nemeth, P.M., Lowry, O.H. & Holloszy, J O. (1996). Mitochondrial enzymes increase in muscle in response to 7-10 days of cycle exercise. Journal of Applied Physiology, 80, 2250–2254.

Spirduso, W.W. & Gronin, D.L. (2001). Exercise dose-response effects on quality of life and independent living in older adults. Medicine & Science in Sports & Exercise, 33,S598–S610.

Stackhouse, S.K., Stevens, J.E., Lee, S.C., Pearce, K.M., Snyder-Mackler, L. & Binder-Macleod, S.A. (2001). Maximum voluntary activation in nonfatigued and fatigued muscle of young and elderly individuals. Physical Therapy, 81, 1102–1109.

Stuart, C.A., Shangraw, R.E., Peters, E.J. & Wolfe, R.R. (1990). Effect of dietary protein on bed-rest-related changes in whole-body-protein synthesis. The American Journal of Clinical Nutrition, 52, 509–514.

Stuewe, S.R., Gwirtz, P.A., Agarwal, N. & Mallet, R.T. (2000). Exercise training enhances glycolytic and oxidative enzymes in canine ventricular myocardium. Journal of Molecular and Cellular Cardiology, 32, 903—913.

Suetta, C., Hvid, L.G., Justesen, L., Christensen, U., Neergaard, K., Simonsen, L., Ortenblad, N.,Magnusson, S.P., Kjaer, M. & Aagaard, P. (2009). Effects of aging on human skeletal muscle after immobilization and retraining. Journal of Applied Physiology, 107, 1172–1180.

Sun, B., Wang, J.H., Lv, Y.Y., Zhu, S.S., Yang, J. & Ma, J.Z. (2008). Proteomic adaptation to chronic high intensity swimming training in the rat heart. Comparative Biochemistry and Physiology. Part D, Genomics & Proteomics, 3, 108–117.

Suominen, H. (2011). Ageing and maximal physical performance. European Review of Aging and Physical Activity, 8, 37–42.

Symons, T.B., Sheffield-Moore, M., Chinkes, D.L., Ferrando, A.A. & Paddon-Jones, D. (2009). Artificial gravity maintains skeletal muscle protein synthesis during 21 days simulated microgravity. Journal of Applied Physiology, 107, 34–38.

Tate, C.A., Helgason, T., Hyek, M.F., McBride, R.P., Chen, M., Richardson, M.A. & Taffet, G.E. (1996). SERCA$_{2a}$ and mitochondrial cytochrome oxidase are increased in hearts of exercise-trained old rats. American Journal of Physiology, 271, 68–72.

Tatsumi, R. (2010). Mechano-biology of skeletal muscle hypertrophy and regeneration: Possible mechanism of stretch-induced activation of resident myogenic stem cells. AnimalScience Journal, 81, 11–20.

Terblanche, S.E., Gohil, K., Packer, L., Henderson, S. & Brooks, G.A. (2001). *The effects of endurance training and exhaustive exercise on mitochondrial enzymes in tissues of the rat (Rattus norvegicus). Comparative Biochemistry and Physiology. Part A, Molecular & Integrative Physiology, 128, 889–896.*

Thomson, D.M., Brown, J.D., Fillmore, N., Ellsworth, S.K., Jacobs, D.L., Winder, W.W.,Fick, C.A. & Gordon, S.E. (2009). *AMP-activated protein kinase response to contractions and treatment with the AMPK activator AICAP in young adult and old skeletal muscle. Journal of Physiology, 587, 2077–2086.*

Toth, M.J. & Tchernof, A. (2000). *Lipid metabolism in the elderly. European Journal of Clinical Nutrition, 54, S121–S125.*

Trappe, T. (2009). *Influence of aging and long-term unloading on the structure and function of human skeletal muscle. Applied Physiology, Nutrition, and Metababolism, 34, 459–464.*

Tyler, C.M., Golland, L.C., Evans, D.L., Hodgson, D.R. & Rose, R.J. (1998). *Skeletal muscle adaptations to prolonged training, overtraining and detraining in horses. Pflügers Archiv – European Journal of Physiology, 436, 391–397.*

van der Vusse, G.J., Glatz, J.F., Stam, H.C. & Reneman, R.S. (1992). *Fatty acid homeostasis in the normoxic and ischemic heart. Physiological Reviews, 72, 881–940.*

van Wessel, T., de Haan, A., van der Laarse, W.J. & Jaspers, R.T. (2010). *The muscle fiber type-fiber size paradox: hypertrophy or oxidative metabolism? European Journal of Applied Physiology, 110, 665–694.*

Verney, J., Kadi, F., Charifi, N., Feasson, L., Saafi, M.A., Castells, J., Piehl-Aulin, K. & Denis, C. (2008). *Effects of combined lower body endurance and upper body resistance training on the satellite cell pool in elderly subjects. Muscle & Nerve, 38, 1147–1154.*

von Bonsdorff, M.B. & Rantanen, T. (2011). *Progression of functional limitations in relation to physical activity: a life course approach. European Review of Aging and Physical Activity, 8, 23–30.*

Weisleder, N., Brotto, M., Komazaki, S., Pan, Z., Zhao, X., Nosek, T., Parness, J., Takeshima, H. & Ma, J. (2006). *Muscle aging is associated with compramised Ca^{2+} spark signaling and segregated intracellular Ca^{2+} release. Journal of Cell Biology, 174, 639–645.*

Welle, S., Bhatt, K. & Thornton, C. (1996). *Polyadenylated RNA, actin mRNA, and myosin heavy chain mRNA in young and old human skeletal muscle. American Journal of Physiology. Endocrinology and Metabolism, 270, E224–E229.*

White, T.P. & Devor, S.T. (1993). *Skeletal muscle regeneration and plasticity of grafts. Exercise and Sport Sciences Reviews, 21, 263–295.*

Wikman-Coffelt, J., Parmley, W.W. & Mason, D.T. (1979). *The cardiac hypertrophy process. Analyses of factors determining pathological vs physiological development. Circulation Research,45, 697–707.*

Willett, T.L., Labow, R.S., Aldous, I.G., Avery, N.C. & Lee, J.M. (2010). *Changes in collagen with aging maintain molecular stability after overload: evidence from an in vitro tendon model. Journal of Biomechanical Engineering, doi:10.1115/1.4000933*

Winder, W.W. & Hardie, D.G.(1996). *Inactivation of acetyl-CoA carboxylase and activation of AMP-activated protein kinase in muscle during exercise. American Journal Physiology. Endocrinology and Metabolism, 270, E299–E304.*

Wisloff, U., Loennechen, J.P., Falck, G., Beisvag, V., Currie, S., Smith, G. & Ellingsen, O. (2001). *Increased conractility and calcium sensitivity in cardiac myocytes isolated from endurance trained rats. Cardiovascular Research, 50, 495–508.*

Wu, Z., Huang, X., Feng, Y., Handschin, C., Feng, Y., Gullicksen, P.S., Bare, O., Labow, M., Spiegelman, B. & Stevenson, S.C. (2006). *Transducer of regulated CREB-binding proteins (TORCs) induce PGC-1α transcription and mitochondrial biogenesis in muscle cells. Proceedings of National Academy of Science of the United States of America, 103, 14379–14384.*

Yarasheski, K.E., Welle, S.L. & Nair, K.S. (2002). *Muscle protein synthesis in younger and older men. The Journal of the American Medical Association, 287, 317–318.*

Spatio-temporal Evolution and Prediction of Action Potential Duration and Calcium Alternans in the Heart

Elena G. Tolkacheva
Department of Biomedical Engineering
University of Minnesota, USA

Ramjay Visweswaran
Department of Biomedical Engineering
University of Minnesota, USA

1   Introduction

The beat-to-beat variation in cardiac action potential durations (APD) is a phenomenon known as electrical alternans (Figure 1A, B). In recent years, alternans has been considered a strong marker of electrical instability and a harbinger for ventricular fibrillation, which is a major cause of sudden cardiac death (Armoundas *et al.*, 2002; Zipes *et al.*, 1981). This beat-to-beat variation in the cardiac APD in the single cell has been shown to correspond to T-wave alternans at the whole heart level, seen in the electrocardiogram (Zipes *et al.*, 1981; Pastore *et al.*, 1999). Moreover, T-wave alternans is recognized as a precursor of ventricular arrhythmia since it was subsequently observed in a wide variety of clinical and experimental conditions associated with such arrhythmias (Salero *et al.*, 1986; Hellerstein *et al.*, 1950; Schwartz & Malliani, 1975; Rosenbaum *et al.*, 1994).

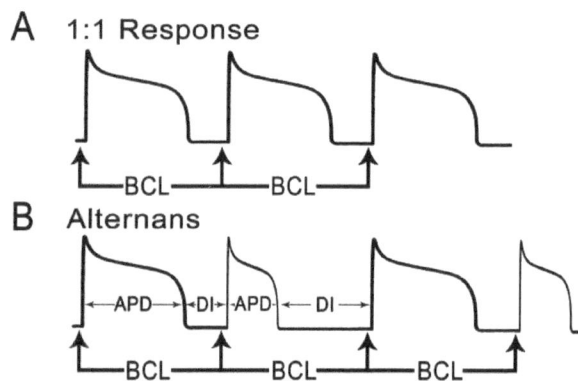

Figure 1: The response of periodically paced cardiac tissue to stimulation (arrows) during **(A)** normal pacing (1:1 response) and **(B)** alternans.

In the heart, membrane voltage and intracellular calcium ($[Ca^{2+}]_i$) are bi-directionally coupled with each exerting an influence on the other during the course of an action potential. $[Ca^{2+}]_i$ transient is influenced by membrane voltage through its effect on the L-type calcium channel, termed calcium-induced-calcium-release (Armoundas *et al*, 2003). On the other hand, $[Ca^{2+}]_i$ amplitude controls APD via its effects on $[Ca^{2+}]_i$ -sensitive membrane currents such as the sodium-calcium exchanger current (Mullins, 1979) and the L-type calcium current (Lee *et al*, 1985). Therefore, APD alternans can be accompanied by alternans $[Ca^{2+}]_i$ transients. $[Ca^{2+}]_i$ transient amplitude alternans has been linked to mechanical alternans (Lee *et al.*, 1988); and the simultaneous occurrence of $[Ca^{2+}]_i$ and APD alternans, termed electromechanical (EM) alternans, is believed to be a substrate for various cardiac arrhythmias (Weiss *et al.*, 2006). It has been postulated that $[Ca^{2+}]_i$ alternans might be responsible for the fluctuations in APD that produce T-wave alternans in the whole heart (Lee *et al.*, 1988; Wan *et al.*, 2005). It is suggested that $[Ca^{2+}]_i$ alternans develops first due to dynamical instabilities in calcium cycling (Shiferaw *et al.*, 2003; Chudin *et al.*, 1998; Morita *et al.*, 2008), which then drives APD alternans, leading to EM alternans in the heart (Lakireddy *et al.*, 2005). Moreover, it was demonstrated that by suppressing $[Ca^{2+}]_i$ cycling and buffering $[Ca^{2+}]_i$ transients, APD alternans under rapid pacing was abolished even though APD was shortened with faster pacing (Goldhaber *et al.*, 2005). These results point towards a primary role for $[Ca^{2+}]_i$ in the genesis of EM alternans. Despite the important role of $[Ca^{2+}]_i$ in the development of EM alternans, no criteria has been proposed to predict the onset of $[Ca^{2+}]_i$ and EM alternans.

Various theories have been put forward to explain how impaired calcium handling can induce calcium and APD alternans. Previous studies have suggested that diminished $[Ca^{2+}]_i$ reuptake and instability in the beat-to-beat feedback control of sarcoplasmic reticulum (SR) content leads to $[Ca^{2+}]_i$ alternans (Eisner et al, 2005). In areas with impaired calcium handling or larger calcium transients, complete reuptake of $[Ca^{2+}]_i$ back into SR may not always be possible before the next activation, leaving the region vulnerable to $[Ca^{2+}]_i$ transient amplitude alternans. This is because the next $[Ca^{2+}]_i$ transient is from a higher diastolic $[Ca^{2+}]_i$ content and vice versa. These beat-to-beat changes in the $[Ca^{2+}]_i$ transient amplitude has a huge effect on the APD due to the aforementioned coupling between membrane voltage and $[Ca^{2+}]_i$. Thus, impaired calcium handling can induce both calcium and APD alternans in the heart.

It has been proposed that the onset of APD alternans in cardiac myocytes can be determined by analysing their responses to periodic stimulation and constructing a restitution curve (Courtemanche, 1996; Guevara et al., 1984; Riccio et al., 1999; Nolasco & Dahlen, 1968), which represents the nonlinear relationship between the APD and the preceding diastolic interval (DI). Furthermore, APD restitution slope has been shown to be an important indicator of wave stability, and it has been proposed theoretically that a slope of the restitution curve equal to one predicts the onset of APD alternans in cardiac myocytes (Nolasco & Dahlen, 1968).

However, the actual dynamics of periodically paced cardiac myocytes are more complex, and the APD usually depends on the entire pacing history (Gilmour, 2002; Goldhaber et al., 2005; de Diego et al., 2008; Koller at al., 1998; Lou et al., 2009; Hall et al., 1999, Tolkacheva et al., 2003), and not only on the preceding DI. One of the main consequences of this phenomenon is a dependence of the restitution curve on the pacing protocol used to obtain it. Several pacing protocols have been used experimentally to construct different restitution curves, where the dynamic and S1-S2 restitution curves are the most common. In a dynamic protocol, steady state APD and DI are measured as the basic cycle length (BCL) decreases. In an S1-S2 protocol, a premature stimulus (S2) is applied at various times relative to the end of a series of paced (S1) beats. Thus, the dynamic and S1-S2 restitution curves describe different aspects of cardiac dynamics: steady state responses and responses to perturbations, respectively. In the presence of memory, these different restitution curves have different slopes, and none of them have been clearly linked to the onset of alternans (Goldhaber et al., 2005; de Diego et al., 2008; Koller et al., 1998). Indeed, several experimental studies demonstrated the existence of alternans for a shallow restitution and no alternans for a steep restitution (Guevara et al., 1984; Riccio et al., 1999; Hall et al., 1999). In addition, the restitution hypothesis has been shown to have little clinical relevance, with studies showing poor correlation between APD alternans, APD restitution, and clinical outcome (Narayan et al., 2007).

One of the possible reasons why the restitution hypothesis does not always hold experimentally is the fact that it does not take into account $[Ca^{2+}]_i$ cycling. Although different mechanisms exist to explain the formation of APD alternans without $[Ca^{2+}]_i$ cycling (Nolasco & Dahlen, 1968), it has been postulated in several numerical and single cell experimental studies that $[Ca^{2+}]_i$ alternans might be responsible for the alternations in APD (Wan et al., 2005; Shiferaw et al., 2003). Even though these results point towards a primary role for $[Ca^{2+}]_i$ in the genesis of EM alternans, no studies have looked into predicting the onset of $[Ca^{2+}]_i$ alternans.

Another reason for the failure of the restitution hypothesis is the complex spatio-temporal evolution of alternans in the heart. Indeed, it has been demonstrated that APD alternans has a local onset in the heart, *i.e.* alternans develops in a small region of the heart, and then occupies the entire surface as the pacing rate increases (Cram *et al.*, 2011). However, not much is known about spatio-temporal evolution of $[Ca^{2+}]_i$ alternans in the heart (Visweswaran *et al.*, 2013).

Recently, a perturbed downsweep pacing protocol was developed theoretically (Tolkacheva *et al.*, 2003) and implemented experimentally (Tolkacheva *et al.*, 2006) leading to the concept of the restitution portrait, which consists of several restitution curves measured simultaneously at various pacing frequencies. It has been shown that the local onset of APD alternans in a small region of an isolated rabbit heart can be predicted by calculating one of the slopes measured in the restitution portrait (Cram *et al.*, 2011). This suggests that the restitution portrait may be a better approach to predict APD alternans compared to individual restitution curves since it captures several aspects of cardiac dynamics simultaneously. Even though the restitution portrait has proved useful in predicting APD alternans, it is still unclear whether it can be applied to predicting the onset of $[Ca^{2+}]_i$ alternans, which might be the primary driving force of EM alternans.

The main objective of this chapter is to discuss the local development of $[Ca^{2+}]_i$ and APD alternans in the isolated rabbit heart using simultaneous recording of both transmembrane voltage and $[Ca^{2+}]_i$. Specifically, we aimed to study the spatio-temporal evolution of both $[Ca^{2+}]_i$ transient amplitude (CaA) and duration (CaD) alternans in relation to APD alternans. In addition, we aim to demonstrate whether the slopes measured in the restitution portrait can predict the onset of APD and $[Ca^{2+}]_i$ alternans in the heart.

2   Methods

2.1   Downsweep Pacing Protocol

All investigations conformed to the Guide for the Care and Use of Laboratory Animals (National Institutes of Health Publication No. 85-23, Revised 1996), and the protocol was approved by the Institutional Animal Care and Use Committee at the University of Minnesota. To determine the development of APD alternans, we used high resolution optical mapping to visualize the electrical activity in N=6 Langendorff-perfused isolated rabbit hearts using the voltage-sensitive dye di-4-ANEPPS, as described previously (Mironov *et al.*, 2008; Cram *et al.*, 2011). Two synchronized CCD cameras were used to record membrane voltage from the left (LV) and right ventricular (RV) epicardial surfaces of the heart. In order to study the spatial and temporal development of $[Ca^{2+}]_i$ and APD alternans, we used simultaneous voltage-calcium optical mapping using voltage-sensitive (RH-237) and calcium-sensitive (Rhod-2AM) dyes in N=8 rabbits, as described previously (Choi & Salama, 2000; Pruvot *et al.*, 2004; Visweswaran *et al.*, 2013). Briefly, the fluorescence signal emitted from the heart upon excitation (532 nm) was split at 630 nm using a dichroic mirror. The split signals were further filtered using a 720 long pass and 585 ± 20nm to obtain the voltage and calcium signals. The choice of dyes was made such that the emission spectra do not overlap. Two cameras were used to measure the calcium and voltage signal simultaneously from the RV surface. A mechanical uncoupler blebbistatin was added to the Tyrode's solution to reduce motion artifacts in both sets of experiments.

The heart was paced at the base and optical mapping movies were recorded at different BCLs *B*. External stimuli (5 ms durations, twice the threshold) were applied to the base of the heart using a perturbed downsweep pacing protocol (Kalb *et al.*, 2004), in which the following steps were applied at each BCL *B*, starting with *B* = 300 ms:

I.   100 stimuli were applied at BCL *B* to achieve a steady state (SS).

II.   One additional stimulus (long perturbation, LP) was applied at a longer BCL $B^{LP} = B + 10ms$.

III.   10 stimuli were applied at BCL B to return to SS.

IV.   One additional stimulus (short perturbation, SP) was applied at a shorter BCL $B^{SP} = B - 10ms$.

V.   10 stimuli were applied at BCL B to return to SS.

After completing steps (I) - (V), the BCL B was progressively reduced in 20 ms decrements until B = 100 ms or until ventricular fibrillation occurred.

At each BCL, APD was measured at 80% repolarization and CaA was calculated as the difference between the local maxima and minima of the same response, representing the systolic and diastolic values of $[Ca^{2+}]_i$, after subtraction of the background fluorescence, as described previously (Qian *et al.*, 2001). The CaD was determined from the maximum first derivative of the $[Ca^{2+}]_i$ upstroke to the time point of 80% recovery of $[Ca^{2+}]_i$ to its original baseline, as was described previously (Choi & Salama, 2000; Lakireddy *et al.*, 2005).

2.2   Alternans Measurements

The amplitudes of APD and CaD alternans were calculated at each pixel as a difference in corresponding values of the SS responses between odd and even beats: $\Delta APD = APD_{even} - APD_{odd}$, and $\Delta CaD = CaD_{even} - CaD_{odd}$. The degree of CaA alternans, ΔCaA, was calculated at each pixel as the alternans ratio, 1-X/Y, where X is the net amplitude of the smaller $[Ca^{2+}]_i$ transient and Y is the net amplitude of the larger $[Ca^{2+}]_i$ transient, as was described previously (Wu & Clusin, 1997). The temporal thresholds for both APD and CaD alternans were set at 5 ms; and for CaA alternans at 0.15. 2D ΔAPD, ΔCaD, and ΔCaA maps were constructed to reveal the spatial distribution and amplitude of each type of alternans for the RV surface of the heart. To eliminate a possibility of inclusion of more complex rhythms or ectopic beats, each movie that was used for alternans analysis was visually inspected to ensure the absence of alternans phase change (long-short to short-long). If such a phase change occurred, the corresponding movie was excluded from the analysis.

The local spatial onset of alternans was defined as the BCL, B^{Onset}, at which at least 10% of the RV surface exhibited alternans separately for APD (B^{Onset}_{APD}), CaA (B^{Onset}_{CaA}), or CaD (B^{Onset}_{CaD}). Two spatial regions of the heart were defined at each B^{Onset}: the *1:1_{alt}* region, which exhibited alternans, and the *1:1* region, which exhibited 1:1 behaviour and no alternans. These two regions were back-projected to all BCLs B preceding B^{Onset}, and the mean values and standard errors for all parameters were calculated and averaged separately for these two regions. The notations $1:1_{alt}$ and 1:1 reflect the fact that both regions exhibit 1:1 behaviour prior to B^{Onset}, and only at B^{Onset} the $1:1_{alt}$ region exhibits alternans. Since alternans occurred at different BCLs during different experiments, a normalized value of BCL according to formula $B_N = B - B^{Onset}$ was introduced.

2.2   Slopes Calculations

The responses at each pixel were used to construct restitution portraits of the heart separately for voltage and $[Ca^{2+}]_i$. Only data from different BCLs prior to B^{Onset} were considered for restitution portrait construction. Specifically, at each pixel, the restitution portrait consists of a dynamic restitution curve measuring SS responses at each BCL B, and several local S1-S2 restitution curves for each BCL B. The following slopes were calculated separately for APD, CaA, and CaD responses at each pixel: 1) slope of dynamic restitution curve, S^{RP}_{dyn}, by fitting SS responses from all B values with a second degree polynomial curve;

and 2) slopes of S1-S2 restitution curve S_{12} (measured at SS) and S_{12}^{Max} (measured at SP) by fitting LP and SP responses from all B values respectively with a second degree polynomial function.

Term	Explanation
B	Basic cycle length (BCL)
B^{onset}	B at which 10% of the heart exhibited alternans
B^{Prior}	B immediately prior to B^{onset}
B_N	Normalized BCL based on the formula $B_N = B - B^{Onset}$

Table 1: Different terms and what each term represents.

Pacing protocol (step)	Responses	Slopes
II	APD and DI after LP	S_{12} - Measured at SS at each B
I	APD and DI after SS	S_{12}^{Max} - Measured at SP at each B
IV	APD and DI after SP	
I	APD and DI after SS	S_{dyn}^{RP} - Measured at SS from all B

Table 2: Different responses and corresponding slopes measured from the pacing protocols.

3   APD Alternans

3.1   Spatio-temporal Evolution of APD Alternans in the Heart

We observed that alternans first appeared locally at $B = B^{onset}$ in ventricles and evolved spatially throughout the heart as the BCL decreased. Figure 2 shows a representative example of the spatiotemporal evolution of alternans in the LV of the rabbit heart at different values of B. The color bar represents the amplitude of alternans ΔAPD. Note the presence of 1:1 behavior (white) at large B, and appearance of alternans (red) as B decreases. For instance, in this particular example, the onset of alternans occurred at $B^{onset} = 170$ ms. At that specific BCL, the two regions, $1:1_{alt}$ and $1:1$, were identified at the surface of the heart and projected back into all prior BCLs (see Figure 2). Note that alternans spread throughout the heart as the BCLs became smaller than B^{onset}, and spatially concordant alternans became spatially discordant, as has been described previously (Weiss *et al.*, 2006; Mironov *et al.*, 2008), and as indicated by the presence of white color (nodal line) at B=150 ms in Figure 2.

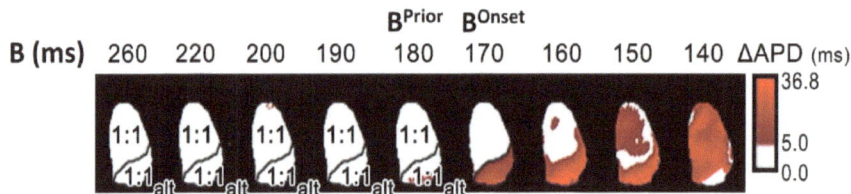

Figure 2: A representative example of the 2D ΔAPD maps in the rabbit LV at different B. The color bar represents amplitude of alternans (red), and 1:1 responses (white). The local spatial onset of alternans occurs at B^{onset} (B_{APD}^{Onset}). At B^{onset}, the two regions, $1:1_{alt}$ and $1:1$ are introduced and projected to all preceding B (black outlines).

3.2   2D Restitution Properties of the Heart

From Figure 2, we notice that alternans develop in a small region of the heart before spreading through-out the epicardial surface as the pacing rate increases. In order to determine whether there are any chang-es in the properties of the myocardium before this local onset of alternans appears, we constructed 2D APD maps for SS, LP, and SP responses at various BCLs. Representative examples of these APD maps are shown in Fig. 3A for large BCL B=200 ms, and for the BCL prior to B^{onset}, B^{Prior}. The color bar repre-sents the duration of the action potentials, and the projected boundaries of the $1:1_{alt}$ and $1:1$ regions are shown as black lines on each APD map. Note, that for large B (top panel in Figure 3A), the spatial distri-butions of APDs measured during LP and SP were similar to the one measured at SS, both for the $1:1_{alt}$ and $1:1$ regions. However, at B^{Prior}, the spatial distribution of APD measured at LP was similar to the one from SS, while the spatial distribution of APD measured at SP was different, both for the $1:1_{alt}$ and $1:1$ regions (see bottom panel in Figure 3A). This shows that, prior to the onset of alternans, all regions of the heart respond similarly both at SS and after perturbation (LP and SP) responses. However, just prior to the onset of alternans, the region of the heart which eventually develops alternans has different restitution properties compared to the region which does not develop alternans.

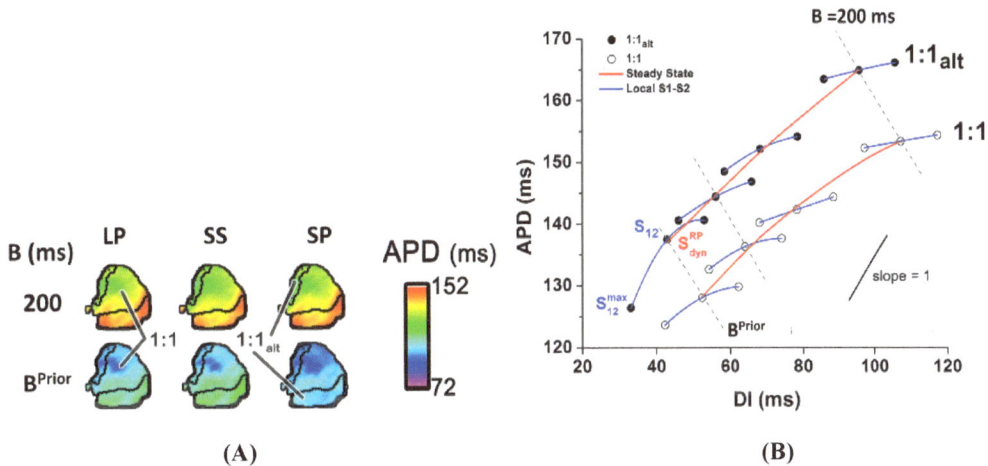

Figure 3: (**A**) Representative examples of 2D APD maps for APDs calculated at LP, SP and SS responses B = 200 ms and B^{Prior}. (**B**) Representative examples of the restitution portraits con-structed for two pixels taken from the $1:1_{alt}$ (solid circles) and $1:1$ (open circles) regions. The SS dynamic restitution curve is shown in red, and the local S1-S2 restitution curves for different B are shown in blue. The gray dotted lines with the slope of -1 represent the equal-BCL lines. The solid line shows the slope of equal one. Three different slopes are present in the restitution por-trait for each B: S_{dyn}^{RP}, S_{12}, and S_{12}^{Max}.

Representative examples of the restitution portraits for two pixels taken from the $1:1_{alt}$ and $1:1$ re-gions are compared in Figure 3B. Here, a unique SS dynamic restitution curve (red) and several local S1-S2 restitution curves for different B (blue) are shown along with the corresponding slopes S_{dyn}^{RP}, S_{12}, and S_{12}^{Max}. The gray dotted lines are the equal BCL lines with the slope = -1, and solid black line show the slope=1. Note that the dynamic restitution curves are almost parallel in both $1:1_{alt}$ and $1:1$ regions, indi-cating the absence of differences in S_{dyn}^{RP} at all B. Similarly, local S1-S2 restitution curves are nearly parallel at large B, indicating that S_{12} and S_{12}^{Max} were similar between $1{:}1_{alt}$ and $1{:}1$ regions as well. However, at B^{Prior}, the difference between local S1-S2 restitution curves is pronounced, and both the S_{12} and S_{12}^{Max} slopes were visually steeper in the $1{:}1_{alt}$ region in comparison to the $1{:}1$ region. Therefore, Fig. 3B indicates that the slopes S_{12} and S_{12}^{Max} correlate with the local onset of alternans in the heart.

3.3   Prediction of the Local Onset of APD Alternans in the Heart

To determine whether the restitution portrait can predict the local onset of APD alternans, we calculated mean values of three slopes measured in the restitution portrait, S_{dyn}^{RP}, S_{12}, and S_{12}^{Max}, over the epicardial surface of the hearts in all experiments separately for the $1{:}1_{alt}$ and $1{:}1$ regions. The data are shown in Fig. 4A – C as a function of B_N.

Note that there is no significant difference between values of S_{dyn}^{RP} calculated both for the $1{:}1_{alt}$ and $1{:}1$ regions at any B_N (Figure 4A). However, the behavior of S_{12} and S_{12}^{Max} slopes are different (Figure 4 B and 4C). At large B_N, both S_{12} and S_{12}^{Max} are similar between the $1{:}1_{alt}$ and $1{:}1$ regions, but as B_N decreases, the values of both slopes becomes significantly larger in the $1{:}1_{alt}$ region compared to the $1{:}1$ region ($p < 0.05$). Note that this significant difference appears first for the S_{12} slope (at $B_N = 20$ ms, Figure 6B) and later for the S_{12}^{Max} slope (at $B_N = 10$ ms, Figure 4C). However, the difference in S_{12}^{Max} values is significantly larger than the difference in S_{12} values between the $1{:}1_{alt}$ and $1{:}1$ regions immediately prior to the onset of alternans, at B^{Prior}. Therefore, both S_{12} and S_{12}^{Max} can serve as an indicator of the local onset of alternans in the heart.

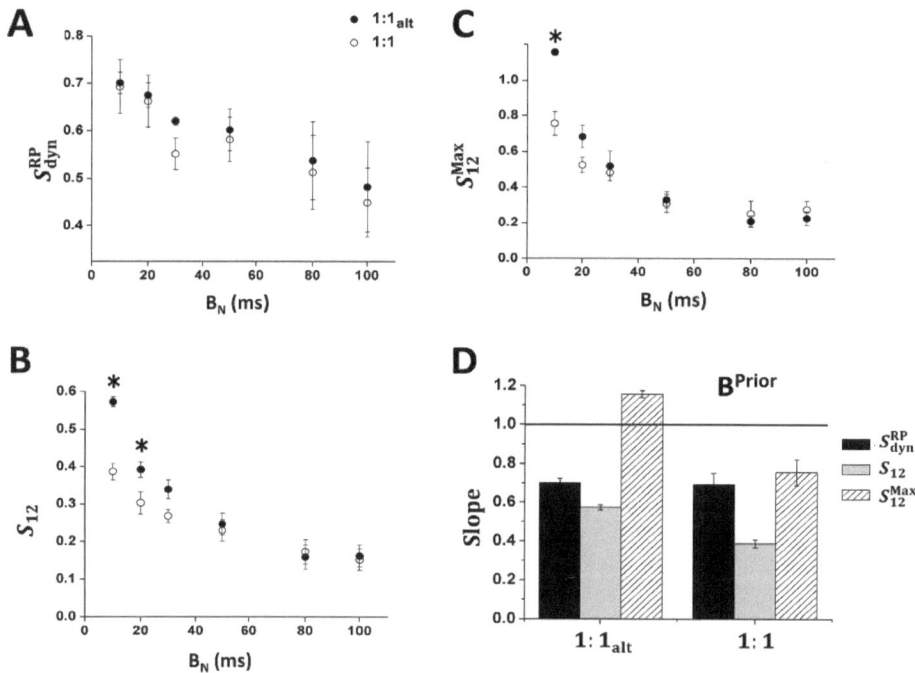

Figure 4: Mean values of **A**, S_{dyn}^{RP}; **B**, S_{12}, **C**, and S_{12}^{Max} as a function of $B_N = B - B^{Onset}$. All slopes were calculated separately for the $1{:}1_{alt}$ (solid circles) and $1{:}1$ (open circles) regions. **D**, Mean values of these slopes measured at B^{Prior} in comparison to the theoretical predicted value of 1. * denotes statistically significant data ($p < 0.05$).

To determine whether any of the slopes measured in our experiments were comparable with the theoretically predicted value of one, we calculated the mean values of S_{dyn}^{RP}, S_{12}, and S_{12}^{Max} immediately prior to the onset of alternans, at B^{Prior}. Figure 4D compares the values of all slopes for both the $1:1_{alt}$ and $1:1$ regions with the value of one. Note that S_{dyn}^{RP}, and S_{12} were less than one in both the $1:1_{alt}$ and $1:1$ regions, while S_{12}^{max} was larger than one in $1:1_{alt}$ and smaller than one in $1:1$ region. Nevertheless, the values of all slopes were significantly different than the theoretically predicted value of one.

4   [Ca^{2+}]$_i$ Alternans

4.1   Spatio-temporal Evolution of [Ca^{2+}]$_i$ Alternans in the Heart

With our simultaneous voltage and calcium optical mapping experiments, we observed that [Ca^{2+}]$_i$ alternans also occurred locally in a small region of the heart and spread to occupy the entire heart as the BCL B decreased, similar to APD alternans. Figure 5 shows the evolution of [Ca^{2+}]$_i$ alternans in relation to APD alternans. Fig. 5 A shows representative examples of the spatiotemporal evolution CaA (top panel), CaD (middle panel), and APD (bottom panel) at different values of B. The color bar represents the amplitude of alternans (red) or the presence of 1:1 responses (white). Note that at large B, there is no alternans in APD, CaD or CaA; but as B decreases, alternans gradually develops in the heart. Note that in this particular example, alternans in CaA develops first at $B_{CaA}^{Onset} = 170$ ms, followed by APD alternans at $B_{APD}^{Onset} = 160$ ms, and CaD alternans occurs last at $B_{CaD}^{Onset} = 150$ ms. Fig. 5 A clearly demonstrates that APD and CaD alternans develop in the same area that was already occupied by CaA alternans. Fig. 5 B shows single pixel traces of [Ca^{2+}]$_i$ transients and action potentials taken from the regions marked as '*','+', and '#' in Fig. 5 A. At large BCL $B = 190$ ms, 1:1 behaviour is seen in both [Ca^{2+}]$_i$ and APD (see '*'); and as the BCL B is decreased to 170 ms (see '+'), note that beat-to-beat changes occur first only in CaA, while 1:1 behaviour is still seen in APD. As the BCL B is further decreased to 150 ms, the alternans in CaA, APD and CaD are seen (see '#'). It is also worth mentioning that CaD alternans, in contrast to CaA and APD alternans, was rarely present and was generally observed only during pacing at a very high frequency.

The spatio-temporal dynamics of alternans illustrated in Fig. 5 A was present across all experiments. Fig. 5 C shows a box plot representation of minimum, median, and maximum values of B_{APD}^{Onset}, B_{CaA}^{Onset}, and B_{CaD}^{Onset}. Note that the onset of CaA alternans, B_{CaA}^{Onset}, always preceded the onset of APD alternans, B_{APD}^{Onset}, while the onset of CaD alternans, B_{CaD}^{Onset} always developed last. Fig. 5D shows the spatial development of CaA, APD, and CaD alternans in all experiments quantified by the percentage of the total RV surface occupied by each type of alternans as a function of B. Note the gradual development of each type of alternans in the heart as the B decreases. Therefore, our results show that CaA and CaD alternans, similar to APD alternans (Cram *et al.*, 2011), has a local onset in the heart, and that the local onset of CaA precedes the local onset of APD and CaD alternans.

Here, we demonstrated that the local onset of [Ca^{2+}]$_i$ alternans always occurs first, which then causes alternations in APD as has been previously demonstrated in numerical investigations and single cell experiments (Shiferaw *et al.*, 2003; Chudin *et al.* 1998). In order for [Ca^{2+}]$_i$ alternans to be considered the cause of accompanying APD alternans, it is necessary to show that, for a given cell within the intact heart, the two phenomena are inexorably linked. Initially, this link has been demonstrated using monophasic action potential electrodes recordings (Lee *et al.*, 1998), and later using more rigorous optical mapping studies (Pruvot *et al.*, 2004). The fact that [Ca^{2+}]$_i$ transient and APD alternans occur together is consistent with the hypothesis that the $[Ca^{2+}]_i$ transient "controls" APD, but this never has been sufficiently proven, because it is possible that purely voltage-dependent currents could produce APD alternans (Clusin, 2008). Our results show that APD alternans occur in the same region that was already occupied by $[Ca^{2+}]_i$ alternans, which seem to indicate that calcium alternans drives APD alternans in the whole heart even with complex spatial factors. This might be due to the steep dependence of the SR Ca^{2+} release on SR Ca^{2+} load (Diaz et al., 2004) and SR Ca^{2+} uptake (Shiferaw et al., 2003), which has been implicated as the primary cause of $[Ca^{2+}]_i$ alternans in single cells. APD alternans can occur passively due to the close dependence between $[Ca^{2+}]_i$ and membrane voltage mediated by the $[Ca^{2+}]_i$ dependent currents.

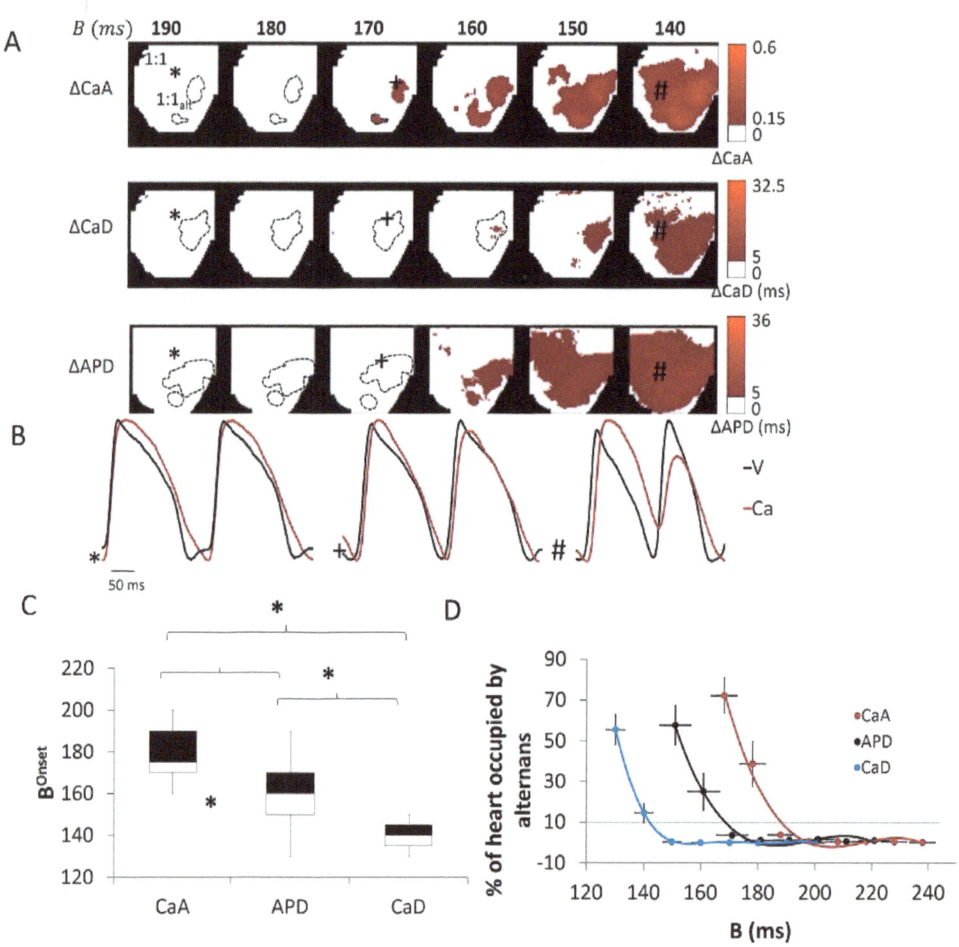

Figure 5: (**A**) Representative example of the 2D ΔCaA, ΔCaD, and ΔAPD maps showing spatio-temporal evolution of alternans at different B values. The color bar represents the amplitude of alternans (*red*) and 1:1 responses (*white*). The local spatial onsets of alternans occur at B^{Onset}. At B^{Onset}, two regions (1:1$_{alt}$ and 1:1) are introduced and back-projected to all prior B values (black outlines). (**B**) Representative traces of $[Ca^{2+}]_i$ (red) and action potential (black) taken from pixels marked as '*', '+', and '#' in **A**. (**C**) Local onset, B^{Onset} of CaA, CaD, and APD alternans and **E**, spatial evolution of alternans as a function of B. Dashed horizontal line indicates spatial threshold for alternans (10% of RV surface).

4.2   Prediction of the Local Onset of CaD and CaA alternans

We then performed a similar analysis to investigate if any of the slopes of the restitution portrait constructed from CaD responses could predict the local onset of CaD alternans. Figure 6A shows representative examples of 2D ΔCaD maps at B_{CaA}^{Onset} and the BCL prior to the onset of CaD alternans, B^{Prior}. The dotted lines indicate the border between 1:1 and 1:1$_{alt}$ regions that was determined at B_{CaA}^{Onset}. Figure 6B shows a representative example of a restitution portrait from the pixel marked as '#' along with the definitions of measured slopes (*top*). The spatial distribution of S_{dyn}^{RP}, S_{12}, and S_{12}^{Max} slopes calculated at B^{Prior} is shown in Figure 6B (*bottom*). In this case, both S_{12}^{Max} and S_{dyn}^{RP} have larger values in the 1:1$_{alt}$ compared to the 1:1 region. The mean S_{dyn}^{RP}, S_{12}, and S_{12}^{Max} slopes calculated at B^{Prior} from all our experiments are shown in Figure 6C separately for 1:1 and 1:1$_{alt}$ regions. Note that in the case of CaD, both S_{12}^{Max} and S_{dyn}^{RP} are significantly larger in 1:1$_{alt}$ region compared to 1:1 region immediately prior to onset of CaD alternans; while the S_{12} slopes remain the same. This indicates that both S_{12}^{Max} and S_{dyn}^{RP} slopes calculated prior to the onset of CaD alternans, at B^{Prior}, can indicate which region of the heart is susceptible to alternans.

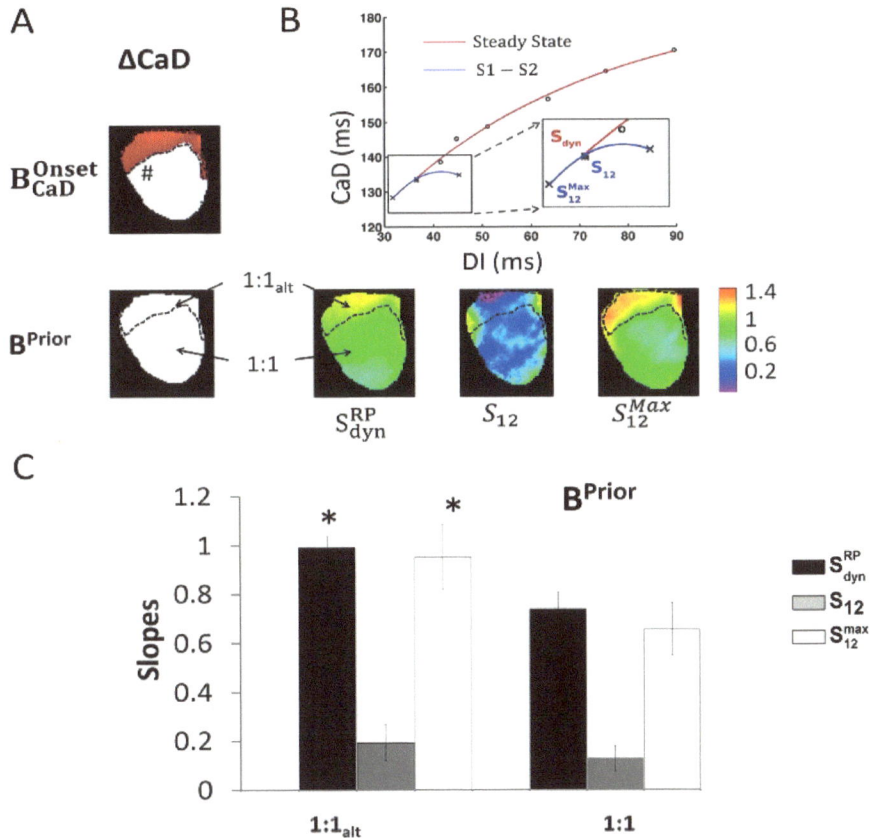

Figure 6: (A) Representative examples of 2D ΔCaD maps at B_{CaA}^{Onset} and B^{Prior}. **(B)** Representative example of CaD restitution portrait for pixel marked as '#' in **A** showing the slopes measured (*top*); 2D distribution of S_{dyn}^{RP}, S_{12}, and S_{12}^{Max} slopes at B^{Prior} (*bottom*). Dashed lines outline the boundary between the 1:1 and 1:1$_{alt}$ regions and **C**, Average S_{dyn}^{RP}, S_{12}, and S_{12}^{Max} slope values at B^{Prior}. '*' indicates statistical significance (p<0.05).

Our experiments demonstrate that the rate dependent shortening/reduction of CaA with BCLs, *i.e.* SS dynamic restitution of CaA, is not present in the isolated hearts. This is in contrast to APD and CaD restitution, as indicated by the red dynamic restitution curves in Figure 3B and 4B, *top*, respectively. However, CaA after SP and LP responses was different from SS responses, especially at lower BCLs. Therefore, the restitution portraits obtained for CaA appear different from the one obtained for APD and CaD. Figure 7A shows representative examples of 2D ΔCaA maps at B_{CaA}^{Onset} and the BCL prior to the onset of CaA alternans, B^{Prior}. The dotted lines indicate the border between 1:1 and 1:1$_{alt}$ regions that was determined at B_{CaA}^{Onset}. Figure 7B shows a representative example of a restitution portrait from a pixel marked in Figure 7A as '#'. Note the presence of the flat dynamic restitution curve indicating that the SS responses are rate-independent, and thus SS CaAs has similar values across all BCLs leading to a very flat dynamic restitution curve. However, the presence of local S1-S2 curves at different BCLs indicates that there are differences between the SS and perturbation (SP and LP) responses. Note that this difference is more pronounced at lower BCLs, closer to the onset of CaA alternans. The spatial distribution of S_{dyn}^{RP}, S_{12}, and S_{12}^{Max} slopes calculated at B^{Prior} is shown in Figure 7B. In this example, both S_{12}^{Max} and S_{12} have larger values in the 1:1$_{alt}$ compared to the 1:1 region, while S_{dyn}^{RP} is close to zero in all regions. The mean S_{dyn}^{RP}, S_{12}, and S_{12}^{Max} slopes calculated at B^{Prior} from all our experiments are shown in Figure 7C separately for 1:1 and 1:1$_{alt}$ regions. Both S_{12} and S_{12}^{Max} are significantly larger in 1:1$_{alt}$ region compared to 1:1 region immediately prior to the onset of CaA alternans at B^{Prior}; while the S_{dyn}^{RP} slopes remain close to zero in both regions. This indicates that both S_{12}^{Max} and S_{12} slopes calculated prior to the onset of CaA alternans, at B^{Prior}, can indicate which region of the heart is susceptible to alternans.

Although previous literature defines $[Ca^{2+}]_i$ alternans as the beat-to-beat variation in the amplitude of the $[Ca^{2+}]_i$ transients, *i.e.* CaA alternans (Qian et al., 2001; Wu & Clusin, 1997), we wanted to investigate CaD alternans as well, since it has received limited attention. Here, we demonstrated that the local onset of CaA and CaD alternans occurred at statistically different values of BCLs. CaD is thought to have similar general features as action potential repolarization and duration maps (Choi & Salama, 2000). The importance of CaD lies in the fact that $[Ca^{2+}]_i$ overload and increases in CaD, due to spontaneous $[Ca^{2+}]_i$ releases from the SR, can be arrhythmogenic. Spontaneous SR $[Ca^{2+}]_i$ releases are thought to be potential sources of early after depolarizations which can result in torsades de pointes, tachycardia, and other arrhythmias (Choi et al., 2002). However, physiological relevance of CaD alternans needs to be further investigated, and it remains unclear whether a combination of CaA and CaD alternans is more arrhythmogenic compared to beat-to-beat variation in CaA only.

It is important to predict the onset of CaA alternans since our results shows that CaA alternans consistently develops ahead of either APD or CaD alternans. Our experiments demonstrate that the rate dependent shortening/reduction of CaA with BCLs, *i.e.* SS dynamic restitution of CaA, is not present in the isolated hearts. However, CaA after SP and LP responses were different from SS responses, especially at lower BCLs. Our analysis of the S1-S2 restitution curves reveals that both S_{12}^{Max} and S_{12} slopes were significantly higher in the 1:1$_{alt}$ region compared to the 1:1 region. Therefore, these slopes are reliable indicators of CaA alternans. Our results are consistent with previous findings in isolated rabbit ventricular myocytes. Specifically, (Tolkacheva *et. al*, 2006) measured the peak L-type calcium current (I_{Ca-L}) during SS, SP and LP, and demonstrated SP does not affect peak I_{Ca-L} for large values of BCL ($\geq$ 350 ms), but significantly reduces it at lower BCLs (200 ms). This is probably due to the complex interplay between reactivation and inactivation kinetics of I_{Ca-L}. I_{Ca-L}, which plays an important role in the upstroke of the cyclic   calcium   transient,   controls   the   amount   of Ca^{2+} present   in   the   intracellular

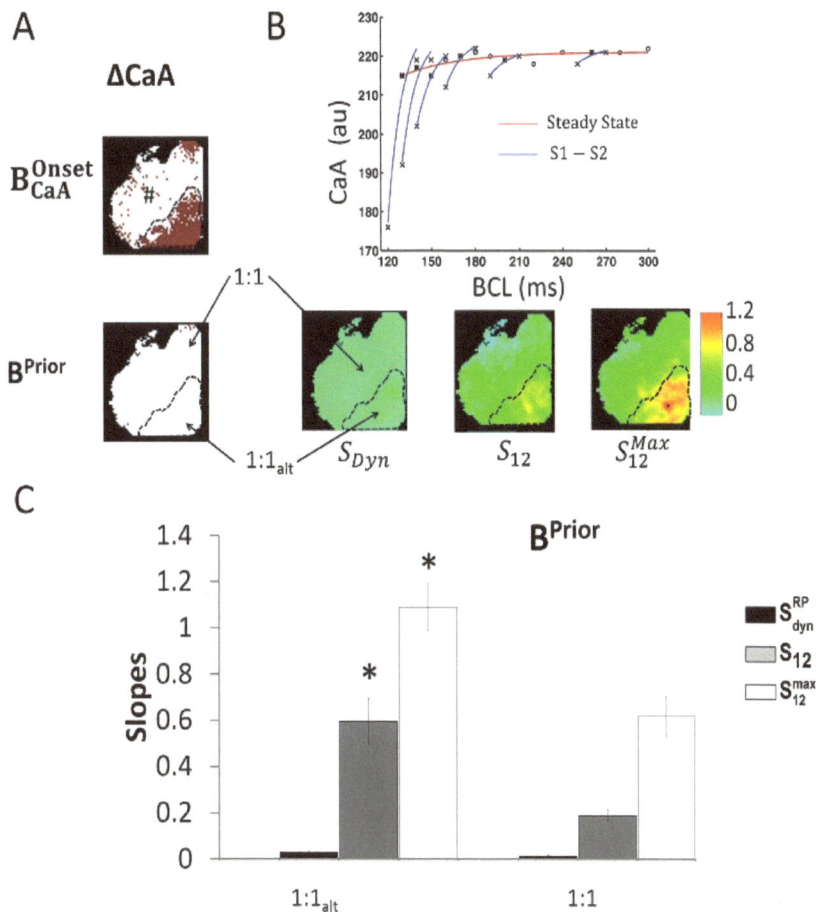

Figure 7: (**A**) Representative examples of 2D ΔCaA maps at B_{CaA}^{Onset} and B^{Prior}. (**B**) Representative example of CaA restitution portrait for pixel marked as '#' in **A** (*top*); 2D distribution of S_{dyn}^{RP}, S_{12} and S_{12}^{Max} slopes at B^{Prior} (*bottom*). Dashed lines outline the boundary between the 1:1 and $1:1_{alt}$ regions and **C**, Average S_{dyn}^{RP}, S_{12}, and S_{12}^{Max} slope values at B^{Prior}. '*' indicates statistical significance ($p < 0.05$).

space during each transient by mediating the entry of the Ca^{2+} into the cell triggering the release of the Ca^{2+} from the SR. The decrease in I_{Ca-L} due to a perturbation at low BCLs would thus lead to smaller amplitude of the calcium transient similar to what is seen during our experiments.

Mechanisms other than impaired calcium handling and electrical restitution have also been implicated as the cause of alternans, specifically spatially discordant APD alternans, in the heart. It has been demonstrated that pre-existing tissue heterogeneity can facilitate alternans formation – changes in pacing rate or an appropriately timed stimulus can induce APD alternans around the locations of heterogeneity (Pastore *et al*, 1999; Chinushi *et al*, 2003; Pastore *et al*, 2006). However, several numerical studies have shown that this is not a primary mechanism and that alternans can be formed in homogeneous tissue (Hayashi *et al*, 2007). Other mechanisms of alternans formation in the heart include steep conduction velocity restitution, *i.e.*, when conduction velocity of a propagating wave has a steep dependence on the preceding DI (Watanabe *et al*, 2001; Fox *et al*, 2002; Fenton *et al,* 2002; Franz, 2003) or short term memory (Mironov *et al*, 2008).

5   Summary

In this Chapter, we discussed a spatio-temporal evolution of both $[Ca^{2+}]_i$ and APD alternans in the isolated rabbit heart, and determined if the local onset of $[Ca^{2+}]_i$ and APD alternans could be predicted using different slopes measured in the restitution portrait. The main results can be summarized as follows. *First*, $[Ca^{2+}]_i$ alternans has a local onset in the heart similar to APD alternans. It initially develops in a small area of the heart, and then evolves to occupy the entire heart. *Second*, the local onset of $[Ca^{2+}]_i$ alternans, specifically CaA alternans, always precedes the local onset of APD alternans, while CaD alternans always follows APD alternans. *Third*, the restitution portrait, can be used to predict the local onset of APD alternans, as well as the local onset of $[Ca^{2+}]_i$ (both CaA and CaD) alternans. Specifically, S_{12} and S_{12}^{Max} measured in the restitution portrait can predict the local onset of APD alternans; S_{dyn}^{RP} and S_{12}^{Max} slopes can be considered as indicators of CaD alternans; while S_{12} and S_{12}^{Max} are indicators of CaA alternans.

References

Armoundas, A. A., Hobai, I. A., Tomaselli, G. F., Winslow, R. L., & O'Rourke, B. (2003). *Role of sodium-calcium exchanger in modulating the action potential of ventricular myocytes from normal and failing hearts. [Comparative Study Research Support, Non-U.S. Gov't Research Support, U.S. Gov't, P.H.S.]. Circulation research, 93(1), 46-53. doi: 10.1161/01.RES.0000080932.98903.D8.*

Armoundas, A. A., Tomaselli, G. F., & Esperer, H. D. (2002). *Pathophysiological basis and clinical application of T-wave alternans. [Research Support, Non-U.S. Gov't Review]. Journal of the American College of Cardiology, 40(2), 207-217.*

Chinushi, M., Kozhevnikov, D., Caref, E. B., Restivo, M., & El-Sherif, N. (2003). *Mechanism of discordant T wave alternans in the in vivo heart. [Comparative Study Research Support, Non-U.S. Gov't Research Support, U.S. Gov't, Non-P.H.S.]. Journal of cardiovascular electrophysiology, 14(6), 632-638.*

Choi, B. R., Burton, F., & Salama, G. (2002). *Cytosolic Ca2+ triggers early afterdepolarizations and Torsade de Pointes in rabbit hearts with type 2 long QT syndrome. [Research Support, Non-U.S. Gov't Research Support, U.S. Gov't, P.H.S.]. The Journal of physiology, 543(Pt 2), 615-631.*

Choi, B. R., & Salama, G. (2000). *Simultaneous maps of optical action potentials and calcium transients in guinea-pig hearts: mechanisms underlying concordant alternans. [In Vitro Research Support, Non-U.S. Gov't Research Support, U.S. Gov't, P.H.S.]. The Journal of physiology, 529 Pt 1, 171-188.*

Chudin, E., Garfinkel, A., Weiss, J., Karplus, W., & Kogan, B. (1998). *Wave propagation in cardiac tissue and effects of intracellular calcium dynamics (computer simulation study). [Research Support, U.S. Gov't, P.H.S. Review]. Progress in biophysics and molecular biology, 69(2-3), 225-236.*

Clusin, W. T. (2008). *Mechanisms of calcium transient and action potential alternans in cardiac cells and tissues. [Historical Article Review]. American journal of physiology. Heart and circulatory physiology, 294(1), H1-H10. doi: 10.1152/ajpheart.00802.2007.*

Courtemanche, M. (1996). *Complex spiral wave dynamics in a spatially distributed ionic model of cardiac electrical activity. Chaos, 6(4), 579-600. doi: 10.1063/1.166206.*

Cram, A. R., Rao, H. M., & Tolkacheva, E. G. (2011). *Toward Prediction of the Local Onset of Alternans in the Heart. Biophysical journal, 100(4), 868-874. doi: DOI 10.1016/j.bpj.2011.01.009.*

de Diego, C., Pai, R. K., Dave, A. S., Lynch, A., Thu, M., Chen, F., . . . Valderrabano, M. (2008). *Spatially discordant alternans in cardiomyocyte monolayers. [Research Support, N.I.H., Extramural Research Support, Non-U.S. Gov't]. American journal of physiology. Heart and circulatory physiology, 294(3), H1417-1425. doi: 10.1152/ajpheart.01233.2007.*

Diaz, M. E., O'Neill, S. C., & Eisner, D. A. (2004). *Sarcoplasmic reticulum calcium content fluctuation is the key to cardiac alternans. [Research Support, Non-U.S. Gov't]. Circulation research, 94(5), 650-656. doi: 10.1161/01.RES.0000119923.64774.72.*

Eisner, D. A., Diaz, M. E., Li, Y., O'Neill, S. C., & Trafford, A. W. (2005). *Stability and instability of regulation of intracellular calcium. [Review]. Experimental physiology, 90(1), 3-12. doi: 10.1113/expphysiol.2004.029231.*

Fenton, F. H., Cherry, E. M., Hastings, H. M., & Evans, S. J. (2002). *Multiple mechanisms of spiral wave breakup in a model of cardiac electrical activity. Chaos, 12(3), 852-892. doi: 10.1063/1.1504242.*

Fox, J. J., Riccio, M. L., Hua, F., Bodenschatz, E., & Gilmour, R. F., Jr. (2002). *Spatiotemporal transition to conduction block in canine ventricle. [In Vitro Research Support, Non-U.S. Gov't Research Support, U.S. Gov't, Non-P.H.S. Research Support, U.S. Gov't, P.H.S.]. Circulation research, 90(3), 289-296.*

Franz, M. R. (2003). *The electrical restitution curve revisited: steep or flat slope--which is better? [Review]. Journal of cardiovascular electrophysiology, 14(10 Suppl), S140-147.*

Gilmour, R. F., Jr. (2002). *Electrical restitution and ventricular fibrillation: negotiating a slippery slope. [Comment Editorial Review]. Journal of cardiovascular electrophysiology, 13(11), 1150-1151.*

Goldhaber, J. I., Xie, L. H., Duong, T., Motter, C., Khuu, K., & Weiss, J. N. (2005). *Action potential duration restitution and alternans in rabbit ventricular myocytes: the key role of intracellular calcium cycling. [Research Support, N.I.H., Extramural Research Support, Non-U.S. Gov't Research Support, U.S. Gov't, P.H.S.]. Circulation research, 96(4), 459-466. doi: 10.1161/01.RES.0000156891.66893.83.*

Guevara, M. R., Ward, G., Shrier, A., & Glass, L. (1984). *Electrical alternans and period-doubling bifurcations. Paper presented at the IEEE Computers in Cardiology, Silver Spring, MD.*

Hall, G. M., Bahar, S., & Gauthier, D. J. (1999). *Prevalence of rate-dependent behaviors in cardiac muscle. Physical review letters, 82(14), 2995-2998. doi: DOI 10.1103/PhysRevLett.82.2995.*

Hayashi, H., Shiferaw, Y., Sato, D., Nihei, M., Lin, S. F., Chen, P. S., . . . Qu, Z. (2007). *Dynamic origin of spatially discordant alternans in cardiac tissue. [In Vitro Research Support, N.I.H., Extramural Research Support, Non-U.S. Gov't]. Biophysical journal, 92(2), 448-460. doi: 10.1529/biophysj.106.091009.*

Hellerstein, H. K., & Liebow, I. M. (1950). *Electrical alternation in experimental coronary artery occlusion. The American journal of physiology, 160(2), 366-374.*

Kalb, S. S., Dobrovolny, H. M., Tolkacheva, E. G., Idriss, S. F., Krassowska, W., & Gauthier, D. J. (2004). *The restitution portrait: a new method for investigating rate-dependent restitution. [Comparative Study Evaluation Studies Research Support, U.S. Gov't, Non-P.H.S. Research Support, U.S. Gov't, P.H.S.]. Journal of cardiovascular electrophysiology, 15(6), 698-709. doi: 10.1046/j.1540-8167.2004.03550.x*

Koller, M. L., Riccio, M. L., & Gilmour, R. F., Jr. (1998). *Dynamic restitution of action potential duration during electrical alternans and ventricular fibrillation. [Research Support, Non-U.S. Gov't]. The American journal of physiology, 275(5 Pt 2), H1635-1642.*

Lakireddy, V., Baweja, P., Syed, A., Bub, G., Boutjdir, M., & El-Sherif, N. (2005). *Contrasting effects of ischemia on the kinetics of membrane voltage and intracellular calcium transient underlie electrical alternans. [In Vitro Research Support, U.S. Gov't, Non-P.H.S.]. American journal of physiology. Heart and circulatory physiology, 288(1), H400-407. doi: 10.1152/ajpheart.00502.2004.*

Lee, H. C., Mohabir, R., Smith, N., Franz, M. R., & Clusin, W. T. (1988). *Effect of ischemia on calcium-dependent fluorescence transients in rabbit hearts containing indo 1. Correlation with monophasic action potentials and contraction. [Research Support, Non-U.S. Gov't Research Support, U.S. Gov't, P.H.S.]. Circulation, 78(4), 1047-1059.*

Lee, K. S., Marban, E., & Tsien, R. W. (1985). *Inactivation of calcium channels in mammalian heart cells: joint dependence on membrane potential and intracellular calcium. [In Vitro Research Support, Non-U.S. Gov't Research Support, U.S. Gov't, P.H.S.]. The Journal of physiology, 364, 395-411.*

Lou, Q., & Efimov, I. R. (2009). *Enhanced susceptibility to alternans in a rabbit model of chronic myocardial infarction. [Research Support, N.I.H., Extramural]. Conference proceedings : ... Annual International Conference of the IEEE Engineering in Medicine and Biology Society. IEEE Engineering in Medicine and Biology Society. Conference, 2009, 4527-4530. doi: 10.1109/IEMBS.2009.5334102.*

Mironov, S., Jalife, J., & Tolkacheva, E. G. (2008). *Role of conduction velocity restitution and short-term memory in the development of action potential duration alternans in isolated rabbit hearts. [In Vitro Research Support, N.I.H., Extramural Research Support, Non-U.S. Gov't]. Circulation, 118(1), 17-25. doi: 10.1161/CIRCULATIONAHA.107.737254.*

Morita, H., Wu, J., & Zipes, D. P. (2008). *The QT syndromes: long and short. [Review]. Lancet, 372(9640), 750-763. doi: 10.1016/S0140-6736(08)61307-0.*

Mullins, L. J. (1979). *The generation of electric currents in cardiac fibers by Na/Ca exchange. [Research Support, U.S. Gov't, Non-P.H.S. Research Support, U.S. Gov't, P.H.S. Review]. The American journal of physiology, 236(3), C103-110.*

Narayan, S. M., Franz, M. R., Lalani, G., Kim, J., & Sastry, A. (2007). *T-wave alternans, restitution of human action potential duration, and outcome. Journal of the American College of Cardiology, 50(25), 2385-2392. doi: DOI 10.1016/j.jacc.2007.10.011.*

Nolasco, J. B., & Dahlen, R. W. (1968). *A graphic method for the study of alternation in cardiac action potentials. Journal of applied physiology, 25(2), 191-196.*

Pastore, J. M., Girouard, S. D., Laurita, K. R., Akar, F. G., & Rosenbaum, D. S. (1999). *Mechanism linking T-wave alternans to the genesis of cardiac fibrillation. [Research Support, Non-U.S. Gov't Research Support, U.S. Gov't, Non-P.H.S. Research Support, U.S. Gov't, P.H.S.]. Circulation, 99(10), 1385-1394.*

Pastore, J. M., Laurita, K. R., & Rosenbaum, D. S. (2006). *Importance of spatiotemporal heterogeneity of cellular restitution in mechanism of arrhythmogenic discordant alternans. [In Vitro Research Support, N.I.H., Extramural Research Support, U.S. Gov't, Non-P.H.S.]. Heart rhythm : the official journal of the Heart Rhythm Society, 3(6), 711-719. doi: 10.1016/j.hrthm.2006.02.1034.*

Pruvot, E. J., Katra, R. P., Rosenbaum, D. S., & Laurita, K. R. (2004). *Role of calcium cycling versus restitution in the mechanism of repolarization alternans. [Comparative Study]*

Research Support, Non-U.S. Gov't Research Support, U.S. Gov't, P.H.S.]. Circulation research, 94(8), 1083-1090. doi: 10.1161/01.RES.0000125629.72053.95.

Qian, Y. W., Clusin, W. T., Lin, S. F., Han, J., & Sung, R. J. (2001). *Spatial heterogeneity of calcium transient alternans during the early phase of myocardial ischemia in the blood-perfused rabbit heart. [In Vitro Research Support, U.S. Gov't, P.H.S.]. Circulation, 104(17), 2082-2087.*

Riccio, M. L., Koller, M. L., & Gilmour, R. F., Jr. (1999). *Electrical restitution and spatiotemporal organization during ventricular fibrillation. [Research Support, Non-U.S. Gov't]. Circulation research, 84(8), 955-963.*

Rosenbaum, D. S., Jackson, L. E., Smith, J. M., Garan, H., Ruskin, J. N., & Cohen, R. J. (1994). *Electrical alternans and vulnerability to ventricular arrhythmias. [Research Support, Non-U.S. Gov't Research Support, U.S. Gov't, P.H.S.]. The New England journal of medicine, 330(4), 235-241. doi: 10.1056/NEJM199401273300402.*

Salero, J. A., Previtali, M., Panciroli, C., Klerbsy, C., Chimienti, M., Regazzi, B. M., . . . Rondanelli, R. (1986). Ventricular arrhythmias during acute myocardial ischemia in man: the role and signifigance of R-ST-T alternans and the prevention of ischemic sudden death by medical treatment. Eur. Heart J, 7, 366-374.

Schwartz, P. J., & Malliani, A. (1975). Electrical alternation of the T-wave: clinical and experimental evidence of its relationship with the sympathetic nervous system and with the long Q-T syndrome. American heart journal, 89(1), 45-50.

Shiferaw, Y., Watanabe, M. A., Garfinkel, A., Weiss, J. N., & Karma, A. (2003). Model of intracellular calcium cycling in ventricular myocytes. [Research Support, Non-U.S. Gov't Research Support, U.S. Gov't, P.H.S.]. Biophysical journal, 85(6), 3666-3686. doi: 10.1016/S0006-3495(03)74784-5.

Tolkacheva, E. G., Anumonwo, J. M. B., & Jalife, J. (2006). Action potential duration restitution portraits of mammalian ventricular myocytes: Role of calcium current. Biophysical journal, 91(7), 2735-2745. doi: DOI 10.1529/biophysj.106.083865.

Tolkacheva, E. G., Schaeffer, D. G., Gauthier, D. J., & Krassowska, W. (2003). Condition for alternans and stability of the 1 : 1 response pattern in a "memory" model of paced cardiac dynamics. Physical Review E, 67(3). doi: Artn 031904 Doi 10.1103/Physreve.67.031904.

Visweswaran, R., McIntyre, S. D., Ramakrishnan, K., Zhao, X., & Tolkacheva, E. G. (2013). Spatio-Temporal Evolution and Prediction of [Ca2+]i and APD Alternans in Isolated Rabbit Hearts. Journal of cardiovascular electrophysiology, n/a-n/a. doi: 10.1111/jce.12200.

Wan, X., Laurita, K. R., Pruvot, E. J., & Rosenbaum, D. S. (2005). Molecular correlates of repolarization alternans in cardiac myocytes. [Comparative Study Research Support, N.I.H., Extramural Research Support, U.S. Gov't, P.H.S.]. Journal of molecular and cellular cardiology, 39(3), 419-428. doi: 10.1016/j.yjmcc.2005.06.004.

Watanabe, M. A., Fenton, F. H., Evans, S. J., Hastings, H. M., & Karma, A. (2001). Mechanisms for discordant alternans. [Research Support, Non-U.S. Gov't Research Support, U.S. Gov't, P.H.S.]. Journal of cardiovascular electrophysiology, 12(2), 196-206.

Weiss, J. N., Karma, A., Shiferaw, Y., Chen, P. S., Garfinkel, A., & Qu, Z. (2006). From pulsus to pulseless: the saga of cardiac alternans. [Research Support, N.I.H., Extramural Research Support, Non-U.S. Gov't Review]. Circulation research, 98(10), 1244-1253. doi: 10.1161/01.RES.0000224540.97431.f0

Wu, Y., & Clusin, W. T. (1997). Calcium transient alternans in blood-perfused ischemic hearts: observations with fluorescent indicator fura red. [Research Support, U.S. Gov't, P.H.S.]. The American journal of physiology, 273(5 Pt 2), H2161-2169.

Zipes, D. P., Heger, J. J., & Prystowsky, E. N. (1981). Sudden cardiac death. [Research Support, U.S. Gov't, P.H.S.]. The American journal of medicine, 70(6), 1151-1154.

Major Bovine Acute Phase Proteins in Relation to Sample Storage Temperature and Time

Csilla Tóthová

Clinic for Ruminants
University of Veterinary Medicine and Pharmacy in Košice, Slovakia

Oskar Nagy

Clinic for Ruminants
University of Veterinary Medicine and Pharmacy in Košice, Slovakia

Gabriel Kováč

Clinic for Ruminants
University of Veterinary Medicine and Pharmacy in Košice, Slovakia

1   Introduction

The acute phase response constitute the non-specific early-defense system of reactions of an organism to the various forms of tissue damage, infection, inflammation, injury, trauma, stress, as well as neoplasia (Gabay & Kushner, 1999). It comprises a wide variety of physiological and biochemical responses, which aim to prevent ongoing tissue damage, isolate and eliminate the cause of the inflammation, and begin the repair processes necessary to restore the normal function (Cray *et al.*, 2009). Usually, the local response is accompanied by a systemic reaction characterized by the fast alteration of the concentrations of several plasma proteins, the acute phase proteins produced mainly by the liver (Baumann & Gauldie, 1994).

Acute phase proteins have been well recognized for their application to human diagnostic medicine and have been described to have value in the diagnosis and prognosis of cardiovascular diseases, various inflammatory diseases, autoimmunity, organ transplant, as well as cancer treatment (Deans & Wigmore, 2005; Ridker, 2007). Due to their high response in affected animals, acute phase proteins may provide an alternative means also for monitoring animal's health (Murata *et al.*, 2004; Petersen *et al.*, 2004). Important points to consider before using acute phase proteins as objective markers of animal health are the possible influences of other factors, including handling, environmental or other types of stress in the absence of disease. Therefore, the objective of this study was to evaluate the effect of storage under various conditions on the concentrations of major bovine acute phase proteins – serum amyloid A (SAA), its mammary isoform (M-SAA), as well as haptoglobin (Hp) and fibrinogen (Fbg).

2   The Acute Phase Response

The acute phase response represents a group of physiological processes occurring soon after the onset of infection, injury, trauma, inflammatory processes, and some malignant processes. It consists of a large number of behavioural, physiologic, biochemical, and nutritional changes. The aim of these reactions is to isolate and destroy the infectious agent(s), prevent ongoing tissue damage and restore the homeostasis (Moshage, 1997, Mackiewicz, 1997).

Cytokines have an important role in the regulation of the production of acute phase proteins during an acute phase response (Koj, 1998). Cytokines are released by activated immune cells at the site of infection, inflammation, and damage. A wide variety of cell types at these sites can produce pro-inflammatory cytokines, including macrophages, neutrophils, mast cells, as well as endothelial cells (Martin *et al.*, 1999). Interleukin-1 (IL-1), IL-8, tumor necrosis factor-alpha (TNF-α) and interferon-gamma (INF-γ) are the major cytokines, which have a profound behavioral, endocrine and metabolic effect. They activate the production of other cytokines and inflammatory mediators, including the IL-6 type of cytokines, which stimulate the production of acute phase proteins from hepatocytes or other tissues (Baigrie *et al.*, 1991).

Cytokines induce a cascade of events which potentiate the appearance of the main clinical changes characterized by fever, anorexia or weight loss (Gabay & Kushner, 1999). In addition, the cytokines activate receptors on different target cells leading to systemic inflammatory reactions, including hormonal or metabolic, and resulting in a number of biochemical changes (Gruys *et al.*, 2005). These symptoms reflect multiple changes in the homeostatic control of the diseased animals, such as increased production of adrenocorticotrophic hormone and glucocorticoids, activation of the complement cascade and blood coagulation system, decreased serum concentrations of calcium, zinc, iron, vitamin A and αtocopherol, and changes in the concentrations of some plasma proteins (Pyörälä, 2000). One of the most important metabolic changes is the strongly increased synthesis of a group of plasma proteins, namely acute phase proteins, by the liver (Raynes, 1994).

3 Acute Phase Proteins

Acute phase proteins are a group of blood proteins synthesized during an acute phase response against several stimuli like infection, inflammation, sress, trauma or tissue damage (Cerón *et al.*, 2005). There are large and varied groups of acute phase proteins released into the blood stream in response to a variety of stressors. All the up-regulated proteins have been called positive acute phase proteins, in order to differentiate them from the so-called negative acute phase proteins (Petersen *et al.*, 2004). They are further classified as major, moderate, or minor, depending on their responsibility. Major proteins represent those that increase 10- to 100-fold, moderate proteins increase 2- to 10-fold, and minor proteins are characterized with only a slight increase (Cerón *et al.*, 2005). Major proteins often are observed to increase markedly within the first 24 – 48 hours after the triggering event and often have a rapid decline due to their very short half-life. Moderate and minor proteins follow in magnitude of response and may both increase more slowly and be more prolonged in duration, depending on the status of the triggering event (Niewold *et al.*, 2003). Moderate and minor acute phase proteins may be observed more often during chronic inflammatory processes (Horadagoda *et al.*, 1999). A few decrease during an acute phase response is observed in the concentrations of negative acute phase proteins. The most studied negative acute phase proteins include albumin, transferrin, and transthyretin.

Another classification of acute phase proteins is based on the amplification of synthesis rate during the acute phase response (Petersen *et al.*, 2004; Eckersall & Bell, 2010). Kushner & Mackiewicz (1987) admitted the existence of first- or second-line proteins. The main first-line acute phase proteins are serum amyloid A and C-reactive protein, which are detected 4 hours after the stimuli, attain the maximum concentrations 1 – 3 days, and quickly return to baseline values. Examples of the second-line acute phase proteins are haptoglobin and fibrinogen, increased concentrations of which are observed 1 – 3 days after the initiation of the disorder or disease, maximum concentrations could be seen 7 – 10 days, and are maintained within 2 or more weeks (Moshage, 1997).

Generally, the main function of acute phase proteins is to defend the host against pathological damage and assist in the restoration of the homeostasis. Some of the acute phase proteins (α_1-antitrypsin, α_2-macroglobulin) have anti-protease activity designed to inhibit proteases released by phagocytes or pathogens to minimize damage to normal tissues (Pyörälä, 2000). Another acute phase proteins (haptoglobin, serum amyloid A, C-reactive protein) have scavenging activities and bind metabolites released from cellular degradation so they can re-enter host metabolic processes rather than be utilized by pathogen (Wagener *et al.*, 2002). Others (α_1-acid glycoprotein) are characterized by anti-bacterial activity and by the ability to influence the course of the immune response (Rossbacher *et al.*, 1999).

3.1 Acute Phase Proteins in Cattle

There are many acute phase proteins applicable as biomarkers in the detection of various diseases and disorders in human medicine (Samols, 2002). However, only some of them can be commonly used in cattle research. The important concept is that each animal species has its own major acute phase proteins that must be considered the markers of choice for diagnostic purposes. Ruminants are significantly different to other species in their acute phase response, in that haptoglobin (Hp) and serum amyloid A (SAA) are the major acute phase proteins (Eckersall & Bell, 2010).

3.1.1   Serum Amyloid A

Serum amyloid A (SAA) is an acute phase protein that belongs to the family of apolipoproteins associated with high density lipoprotein in plasma (Uhlar *et al.*, 1994). Serum amyloid A in mammals has a molecular weight of 12 kDa (Malle *et al.,* 1993). Different isoforms of SAA are expressed constitutively at different levels in response to inflammatory stimuli (Uhlar & Whitehead, 1999; Takahashi *et al.,* 2009). During inflammation, SAA1 and SAA2 are expressed principally in the liver, whereas SAA3 is induced in many distinct tissues, including the adipose tissue, mammary gland and intestinal epithelial cells (Ametaj *et al.*, 2011; Eckhardt *et al.*, 2010). The fourth isoform, SAA4, does not respond to external stimuli (de Beer *et al.,* 1995).

The main functions of serum amyloid A are the reverse transport of cholesterol from tissue to hepatocytes, opsonisation, inhibition of phagocyte oxidateive burst and platelet activation (Mukesh *et al.*, 2010; van der Westhuyzen *et al.*, 2007). The SAA3 isoform found in colostrum stimulates the production of mucin from intestinal cells assisting the initiation of secretions from the neonatal intestine and helping to prevent bacterial colonization (Mack *et al.*, 2003).

Serum amyloid A is a rapidly reacting acute phase protein characterized by a high increase in serum concentrations after the inflammatory stimulus, with higher increase in cases of acute compared to chronic inflammation (Horadagoda *et al.*, 1999). However, some results indicate that serum concentrations of SAA may be elevated also in cases of chronic inflammation (Chan *et al.*, 2010; Tóthová *et al.*, 2010). In cattle, SAA was raised following experimental infection with *Mannheimia haemolytica,* bovine respiratory syncytial virus and natural or experimental cases of mastitis (Heegaard, 2000). Cardiovascular diseases are also accompanied by the elevation of several acute phase proteins, including serum amyloid A, and its concentrations vary according to the severity of the cardiovascular disorder (Hirschfield & Pepys, 2003).

3.1.2   Haptoglobin

Haptoglobin (Hp) has been found in all mammals, as well as some birds (Bowman & Kurosky, 1982). Haptoglobin, in its simplest form, consists of two α and two β chains, connected by disulfide bridges (Kurosky *et al.*, 1980). Hp exists in two allelic forms in the human population, so called Hp1 and Hp2, the latter one having arisen due to the partial duplication of Hp1 gene (Carter & Worwood, 2007). Haptoglobin in cattle contains an α chain, the structure of which is similar to that of the human Hp2 α-chain (Wicher & Fries, 2007).

In the blood plasma, Hp binds free hemoglobin (Hb) released from erythrocytes with high affinity and thereby inhibits its oxidative activity (Yang *et al.*, 2003). The Hp-hemoglobin complex will then be removed by the reticuloendothelial system, mostly the spleen. This binding also reduces the availability of the heme residue from bacterial growth and therefore Hp has an indirect anti-bacterial activity (Murata *et al.*, 2004). Many studies have indicated the significance of Hp as a clinically useful parameter for measuring the occurrence and severity of inflammatory responses in cattle with mastitis, pneumonia, enteritis, peritonitis, endocarditis, abscesses, endometritis and other natural or experimental infectious conditions (Eckersall, 2000).

3.1.3   Fibrinogen

Fibrinogen (Fbg), a precursor of fibrin, is also an acute phase protein, which has been used for many years to evaluate inflammatory and traumatic diseases in cattle, and is characterized by markedly increased synthesis in response to infection (Hirvonen & Pyörälä, 1998). Fibrinogen is a β-globulin present in the plasma. It is composed of 3 polypeptide chains linked by disulfide bridges and a glycoprotein (Gentry, 1999). Fibrinogen is involved in homeostasis, providing a substrate for fibrin formation, and in tissue repair, providing a matrix for the migration of inflammatory-related cells (Thomas, 2000).

3.1.4   Ceruloplasmin

Ceruloplasmin (Cp) is a ferroxidase enzyme that is the major copper-carrying protein in the blood, and plays a role in iron metabolism (Lovstad, 2006). Ceruloplasmin is synthesized mainly in the liver, but may be released also from other tissues including spleen, lung, uterus and mammary gland (Aldred *et al.*, 1987; Thomas *et al.*, 1989). Ceruloplasmin carries about 70 % of the total copper in human plasma, thus might play a role in Cu homeostasis (Martinez-Subiela *et al.*, 2007). It exhibits a copper-dependent oxidase activity, which is associated with possible oxidation of Fe^{2+} into Fe^{3+}, therefore assisting in its transport in the plasma in association with transferrin, which can carry iron only in the ferric state (Fleming *et al.*, 1991). In humans, ceruloplasmin has been utilized diagnostically for a variety of clinical and pathological conditions, including rheumatoid arthritis, liver disease, copper deficiency (Sogawa *et al.*, 1994). In animals, ceruloplasmin has been evaluated as a marker of animal health and welfare (Skinner, 2001). From a diagnostic perspective, ceruloplasmin may have applications in several disease conditions in cattle, including mastitis and pneumonic pasteurellosis (Chassagne *et al.*, 1998; Fagliari *et al.*, 2003).

3.1.5   Alpha-1 acid Glycoprotein

Alpha-1 acid glycoprotein (AGP) is highly glycosylated protein with a molecular mass of around 43 kD of which about 45 % is carbohydrate and the composition of the glycan residues is known to alter during an acute phase response (Fournier *et al.*, 2000). It has a moderate acute phase response in most species and is more likely associated with chronic conditions. The serum concentration of AGP is a valuable differential diagnostic analyte in identification of infectious peritonitis (Bence *et al.*, 2005).

3.1.6   Lactoferrin

Lactoferrin (Lf), also known as lactotransferrin, is a multifunctional glycoprotein that is widely represented in various secretory fluids, such as milk, saliva, and nasal secretions (Susana *et al.*, 2009). It is one of the transferrin proteins that transfer iron to the cells and control the concentrations of free iron in the blood and external secretions (Moore *et al.*, 1997). Lactoferrin forms reddish complex with iron, its affinity for iron is 300 times higher than that of transferrin, and increases in weakly acidic medium. This facilitates the transfer of iron from transferrin to lactoferrin during inflammations, when the pH of tissues decreases due to accumulation of lactic and other acids (Brock, 1980). Apart from its main biological function, lactoferrin also has antimicrobial activities and regulate the cellular growth (Ward *et al.*, 2002).

Human colostrums has the highest concentration of lactoferrin, followed by human milk, then cow's milk (from 0.1 – 1.0 mg/ml in healthy cows). Its concentrations may rapidly increase in cows with sub-clinical and clinical mastitis and are positively correlated with somatic cell count (SCC) (Kawai *et al.*, 1999; Hagiwara *et al.*, 2003). According to Kutila *et al.* (2003), the concentrations of lactoferrin are 100-fold higher in cows during drying off and early mammary involution period than during lactation.

Harmon *et al.* (1975) evaluated the concentrations of lactoferrin in cows with *Escherichia coli* mastitis and found a 30-fold increase of its values in the mammary secretion by 90 hours post inoculation.

3.1.7   Albumin

Serum albumin is the major negative acute phase protein. During the acute phase response the demand for amino acids for synthesis of the positive acute phase proteins is markedly increased, which necessitates reprioritization of the hepatic protein synthesis: albumin synthesis is down-regulated and amino acids are shunted into synthesis of positive acute phase proteins (Aldred & Schreiber, 1993). It has been reported that during the acute phase response 30 to 40 % of the hepatic protein synthesizing capacity is used for production of positive acute phase proteins and the production of other proteins thus need to be diminished (Mackiewicz, 1997). Albumin is responsible for about 75 % of the osmotic pressure of plasma and is a major source of amino acids that can be utilized by the animal's body when necessary.

4   The Diagnostic Utility of Acute Phase Proteins in the Veterinary Practice

It is important to recognize that acute phase protein concentrations are elevated in animals with many different diseases, having very poor diagnostic specificity in detecting the cause, so they can not be used as the primary diagnostic test for a particular disease. However, they have very high sensitivity in detecting many conditions that alter the health of the animal and in providing evidence that an animal has subclinical inflammation or infection (Cerón *et al.*, 2005). It was reported by Kent (1992) that acute phase proteins quickly and precisely demonstrate the presence of infectious and inflammatory conditions, but not the cause. A very interesting characteristic of the acute phase proteins is the possibility of detecting subclinical diseases (Cerón *et al.*, 2005). Petersen *et al.* (2004) stated also that acute phase proteins can detect the presence of subclinical disease which is the cause of reduced growth rate and losses in the production. In the clinical field, acute phase proteins may serve as indicators of prognosis and effect of treatment. The magnitude and duration of the acute phase response reflect the severity of the infection and underlying tissue damage (Heegaard *et al.*, 2000).

There is an increasing body of evidence to support utilization of acute phase proteins as biomarkers of inflammation in cattle. Different investigators have reported enhanced concentrations of some acute phase proteins in various metabolic, inflammatory and infectious diseases, including mastitis, metritis, laminitis, several bacterial and viral diseases, as well as fatty liver, milk fever, ruminal acidosis, milk fat depression (Eckersall *et al.*, 2000; Petersen *et al.*, 2004). However, further research is needed to establish the effect of other factors not related to diseases on the concentrations of acute phase proteins in cattle.

5   Acute Phase Proteins and the Effect of Factors not Related to Diseases

Measurement of the acute phase proteins is a potentially useful clinical tool in veterinary medicine, but further studies are required to assess the influence of other factors not associated with diseases on their concentrations, including, sample collection, processing, as well as handling. Moreover, the concentrations of acute phase proteins must be interpreted in the view of many other physiological influences not associated with diseases. The age of evaluated animals, parturition, the transition of pregnancy to lactation are important factors that may affect the concentrations of frequently analyzed biochemical variables, including the concentrations of acute phase proteins (Tóthová *et al.*, 2011).

6   The Effect of Storage Temperature and Time on the Concentrations of Some Acute Phase Proteins

Biochemical investigations are used extensively in medicine, both in relation to diseases that have an obvious metabolic basis, and those in which biochemical changes are a consequence of the disease. The principal uses of biochemical investigations are for diagnosis, prognosis, monitoring, and screening of diseases. It is therefore critical that the results generated by the laboratory be accurate, relevant, and interpreted correctly (McCudden *et al.*, 2010). The specimen for analysis must be collected and transported to the laboratory according to a specified procedure, and every step in the process of sample handling and analysis requires careful attention if the data are to be of clinical value (Bonini *et al.*, 2002). In some cases, when the requested tests are not available, the analysis is delayed, or the specimens are sent to distant laboratories for analysis, there is a need to use stored samples. Moreover, the planning for multiple experimental time points often results in samples that will be analyzed together at a later date, and thus subjected to different periods of storage before analysis (Sharma, 2009). In such cases, degradation of labile analytes must be prevented by refrigerating or freezing the samples. A lot of authors stated that not only physiological conditions and factors (e.g. age, sex, pregnancy, nutritional status), but also inadequate biological sample storage, as a potential source of preanalytical errors, may markedly affect the concentrations of many biochemical variables (Jakubowski *et al.*, 1998; Ehsani *et al.*, 2008; Cray *et al.*, 2009). However, the influence of sample storage on the concentrations of less frequently measured biochemical variables, including acute phase proteins, and their stability during storage in veterinary medicine is less well documented. In bovine practice, an increased focus on the application of acute phase proteins has recently been developed. Stability and storage study is one of the most important studies that should be performed during the course of the introduction of the method of the acute phase protein determination. For this reason, the main objective of the present study is to evaluate the effect of storage under various conditions on the concentrations of the diagnostically most important bovine acute phase proteins – serum amyloid A, milk amyloid A, haptoglobin and fibrinogen.

6.1   Material and Methods

6.1.1   Sample Collection

The effect of storage at freezer and refrigerator temperatures on the concentrations of serum amyloid A (SAA, μg/ml) during storage was investigated in blood samples from seven clinically healthy female calves from a conventional dairy farm. The calves were of a Slovak spotted breed and its crossbreeds at the age of 4 – 6 months, and their body weight was 85 – 140 kg. For the evaluation of the concentrations of haptoglobin (Hp, mg/ml) and fibrinogen (Fbg, g/l), blood samples from another seven clinically healthy calves of the same age and breed were included into this study. The same feeding and management regimes were applied to calves used in this study. The evaluated animals were housed loosely in larger groups, and fed hay and grain with free access to water.

Blood samples for the analyses were collected by direct puncture of *v. jugularis* into serum gel separator tubes without anticoagulant. For the determination of the concentrations of fibrinogen, blood samples were taken into special tubes with sodium citrate. Blood samples were allowed to clot at room temperature and within two hours after withdrawal serum samples were prepared. The blood samples were centrifuged at 3000 g for 30 minutes to separate serum. The harvested blood serum and plasma were fractioned into aliquots. One aliquot was analyzed for the concentrations of the evaluated acute phase proteins immediately after the separation without storage, and these results obtained at time 0 were considered as initial concentrations. The second aliquots of the separated serum and plasma were stored in refrigerator at 4 °C for 1 day, and then analyzed. The remaining aliquots were kept frozen at -18 °C, and the concentrations of acute phase proteins were determined after 2, 7, 14, and 21 days of storage. On these days the samples were kept at room temperature for 2 hours to thaw the serum, and then the measurements were performed. The time and temperature during the sample preparation and storage was monitored for consistency.

For the evaluation of the changes in the concentrations of mammary isoform of SAA (M-SAA, ng/ml) during storage, milk samples from six clinically healthy dairy cows from a conventional dairy farm were included into this study. The cows were of the Slovak spotted breed and its crossbreeds between 3 – 5 years of age. The evaluated cows were fed twice a day individual feeding rations according to the milk production, and had *ad libitum* access to water. Composite milk samples were collected into plastic tubes by hand-stripping. Forestrips were milked out, and then approximately equal parts of milk from each quarter were taken and mixed together. The collected milk samples were fractioned into aliquots. One aliquot was analyzed for the concentrations of M-SAA on the day of sample collection without storage. The second aliquot of milk samples was stored in refrigerator at 4 °C for 1 day, and then analyzed. The remaining aliquots were stored at -18 °C, and were analyzed for M-SAA concentrations after 2, 7, 14, and 21 days of storage.

6.1.2   Laboratory Analyses

The serum concentrations of SAA were analyzed by method of sandwich enzyme linked immunosorbent assay using commercial ELISA kits (Tridelta Development, Ireland) according to the procedure described by the manufacturer. The concentrations of Hp were assessed using commercial colorimetric kits (Tridelta Development, Ireland) in microplates, based on Hp-haemoglobin binding and preservation of the peroxidase activity of the bound haemoglobin at low pH. All the samples, including the standards, were tested in duplicate. The optical densities were read on automatic microplate reader Opsys MR (Dynex Technologies, United Kingdom) at 630 nm for Hp, and at 450 nm using 630 nm as reference for SAA. The determination of fibrinogen was performed on semi-automatic 4-channel coagulometer Behnk CL-4 (Behnk Elektronik GmbH & Co., Germany) using commercial diagnostic kits (Diagon Kft, Hungary), based on the principle of electromagnetic detection of fibrin formation.

The concentrations of M-SAA were determined by ELISA method using commercial diagnostic kits (Tridelta Development, Ireland) according to the method described for SAA, modified by the manufacturer for the determination of M-SAA in milk samples.

6.1.3   Statistical Analyses

Arithmetic means (x), standard deviations (SD), and medians for the concentrations of evaluated acute phase proteins in serum, as well as milk samples were calculated using descriptive statistical procedures. The effect of time on the concentrations of evaluated variables during the storage of the samples frozen at -18 °C was evaluated by Friedman`s rank sum test. The comparison between the initial concentrations and the values determined on day 2, 7, 14, and 21 of storage at -18 °C was performed using Wilcoxon matched pairs test. The Wilcoxon test was also used for the evaluation of the differences between the initial concentrations of measured parameters and the values quantified in samples stored 1 day at 4 °C. All statistical analyses were performed using the programme GraphPad Prism V5.02 (GraphPad Software Inc., California, USA).

6.2   Results

The data referring to the concentrations of evaluated acute phase proteins in bovine serum, and the values of M-SAA in milk samples during storage expressed as average values, standard deviations, and medians, including the significance of differences between measured concentrations are presented in Tables 1 and 2. The changes in the concentrations of measured acute phase proteins expressed as percentages relative to the values measured at day 0 are shown on Figures 1 – 4.

Parameter		Time of analysis (days)					P <
		0	2	7	14	21	
SAA (µg/ml)	x	30.30	17.89*	17.42*	13.77*	13.94*	0.001
(n = 7)	± SD	17.19	12.32	10.10	10.94	12.07	
	median	30.50	15.60	17.10	12.00	17.30	
M-SAA (ng/ml)	x	5945.1	4822.8	4261.2*	4162.3*	4149.2*	0.01
(n = 6)	± SD	1765.7	1819.7	1559.0	1641.6	1532.6	
	median	6439.6	5471.7	4631.2	4685.9	4483.2	
Hp (mg/ml)	x	0.12	0.12	0.13	0.12	0.12	n. s.
(n = 7)	± SD	0.24	0.26	0.22	0.22	0.25	
	median	0.03	0.02	0.05	0.03	0.03	
Fbg	x	2.71	2.62*	2.60*	2.44*	2.40*	0.001
(g/l)	± SD	0.27	0.32	0.32	0.23	0.29	
(n = 7)	median	2.81	2.69	2.60	2.46	2.48	

Table 1: The changes in the concentrations of SAA, M-SAA, Hp, and Fbg with time during freezer storage. P – significance of Friedman's test; n.s. – non significant; * superscripts in rows mean statistically significant difference compared with the initial concentration (Wilcoxon test, P < 0.05).

The evaluation of the serum concentrations of SAA over time showed a tendency of highly significant decrease of values during storage at -18 °C (P < 0.001, Table 1). The samples stored in a freezer had more markedly reduced concentrations from day 2 onward, with the significantly lowest concentrations on day 14 of storage compared with the initial values (P < 0.05, Figure 1). More detailed analysis of the serum SAA concentrations showed that by the analysis of samples without storage (day 0) 50 % values ranged from 11.70 to 42.10 µg/ml, with median concentration of 30.50 µg/ml. The median SAA concentration recorded on day 2 of storage was about half as lower (15.60 µg/ml) than the initial median value, and 50 % of measured values were in the range of 6.89 – 29.70 µg/ml. Similar trend of lower values was found in the next period of freezer-storage, with the lowest median concentration of SAA on day 14 of storage (12. 00 µg/ml).

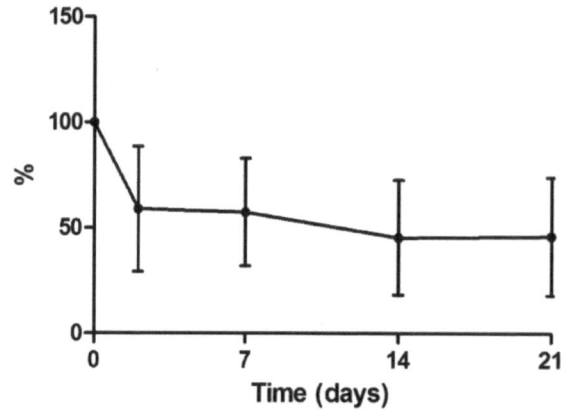

Figure 1: Changes of the concentrations of SAA (mean ± SD; %) in bovine serum samples (n=7) relative to the value at t=0 of freezer-storage (-18°C).

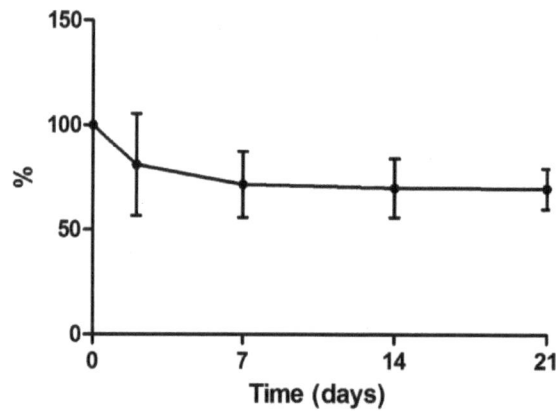

Figure 2: Changes of the concentrations of M-SAA (mean ± SD; %) in bovine milk samples (n=6) relative to the value at t=0 of freezer-storage (-18°C).

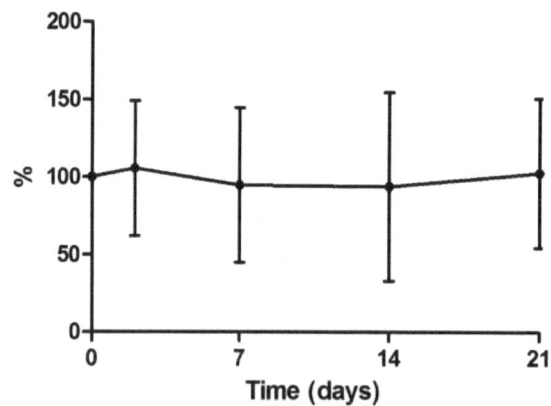

Figure 3: Changes of the concentrations of Hp (mean ± SD; %) in bovine serum samples (n=7) relative to the value at t=0 of freezer-storage (-18°C).

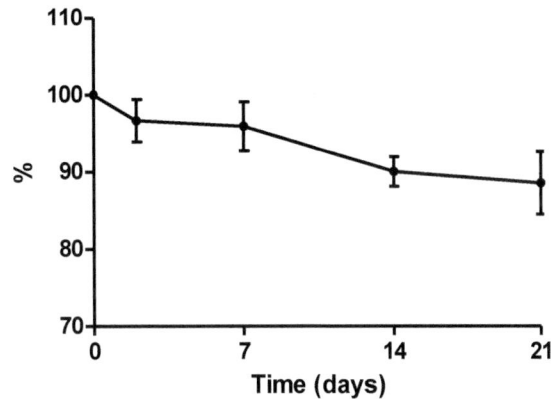

Figure 4: Changes of the concentrations of Fbg (mean ± SD; %) in bovine plasma samples (n=7) relative to the value at t=0 of freezer-storage (-18°C).

The changes in the concentrations of M-SAA in milk samples in relation to the time of storage at the temperature of -18 °C were significant (P < 0.01, Table 1). For the concentrations of M-SAA in milk samples determined on day 2 of freezer-storage, a more marked but statistically insignificant decrease of values was found compared with initial values (Table 1). Significantly reduced M-SAA concentrations we recorded on day 7 of storage (P < 0.05), and then the values remained relatively stable for the evaluated period of freezer-storage (Figure 2). In the median concentrations of M-SAA we observed a gradual decrease of values during freezer-storage, with the lowest median concentration determined on day 21 of storage (4483.2 ng/ml). By more detailed evaluation of individual M-SAA concentrations we found that during the initial analysis of milk samples 50 % of measured values ranged from 3936 to 7326 ng/ml, and in samples analyzed on day 2 of storage we already recorded lower concentrations with the range of 50 % of measured values between 3371 – 6091 ng/ml.

On the other hand, in the concentrations of Hp during the time under study, no significant variations were observed, and the values determined in serum samples stored at -18 °C were roughly uniform (Table 1, Figure 3).

The changes in the concentrations of Fbg in blood plasma in relation to the time of storage at the temperature of -18 °C were significant (P < 0.001). A significant decrease of Fbg concentrations compared with initial values was found already in samples determined on day 2 of freezer-storage (P < 0.05), with further decrease of measured values in the next period of storage (Figure 4). For the median concentrations of Fbg, a similar trend of gradually decreasing values was observed during freezer storage. The significantly lowest mean value was recorded on day 21 of freezer storage.

The mean concentration of SAA obtained in bovine serum stored at 4 °C for 1 day was nonsignificantly lower than the value recorded by the evaluation of samples analyzed immediately (Table 2). Similarly, when analyzing the concentrations of M-SAA in milk samples after the storage in refrigerator, no significant differences were found between the concentrations determined in samples without storage and in samples stored 1 day at 4 °C. In the concentrations of haptoglobin we observed no significant differences between the two analyses. On the other hand, the concentrations of fibrinogen in samples after storage in refrigerator for 1 day were significantly lower than in samples without storage (P < 0.05).

Parameter		Samples		P <
		without storage	stored at 4 °C for 1 day	
SAA	x	30.30	26.24	n. s.
(µg/ml)	± SD	17.19	14.97	
(n=7)	median	30.50	30.80	
M-SAA (ng/ml)	x	5945.1	5376.9	n. s.
(n=6)	± SD	1765.7	1796.9	
	median	6439.6	5906.9	
Hp	x	0.12	0.13	n. s.
(mg/ml)	± SD	0.24	0.23	
(n=7)	median	0.03	0.04	
Fbg	x	2.71	2.62	0.05
(g/l)	± SD	0.27	0.31	
(n=7)	median	2.81	2.66	

Table 2: Comparison of the concentrations of SAA, M-SAA, Hp, and Fbg analyzed in samples without storage and stored at 4 °C for 1 day. P – significance of Wilcoxon test; n.s. – non significant

6.3   Discussion

Many clinical trials and research studies depend on delayed batch analyses of collected blood samples. To accomplish these analyses, blood samples are separated by centrifugation, and the harvested serum or plasma is quickly frozen (Ridker *et al.*, 1999). At specific follow-up times, the samples are thawed and analyzed as designated by the study protocol. The stability of routine clinical biochemistry parameters (total proteins, albumin, lactate dehydrogenase, creatine kinase, trace elements, and hormones) was tested in human and in a range of animal species under different laboratory storage conditions (Reimers *et al.*, 1991; Jakubowski *et al.*, 1998; Boyanton & Blick, 2002). These studies stated that the temperature and the duration of the storage are important factors, which may impact the results of biochemical analyses. Tanner *et al.* (2008) stated that potassium, glucose, phosphate, creatinine, urea, iron, lactate-dehydrogenase, magnesium and calcium are not stable and are significantly affected during storage.

Studies of human blood samples, including stability analyses for refrigeration and the effects of freeze-thawing, have resulted in guidelines for storage (Comstock *et al.*, 2001; Clark *et al.*, 2003; O'Keane & Cunningham, 2006). Surprisingly, data from such reports in veterinary medicine, particularly regarding the stability of acute phase proteins, are rather scarce, with only a few reports on the effects of storage on canine and avian samples (Thoresen *et al.*, 1995; Hawkins *et al.*, 2006; Reynolds *et al.*, 2006). Stability and storage studies were performed to determine the effect of storage on the concentrations of C-reactive protein, as the diagnostically most important acute phase protein in humans (Aziz *et al.*, 2003; Ledue & Rifai, 2003). On the other hand, data on storage stability of acute phase proteins, and the effect of the temperature and duration of storage on their concentrations in veterinary medicine are still limited. Because acute phase protein determination may become of importance in laboratory testing also in cattle, it is important to collect information about their biological variation and the effect of storage on their values, as one of the pre-analytical factors that may influence the results of the assay.

In the presented study, we observed a marked effect of sample storage at lower temperatures on the concentrations of serum amyloid A, characterized by different intensities of changes in its concentrations at freezer or refrigerator temperatures. In frozen serum samples, the results showed a trend of significantly decreasing SAA concentrations over time. Significantly lower concentrations of SAA were found already after 2 days of storage. The SAA concentrations determined in serum samples stored at refrigerator temperatures differed non-significantly from the values measured in samples without storage, but its mean value was lower. These differences were less marked than those evaluated during longer lasting freezer-storage. Storage stability of SAA was investigated by Hillström *et al.* (2010) in equine serum samples. The authors observed no significant changes in SAA concentrations over time in serum samples stored at 4 °C, and the variance between days was not higher than could be explained by the imprecision of the method. Similarly, in another study, where an equine SAA standard pool was stored at 4 °C over a period of up to two months, no significant changes in SAA concentrations were noted (Pepys *et al.*, 1989). These authors observed only a slight fluctuation in measured values that they explained by the imprecision of the method. In addition, no influence on the stability of human SAA and C-reactive protein was found for the samples that were stored at -20 °C for 2 months until actual measurement (Rothkrantz-Kos *et al.*, 2003). According to our findings, bovine SAA appears to be less stable during storage at lower temperatures, predominantly at freezing. Diminished concentrations of SAA at lower temperatures, obtained in our study during freezer, as well as refrigerator storage, may be related to the lability and degradation of this protein resulting from the changes in its molecular configuration during storage. Another reason for variations in the stability of SAA during storage could be its biological behavior (Hillström *et al.*, 2010). However, the aforementioned contradictory data indicate that further investigations are needed to clarify the possible influence of the temperature and duration of storage on the concentrations of bovine serum amyloid A, and to explain the changes in its concentrations during storage at lower temperatures.

The effect of storage temperature and duration on the concentrations of mammary isoform of SAA in milk samples of dairy cows is less well documented. According to the manufacturer's data, milk samples collected for the determination of M-SAA can be stored for up to 2 days at 4 °C or stored frozen at -20 °C for longer periods (Tridelta Development, Ireland). However, to our knowledge, no published studies have been reported on the effect of sample storage on the concentrations of M-SAA in relation to the temperature and duration of storage. In the presented study, we observed a trend of significantly progressively decreasing values of M-SAA during storage at freezer temperatures from day 2 onward. Similarly, non-significantly diminished M-SAA concentrations were found in milk samples maintained at refrigerator temperatures. The aforementioned reduction in the concentrations of M-SAA in milk samples after storage might be caused by degradation of this mammary isoform of SAA, as several factors have been found to affect milk components during storage at various temperatures and time (Barbano *et al.*, 2006).

Presented study showed no significant variations in the concentrations of haptoglobin during freezer storage. Similarly, its values determined in samples without storage and in samples stored one day at 4 °C were roughly uniform. Solter *et al.* (1991) and Cerón *et al.* (2005) reported that acute phase proteins, including haptoglobin and C-reactive protein, are more stable than the cellular components of blood, and assays can be performed on frozen serum samples. Jansen *et al.* (2013) evaluated the stability of biomarkers of the iron status, including haptoglobin, ceruloplasmin, as well as transferrin, up to 1 year of freezer-storage, and the concentrations of all biomarkers tested remained constant upon storage at -20, -70 and -196 °C. Aziz *et al.* (2003) indicated that the effect of different specimen processing and storage conditions on the concentrations of acute phase proteins may vary depending on the assay configuration, and should be validated at the beginning of any research project.

Clinical trials often involve batch laboratory analyses of coagulation tests, including fibrinogen, which requires freezing of the plasma samples. Although rapid freezing by immersion of sample tubes into liquid nitrogen and storage at -70 °C is recommended, plasma samples are often stored at -20 °C (Alesci et al., 2009). Therefore, the aim of the present study was to assess the effect of different storage conditions on fibrinogen concentrations in samples from healthy calves. In the presented study, we observed a trend of significantly progressively decreasing values of Fbg during storage at freezer temperatures from day 2 onward. Similarly, significantly diminished Fbg concentrations were found in plasma samples maintained at refrigerator temperatures. Casella et al. (2009) reported also a significant effect of storage on coagulation parameters in healthy horses, including fibrinogen. The aforementioned authors concluded that coagulation tests can be done within 6 hours when samples are stored at 8 °C, storage at -20 °C is acceptable only after 24 hours for fibrinogen measurements, because after 48 hours, freezing alters the values of clotting parameters. In contrast, the results presented by Iazbik et al. (2001) and Alesci et al. (2009) showed only a little effect of freezing on fibrinogen concentrations. The reduction in the concentrations of fibrinogen in plasma samples after storage, presented in our study, might be caused by degradation of this protein, as several factors may affect blood components during storage at various temperatures and time. Woltersdorf et al. (2001) reported that the freezing process and the resulting time delay of the analysis may result in physical changes in the sample, which may affect the concentration of the analytes.

The concentrations of acute phase proteins are quantified to get information for diagnostic or monitoring purposes (Eckersall et al., 2001; Akerstedt et al., 2009). This demands precise measurement of acute phase protein concentrations and analytical stability. According to the presented results, fresh serum or plasma samples are recommended for acute phase protein analyses in cattle, predominantly for the determination of SAA and Fbg, because the protein degradation during storage at lower temperatures may cause alterations in their concentrations. On the other hand, in the presented study only samples from clinically healthy calves were used. Samples from sick animals, with higher acute phase protein concentrations might behave differently. Seeing that published data on the stability of acute phase proteins during storage under various conditions in cattle are still limited, further studies may be helpful, including studies dealing with the effect of storage at low temperatures (i.e. -70 °C) on the concentrations of these proteins.

7   Conclusions

The objective determination of animal health is important due to the increasing focus of consumers and farmers on the welfare of animals. As non-specific markers of inflammation, acute phase protein testing is a useful tool for the assessment of health in general, to monitor the health state, the spread of infection or the efficacy of treatment. The measurement of acute phase proteins may also be useful in defining the objective health status of an animal or a herd. They are reliable biomarkers that can be used both in diagnostic approaches and for research purposes.

Practical uses and advantages of acute phase protein assays have been described in a large number of scientific reports published in the last few years. Clinical application of acute phase proteins has not been extensive in routine clinical animal practice due to practical limitations associated with their analysis. The most of the methods available for measuring specific acute phase proteins are immunological methods, which are time-consuming and relatively expensive, so limiting the wide-scale use of acute phase proteins in routine practice. Seeing that there is a broad spectrum of possible applications of acute phase protein based diagnostics for the use in cattle, it is necessary to develop and optimise rapid field tests that allow the determination of acute phase proteins in a short time period.

Despite the challenges in the determination of acute phase proteins, with the insights provided by ongoing research in this area, it is likely that these analytes will be increasingly used in the diagnosis and prognosis of diseases also in farm animal medicine. Acute phase proteins have proven to be very useful in the early detection of sub-clinical diseases or alterations of the health status of an animal, with predictive information regarding the development of disease. Changes in the serum concentrations of acute phase proteins indicate the need for a more detailed clinical evaluation of a patient. In addition, acute phase proteins can be a powerful tool in the monitoring of treatment.

Although many prior studies have resulted in well-established procedures for the proper collection, processing, and storage of blood and blood fractions, additional studies are needed. For example, among future trends in blood collection, smaller volumes will be required as laboratory analyses become more sophisticated and sensitive. Although some effects of blood collection tube additives have been studied and documented, the advent of new collection tubes with new variations of additives will require additional studies to assure that they do not affect certain assays. The stability of blood fractions with respect to a variety of assays has not been well documented. For each assay, including acute phase proteins, it must be determined if the blood or blood fraction sample is stable under the planned storage conditions (i.e. length of time and temperature).

In conclusion, our results indicate that proper sample handling, and the temperature and duration of storage are important factors also for acute phase protein analyses. In our study, the presented results showed marked effect of sample storage, predominantly at freezer temperatures, on the concentrations of bovine serum amyloid A, milk amyloid A and fibrinogen with progressively decreasing values over time. Thus, after storage at lower temperatures, the measurement of their concentrations in serum, plasma or milk samples may not be accurate, potentially causing erroneous interpretations. Therefore, issues related to the pre-analytical factors of acute phase protein measurement should be considered to avoid potential misclassification between sick and healthy animals.

Acknowledgement

This work was supported by VEGA Scientific Grants No 1/0447/14 and 1/0812/12 from the Ministry of Education, and by Slovak Research and Development Agency under contract No. APVV-0475-10.

References

Äkerstedt, M., Persson Waller, K., & Sternesjö, Å. (2009). Haptoglobin and serum amyloid A in bulk tank milk in relation to raw milk quality. Journal of Dairy Research, vol. 76, 483-489.

Alayash, A. I. (2004). Oxygen therapeutics: can we tame hemoglobin? Nature Reviews, Drug Discovery, 3(2), 152-159.

Aldred, A. R., Grimes, A., Schreiber, G., & Mercer, J. F. (1987). Rat ceruloplasmin. Molecular cloning and gene expression in liver, choroid plexus, yolk sac, placenta, and testis. The Journal of Biological Chemistry, 262(6), 2875-2878.

Aldred, A. R. & Schreiber, G. (1993). The negative acute phase protein. In: Mackiewicz, I., Kushner, I., & Baumann, H. (Eds.): Acute phase proteins. Molecular biology, biochemistry, and clinical applications. Boca Raton, Florida: CRC Press, 21-37.

Alesci, S., Borggrefe, M., & Dempfle, C.-E. (2009). Effect of freezing method and storage at -20 °C and -70 °C on pro-thrombin time, aPTT and plasma fibrinogen levels. Thrombosis Reearchs, 124, 121-126.

Ametaj, B. M., Hosseini, A., Odhiambo, J.F., Iqbal, S., Sharma, S., Deng, Q., Lam, T.H., Farooq, U., Zebeli, Q. & Dunn, S.M. (2011). Application of acute phase proteins for monitoring inflammatory states in cattle. In: Veas, F. (ed.): Acute phase proteins as early non-specific biomarkers of human and veterinary diseases. InTech, Rijeka, Croatia, 299-354, ISBN 978-953-307-873-1.

Aziz, N., Fahey, J.L., Detels, R., & Butch, A.W. (2003). Analytical Performance of a Highly Sensitive C-Reactive Protein-Based Immunoassay and the Effects of Laboratory Variables on Levels of Protein in Blood. Clinical and Diagnostic Laboratory Immunology, 10, 652-657.

Baigrie, R. J., Lamont, P. M., Dallamn, M., & Morris, P. J. (1991). The release of interleukin-1B (IL-1) precedes that of interleukin-6 (IL-6) in patients undergoing major surgery. Lymphokine Cytokine Research, 10(4), 253-256.

Barbano, D. M., Ma, Y., & Santos, M. V. (2006). Influence of row milk quality on fluid milk shelf life. Journal of Dairy Science, 89(Suppl. E), E15-E19.

Baumann, H. & Gauldie, J. (1994). The acute phase response. Immunology Today, 15(2), 74-80.

Bence, L. M., Addie, D. D., & Eckersall, P. D. (2005). An immunoturbidimetric assay for rapid quantitative measurement of feline alpha-1-acid glycoprotein in serum and peritoneal fluid. Veterinary Clinical Pathology, 34, 335-340.

Bonini, P., Plebani, M., & Ceriotti, F. (2002). Errors in laboratory medicine. Clinical Chemistry, 48, 691-698.

Bowman, B. H. & Kurosky, A. (1982). Haptoglobin: the evolutionary product of duplication, unequal crossing over, and point mutation. Advances in Human Genetics. 12, 189-261.

Boyanton, B., & Blick, K. E. (2002). Stability studies of twenty-four analytes in human plasma and serum. Clinical Chemistry, 48, 2242-2247.

Brock, J.H. (1980). Lactoferrin in human milk: Its role in iron absorption and protection against enteric infection in the newborn infant. Archives of Disease in Childhood, 55(6), 417-421.

Carter, K. & Worwood, M. (2007). Haptoglobin: a review of the major allele frequences worlwide and their association with disease. International Journal of Laboratory Hematology, 29(2), 92-110.

Casella, S., Giannetto, C., Fazio, F., Giudice, E., & Piccione, G. (2009). Assessment of prothrombin time, activated partial thromboplastin time, and fibrinogen concentration on equine plasma samples following different storage conditions. Journal of Veterinary Diagnostic Investigation, 21(5), 674-678.

Cerón, J. J., Eckersall, P. D., & Martinez-Subiela, S. (2005). Acute phase proteins in dogs and cats: current knowledge and future perspectives. Veterinary Clinical Pathology, 34, 85- 99.

Chan, J. P. W., Chang, C.-C., Hsu, W.-I., Liu, W.-B., & Chen, T.-H. (2010). Association of increased serum acute-phase protein concentrations with reproductive performance in dairy cows with postpartum metritis. Veterinary Clinical Pathology, 39(1), 72-78.

Chassagne, M., Barnouin, J., & Chacornac, J. P. (1998). Biological predictors of early clinical mastitis occurence in Holstein cows under field conditions in France. Preventive Veterinary Medicine, 35, 29-38.

Clark, S., Youngman, L. D., Palmer, A., Parish, S., Peto, R., & Collins, R. (2003). Stability of plasma analytes after delayed separation of whole blood: implications for epidemiological studies. Internal Journal of Epidemiology, 32, 125-130.

Comstock, G. W., Burke, A. E., Norkus, E. P., Gordon, G. B., Hoffman, S. C., & Helzlsouer, K. J. (2001). Effects of repeated freeze-thaw cycles on concentrations of cholesterol, micronutrients, and hormones in human plasma and serum. Clinical Chemistry, 47, 139-142.

Cray, C., Rodriguez, M., Zaias, J., & Altman, N. (2009). Effects of storage temperature and time on clinical biochemical parameters from rat serum. Journal of the American Association of Laboratory Animal Science, 48, 202-204.

Deans, C. & Wigmore, S. J. (2005). Systemic inflammation, cachexia, and prognosis in patients with cancer. Current Opinion in Clinical Nutrition and Metabolic Care, 8, 265-269.

De Beer, M. C., Yuan, T., Kindy, M. S., Asztalos, B. F., Roheim, P. S., & de Beer, F. C. (1995). Characterization of constitutive human serum amyloid A protein (SAA4) as an apolipoprotein. Journal of Lipid Research, 36(3), 526-534.

Eckersall, P. D. (2000). Recent advances and future prospects for the use of acute phase proteins as markers of disease in animals. Revue Médicine Véterinarie, 151, 577-584.

Eckersall, P.D., F. J. Young, C. McComb, C. J. Hogarth, S. Safi, A. Weber, T. McDonald, A. M. Nolan, and J. L. Fitzpatrick, „Acute phase proteins in serum and milk from dairy cows with clinical mastitis,“ Veterinary Record, vol. 148, pp. 35-41, 2001.

Eckersall, P. D. & Bell, R. (2010). Acute phase proteins: biomarkers of infection and inflammation in veterinary medicine. The Veterinary Journal, 185, 23-27.

Eckhardt, E. R., Witta, J., Zhong, J., Arsenescu, R., Arsenescu, V., Wang, Y., Ghoshal, S., de Beer, M. C., de Beer, F. C., & de Villiers, W. J. (2010). Intestinal epithelial serum amyloid A modulates bacterial growth in vitro and proinflammatory responses in mouse experimental colitis. BiomMed Central Gastroenterology, 10, 133-141.

Ehsani, A., Afshari, A., Bahadori, H., Mohri, M., & Seifi, H. A. (2008). Serum constituents analyses in dairy cows: Effects of duration and temperature of the storage of clotted blood. Research in Veterinary Science, 85, 473-475.

Fagliari, J. J., Weiss, D. J., McClenanhan, D., & Evanson, O. A. (2003). Serum protein concentrations in calves with experimentally induced pneumonic pasteurellosis. Arquivo Brasileiro de Medicina Veterinária e Zootecnia, 55, 4.

Fleming, R. E., Whitman, I. P., & Gitlin, J. D. (1991). Induction of ceruloplasmin gene expression in rat lung during inflammation and hyperoxia. The American Journal of Physiology, 260(2), L68-74.

Fournier, T., Medjoubi, N., & Porquet, D. (2000). Alpha-1-acid glycoprotein. Biochimica et Biophysica Acta, 1482(1-2), 306-311.

Gabay, C. & Kushner, I. (1999). Acute-phase proteins and other systemic responses to inflammation. New England Journal of Medicine, 340, 448-454.

Gentry, P. A. (1999). Acute phase proteins. In: Loeb, W. F. & Quimby, F. W. (eds.): Clinical chemistry of laboratory animals. Philadelphia: Taylor & Francis, 336-398.

Gruys, E., Toussaint, M. J. M., Niewold, T. A., & Koopmans, S. J. (2005) Acute phase reaction and acute phase proteins. Journal of Zhejiang University Science, 6B(11), 1045-1056.

Hagiwara, S., Kawai, K., Anri, A., & Nagahata, H. (2003). Lactoferrin concentrations in milk from normal and subclinical mastitic cows. The Journal of Veterinary Medical Science, 65(3), 319-323.

Harmon, R. J., Schanbacher, F. L., Ferguson, L. C., & Smith, K. L. (1975). Concentration of lactoferrin in milk of normal lactating cows and changes occuring during mastitis. American Journal of Veterinary Research, 36(7), 1001-1007.

Hawkins, M. G., Kass, P. H., Zinkl, J. G., & Tell, L. A. (2006). Comparison of biochemical values in serum and plasma, fresh and frozen plasma, and hemolyzed samples from orange-winged amazon parrots (Amazona amazonica). Veterinary Clinical Pathology, 35, 219-225.

Heegaard, P. M. H., Godson, D. L., Toussaint, M. J. M., Tjornehoj, K., Larsen, L. E., Viuff, B., & Ronsholt, L. (2000). The acute phase response of haptoglobin and serum amyloid A (SAA) in cattle undergoing experimental infection with bovine respiratory syncytial virus. Veterinary Immunology and Immunopathology, 77, 151-159.

Hillström, A., Tvedten, H., & Lilliehöök, I. (2010). Evaluation of an in-clinic Serum Amyloid A (SAA) assay and assessment of the effects of storage on SAA samples. Acta Veterinaria Scandinavica, 52, 8-13.

Hirschfield, G. M. & Pepys, M. B. (2003). C-reactive protein and cardiovascular disease: new insights from an old molecule. Quarterly Journal of Medicine, 96, 793-807.

Hirvonen, J. & Pyörälä, S. (1998). Acute-phase response in dairy cows with surgically treated abdominal disorders. Veterinary Journal, 155, 53-61.

Horadagoda, N. U., Knox, K. M., Gibbs, H. A., Reid, S. W., Horadagoda, A., Edwards, S. E., & Eckersall, P. D. (1999). Acute phase proteins in cattle: discrimination between acute and chronic inflammation. Veterinary Record; 144, 437–441.

Iazbik, C., Couto, G., Gray, T. L., & Kociba, G. (2001). Effect of storage conditions on hemostatic parameters of canine plasma obtained for transfusion. American Journal of Veterinary Research, 6(5), 734-735.

Jakubowski, J., Luetzelschwab, J., Aebischer, V., Vogel, B., Donatsch, P., & Cordier, A. (1998). Stability of clinical chemistry parameter values in minipig serum under different storage conditions. Scandinavian Journal of Animal Science, 25(Suppl. 1), 197-204.

Jansen, E.H.J.M., Beekhof, P.K., & Schenk, E. (2013). Long-term stability of biomarkers of the iron status in human serum and plasma. Biomarkers, 18 (4), 365-368.

Kawai, K., Hagiwara, S., Anri, A., & Nagahata, H. (1999). Lactoferrin concentration in milk of bovine clinical mastitis. Veterinary Research Communications, 23(7), 391-398.

Kent, J. (1992). Acute phase proteins: their use in veterinary diagnosis. British Veterinary Journal, 148, 279-281.

Koj, A. (1998). Termination of acute-phase response: role of some cytokines and anti-inflammatory drugs. General Pharmacology, 31(1), 9-18.

Kurosky, A., Barnett, D. R., Lee, T. H., Touchstone, B., Hay, R. E., Arnott, M. S., Bowman, B. H., & Fitch, W. M. (1980). Covalent Structure of human haptoglobin: a serin protease homolog (amino acid sequence/plasmonigen/prothrombin/protein evolution). Proceedings of the National Academy of Sciences of the United States of America, 77(6), 3388-3392.

Kushner, I. & Mackiewicz, A. (1987) Acute phase protein as disease markers. Disease Markers, 5(1), 1-11.

Kutila, T., Pyörälä, S., & Kaartinen, L. (2003). Lactoferrin and citrate concentrations at drying-off and during early mammary involution in dairy cows. Journal of Veterinary Medicine Series A, 50(7), 350-353.

Ledue, T. B. & Rifai, N. (2003). Preanalytic and Analytic Sources of Variations in C-Reactive Protein Measurement: Implications for Cardiovascular Disease Risk Assessment. Clinical Chemistry, 49, 1258-1271.

Loøvstad, R. A. (2006). A kinetic study on the phenothiazine dependent oxidation of NADH by bovine ceruloplasmin. Biometals, 19(1). 1-5.

Mack, D. R., McDonald, T. L., Larson, M.-A., Wei, S., & Weber, A. (2003). The conserved TFLK motif of mammary-associated serum amyloid A is responsible for up-regulation of intestinal MUC3 mucin expression in vitro. Pediatric Research, 53, 137-142.

Mackiewicz, A. (1997). Acute phase proteins and transformed cells. International Review of Cytology, 170, 225-300.

Malle, E., Steinmetz, A., & Raynes, J. G. (1993). Serum amyloid A (SAA): an acute phase protein and apolipoprotein. Atherosclerosis, 102(2), 131-146.

Martin, F., Santolaria, F., Batista, N., Milena, A., Gonzalez-Reimers, E., Brito, M. J., & Oramas, J. (1999). Cytokine levels (IL-6 and ING-gamma), acute phase response and nutritional status as prognostic factors in lung cancer. Cytokine, 11(1), 80-86.

Martinez-Subiela, S., Tecles, F., & Ceron, J. J. (2007). Comparison of two automated spectrophotometric methods for ceruloplasmin measurement in pigs. Research in Veterinary Science, 83(1), 12-19.

McCudden, C. R., Rogers, M., Erickson, J., Erickson, R., & Willis, M. S. (2010). Method evaluation and quality management. In: Bishop, M. L., Fody, E. P., & Schoeff, L. E. (eds.): Clinical chemistry: Techniques, principles, correlations. Lippincott Williams & Wilkins, Philadelphia, USA, 88-129.

Moore, S. A., Anderson, B. F., Groom, C. R., Haridas, M., & Baker, E. N. (1997). Three-dimensional structure of diferric bovine lactoferrin at 2.8 A resolution. Journal of Molecular Biology, 274(2), 222-236.

Moshage, H. (1997). Cytokines and the hepatic acute phase response. Journal of Pathology, 181, 257-266.

Mukesh, N., Bionaz, M., Graugnard, D. E., Drackley, J. K., & Loor, J. J. (2010). Adipose tissue depots of Holstein cows are immune responsive: inflammatory gene expression in vitro. Domestic Animal Endocrinology, 38(3), 168-178.

Murata, H., Shimada, N., & Yoshioka, M. (2004). Current research on acute phase proteins in veterinary diagnosis: an overview. Veterinary Journal, 168, 28-40.

Niewold, T. A., Toussaint, M. J. M., & Gruys, E. (2003). Monitoring health by acute phase proteins. Proceedings of the Fourth European Colloquium on Acute Phase Proteins. Segovia, Spain, 2003, 57-67.

O'Keane, M. P. & Cunningham, S. K. (2006). Evaluation of three different specimen types (serum, plasma lithium heparin, and serum gel separator) for analysis of certain analytes: clinical significance of differences in results and efficiency in use. Clinical Chemistry and Laboratory Medicine, 44, 662-668.

Pepys, M. B., Baltz, M. L., Tennent, G. A., Kent, J., Ousey, J., & Rossdale, P. D. (1989). Serum amyloid A protein (SAA) in horses: objective measurement of the acute phase response. Equine Veterinary Journal, 21, 106-109.

Petersen, H. H., Nielsen, J. P., & Heegaard, P. M. H. (2004). Application of acute phase protein measurements in veterinary clinical chemistry. Veterinary Research, 35, 136-187.

Pyörälä, S. (2000). Hirvonen's thesis on acute phase response in dairy cattle. PhD thesis. University of Helsinki, Helsinki, Finnland, ISBN 951-45-9104-6.

Raynes, J.G. (1994). The acute phase response. Biochemical Society Transactions, 22, 69-74.

Reimers, T. J., Lamb, S. V., Bartlett, S. A., Matamoros, R. A., Cowan, R. G., & Engle, J. S. (1991). Effects of hemolysis and storage on quantification of hormones in blood samples from dogs, cattle, and horses. American Journal of Veterinary Research, 52, 1075-1080.

Reynolds, B., Taillade, B., Medaille, C., Palenche, F., Trumel, C., & Lefebvre, H. P. (2006). Effect of repeated freeze-thaw cycles on routine plasma biochemical constituents in canine plasma. Veterinary Clinical Pathology, 35, 339-340.

Ridker, P. M. (2007). Inflammatory biomarkers and risks of myocardial infarction, stroke, diabetes, and total mortality: implications for longevity. Nutrition Review, 65, S253-S259.

Ridker, P. M., Rifai, N., Pfeffer, M. A., Sacks, F., & Braunwald, E. (1999). Long-term effects of pravastatin on plasma concentration of C-reactive protein. Circulation, 100, 230-235.

Rossbacher, J., Wagner, L., & Pasternack, M. S. (1999). Inhibitory effect of haptoglobin on granulocyte chemotaxis, phagocytosis and bactericidal activity. Scandinavian Journal of Immunology, 50, 399-404.

Rothkrantz-Kos, S., van Dieijen-Visser, M. P., Mulder, P. G. H, & Drent, M. (2003). Usefulness of inflammatory markers to depict respiratory functional impairment in sarcoidosis. Clinical Chemistry, 49, 1210-1517.

Samols, D., Agrawal, A., & Kushner, I. (2002). Acute phase proteins. In: Oppenheim, J. J. & Feldman, M. (eds.): Cytokine reference on-line. Academic Press, Harcourt, London, United Kingdom.

Sharma, P. (2009). Preanalytical variables and laboratory performance. Indian Journal of Clinical Biochemistry, 24, 109-110.

Sheldon, I. M., Noakes, D. E., Rycroft, A. N., & Dobson, H. (2002). Effect of pospartum manual examination of the vagina on uterine bacterial contamination in cows. Veterinary Record, 151(18), 531-534.

Skinner, J.G. (2001). International standardization of acute phase proteins. Veterinary Clinical Pathology, 30(1), 2-7.

Sogawa, K., Yamada, T., Suzuki, Y., Masaki, T., Watanabe, S., Uchida, Y., Arima, K., Nishioka, M. & Matsumoto, K. (1994). Elevation of ceruloplasmin activity involved in changes of hepatic metal concentration in primary biliary cirrhosis. Research Communications in Chemical Pathology and Pharmacology, 84 (3), 367-370.

Solter, P. F., Hoffmann, W. E., Hungerford, L. L., Siegel, J. P., St Denis, S. H., & Dorner, J.L. (1991). Haptoglobin and ceruloplasmin as determinants of inflammation in dogs. American Journal of Veterinary Research, 52, 1738-1742.

Susana, A., Chavez, G., Gallegos, S. A., & Cruz, Q. R. (2009). Lactoferrin: structure, function and application. International Journal of Antimicrobial Agents, 33(4), 301.e1-301.e8.

Takahashi, E., Kuwayama, H., Kawamoto, K., Matsui, T., & Inokuma, H. (2009). Detection serum amyloid A isoforms in cattle. Journal of Veterinary Diagnostic Investigation, 21(6), 874-877.

Tanner, M., Kent, N., Smith, B., Fletcher, S., & Lewer, M. (2008). Stability of common biochemical analytes in serum gel tubes subjected to various storage temperatures and times pre-centrifugation. Annals of Clinical Biochemistry, 45, 375-379.

Thomas, J. S. (2000). Overview of plasma proteins. In: Feldman, B. F., Zinkl, J, G., & Jain, N. C. (eds.): Schalm's Veterinary Hematology. Philadelphia: Lippincott Williams & Wilkins; 891-898.

Thomas, T., Schreiber, G., & Jaworowski, A. (1989). Developmental patterns of gene expression of secreted proteins in brain and choroid plexus. Developmental Biology, 134(1), 38-47.

Thoresen, S. I., Tverdal, A., Havre, G., & Morberg, H. (1995). Effects of storage time and freezing temperature on clinical chemical parameters from canine serum and heparinized plasma. Veterinary Clinical Pathology, 24, 129-133.

Tóthová, Cs., Nagy, O., Seidel, H., & Kováč, G. (2010). The effect of chronic respiratory diseases on acute phase proteins and selected blood parameters of protein metabolism in calves. Berliner und Munchener Tierarztliche Wochenschrift, 123, 307-313.

Tóthová, Cs., Nagy, O., Seidel, H., & Kováč, G. (2011). Age-related changes in the concentrations of acute phase proteins and some variables of protein metabolism in calves. Wiener Tierärztliche Monatschrift – Veterinary Medicine Austria; 98, 33-44.

Uhlar, C. M., Burgess, C. J., Sharp, P. M., & Whitehead, A. S. (1994). Evolution of the serum amyloid A (SAA) protein superfamily, Genomics, 19(2), 228-235.

Uhlar, C. M. & Whitehead, A. S. (1999). Serum amyloid A, the major vertebrate acute phase reactant. European Journal of Biochemistry, 265(2), 501-523.

Van der Westhuyzen, D. R., de Beer, F. C., & Webb, N. R. (2007). HDL cholesterol transport during inflammation. Current Opinion in Lipidology, 18(2), 147-151.

Wagener, F. A., Eggernt, A., Boerman, O. C., Oyen, W. J., Verhofstad A., Abraham N. G., Adema G., van Kooyk Y., de Witte T., & Figdor C. G. (2002). Heme is a potent inducer of inflammation in mice and is countected by heme oxygenase. Blood, 98, 1802-1811.

Ward, P. P., Uribe-Luna, S., & Conneely, O. M. (2002). Lactoferrin and host defense. Biochemistry and Cell Biology, 80(1), 95-102.

Wicher, K. B., & Fries, E. (2007). Convergent evolution of human and bovine haptoglobin: partial duplication of the genes. Journal of Molecular Evolution, 65(4), 373-379.

Woltersdorf, W. W., Bayly, G. R., & Day, A. P. (2001). Practical implications of in vitro stability of cardiac markers. Annals of Clinical Biochemistry, 38, 61-63.

Yang, F. M., Haile, D. J., Berger, F. G., Herbert, D. C., Van Beveren, E., & Ghio, A. J. (2003). Haptoglobin reduces lung injury associated with exposure to blood. American Journal of Physiology and Lung Cell Molecular Physiology, 284, L402-L409.

Overview of Hypertrophic Cardiomyopathy (HCM) Genomics and Transcriptomics: Molecular Tools in HCM Assessment for Application in Clinical

Susana Rodrigues Santos
Centro Química Estrutural, Instituto Superior Técnico
Universidade de Lisboa, Portugal
Faculdade de Engenharia
Universidade Lusófona de Humanidades e Tecnologias, Portugal

Ana Teresa Freitas
Instituto de Engenharia de Sistemas e Computadores, Instituto Superior Técnico
Universidade de Lisboa, Portugal

Alexandra Fernandes
Departamento Ciências da Vida, Faculdade de Ciências e Tecnologia
Universidade Nova de Lisboa, Caparica, Portugal
Centro Química Estrutural
Instituto Superior Técnico, Universidade de Lisboa, Portugal

1   Inherited Cardiomyopathies

Inherited cardiomyopathies are a group of cardiovascular disorders classified based on the morphology and function of the ventricle and include hypertrophic cardiomyopathy (HCM), arrhythmogenic right ventricular cardiomyopathy (ARVC), dilated cardiomyopathy (DCM), left ventricular noncompaction (LVNC), and restrictive cardiomyopathy (RCM) (Teekakirikul *et al.,* 2013).

In this book chapter we will review current status of HCM molecular genetics and the importance of transcriptomics for revealing new diagnostic and therapeutic biomarkers and bioinformatic approaches to improve the translation between the bench and the clinic.

2   Physiopathological, Pathological, and Clinical Characteristics of HCM

HCM is a primary disorder of the myocardium classically characterized by unexplained left ventricular hypertrophy (LVH) (Figure 1) in the absence of an underlying systemic condition or other cardiac disease (such as hypertension or valvular heart disease), and by distinctive histopathologic features of cardiomyocyte hypertrophy, disarray and increased myocardial fibrosis (Figure 2) (Teekakirikul *et al.,* 2013; Spirito *et al.,* 2000, McKenna & Behr, 2002; McKenna *et al.,* 2003, Yaxin *et al.,* 2013). Apart from LVH, due to mitral valve systolic anterior motion and mitral-septal contact, LV outflow tract obstruction occurs in approximately 70% of HCM cases at rest and/or with physiologic provocation (Maron *et al.,* 2006). Other HCM common phenotypic features include shortness of breath, chest pain, palpitations, presyncope or syncope and orthostasis (Teekakirikul *et al.,* 2013). Despite these more common phenotypic features, HCM clinical manifestations are highly variable ranging from being completely asymptomatic to progressive heart failure and sudden cardiac death (SCD) caused by mechanical or electric defects (Teekakirikul *et al.,* 2013; Tian *et al.,* 2013, Lopes *et al.,* 2013; Spirito *et al.,* 2000, McKenna & Behr, 2002; McKenna *et al.,* 2003). Indeed, HCM is the leading cause of sudden nontraumatic death in young adults and competitive athletes in the United States (Maron *et al.,* 2003). HCM has an estimated prevalence of 1 in 500 in the general population (Gersh *et al.,* 2011; Lopes *et al.,* 2013; Maron *et al.,* 1995).

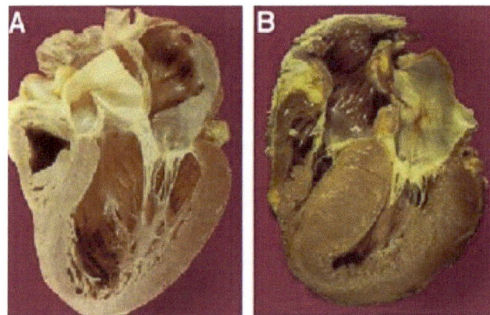

Figure 1: Morphologic features of the normal heart (A), compared to hypertrophic cardiomyopathy (B).We can observe the hypertrophied interventricular septum (arrow) (adapted from Ahmad *et al.,* 2005).

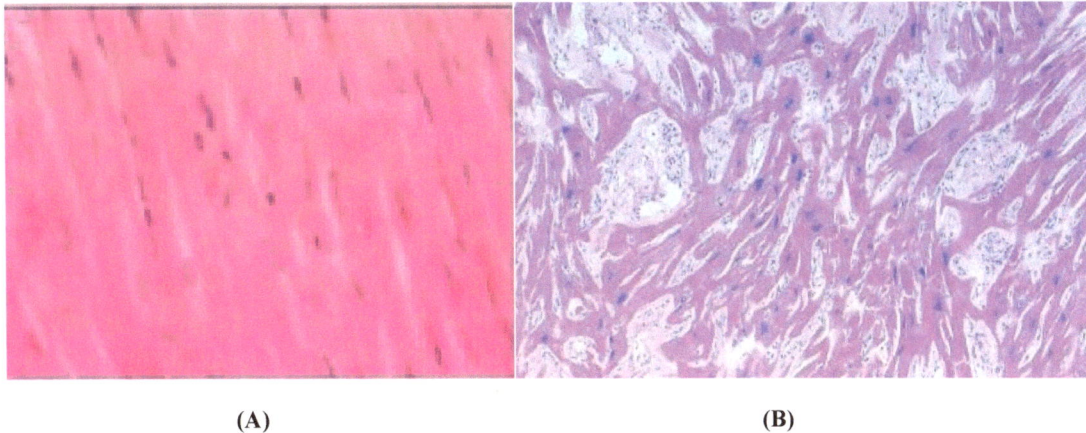

(A)   **(B)**

Figure 2: Histological images of a heart tissue from A. Normal individual; B. Patient with HCM showing the disarray and increased fibrosis (adapted from Ahmad *et al*., 2005).

HCM is usually diagnosed by a maximal LV wall thickness $\geq$ 15mm (13-14 mm=borderline, most commonly asymmetric septal and less frequently concentric and apical) through cardiac imaging, commonly done with two-dimensional echocardiography (ECHO) (the "gold standard" technique) but increasingly with cardiac magnetic resonance (CMRI) (Gersh *et al*., 2011). Some characteristic ECHO findings include systolic anterior motion of the mitral valve with associated left ventricular outflow tract obstruction and mitral regurgitation; midventricular obstruction as a result of systolic cavity obliteration; diastolic dysfunction including restrictive physiology (Teekakirikul *et al*., 2013). More recently, contrast-enhanced CMRI with gadolinium (Gd-CMRI) can reliably detect myocardial fibrosis *in vivo* and has been reported to be useful for the differential diagnosis of HCM (Miller *et al*., 2009).

The broad spectrum of HCM clinical manifestations described above and the age-dependent expression of hypertrophy make HCM clinical diagnosis difficult (Tian *et al*., 2013; Lopes *et al*., 2013; Spirito *et al*., 2000, McKenna & Behr, 2002; McKenna *et al*., 2003). A prior history of sudden cardiac arrest, syncope caused by cardiac arrhythmias, repetitive non-sustained or sustained ventricular tachycardia, severe cardiac hypertrophy and a strong family history of SCD are considered important risk factors and can be crucial for an early diagnosis (Elliot *et al.,* 2000, Spirito *et al*., 2000, Marian, 2003, Frenneaux, 2004). Also extremely important is the differential diagnosis of HCM due to HCM phenocopies. HCM phenocopies mimic the phenotypic and clinical features of sarcomeric HCM and include several syndromes that typically manifest with multiorgan involvement but that can also present with isolated or predominant LVH. These syndromes include metabolic cardiomyopathies, such as Danon disease and Wolf-Parkinson-White syndrome (Arad *et al.,* 2005) and the lysosomal storage disorder, Fabry disease (Sachdev *et al*., 2002). LVH in these conditions is not accompanied by myocyte disarray or fibrosis but by a characteristic accumulation of glycogen or glycosphingolipids in cellular vacuoles (Arad *et al*., 2005). LVH is also a part of the phenotypic spectrum of Noonan syndrome (Nishikawa *et al*., 1996) and Friedreich ataxia (Osterziel *et al*., 2002). The incidence of phenocopies in patients with the clinical diagnosis of HCM is unknown but is estimated at 10% (Marian, 2010).

3 HCM as a Genetic Disease: Importance of Genetic Diagnosis

Genetic studies established the paradigm that HCM is a disease of the sarcomere, caused by dominant mutations in genes encoding components of the contractile apparatus (Figure 3) with most of them (80%) present in the *MYH7* and *MYBPC3* genes (Table 1) (Seidman CE & Seidman JG, 2011). Until now more than 900 mutations in sarcomeric and more recently also in nonsarcomeric genes (for example in genes encoding Z-disk proteins and genes encoding proteins located in the sarcoplasmic reticulum and plasma membrane) have been described in HCM patients (Lopes *et al.*, 2013; Teekakirikul *et al.*, 2013; Santos *et al.*, 2011; Santos *et al.*, 2012) (Table 1). However, variants in these nonsarcomeric genes are rare (Table 2), and most studies do not provide complete evidence of their role in HCM. Segregation with disease or *in vivo* functional data are necessary for most of these rare variants (Teekakirikul *et al.*, 2013).

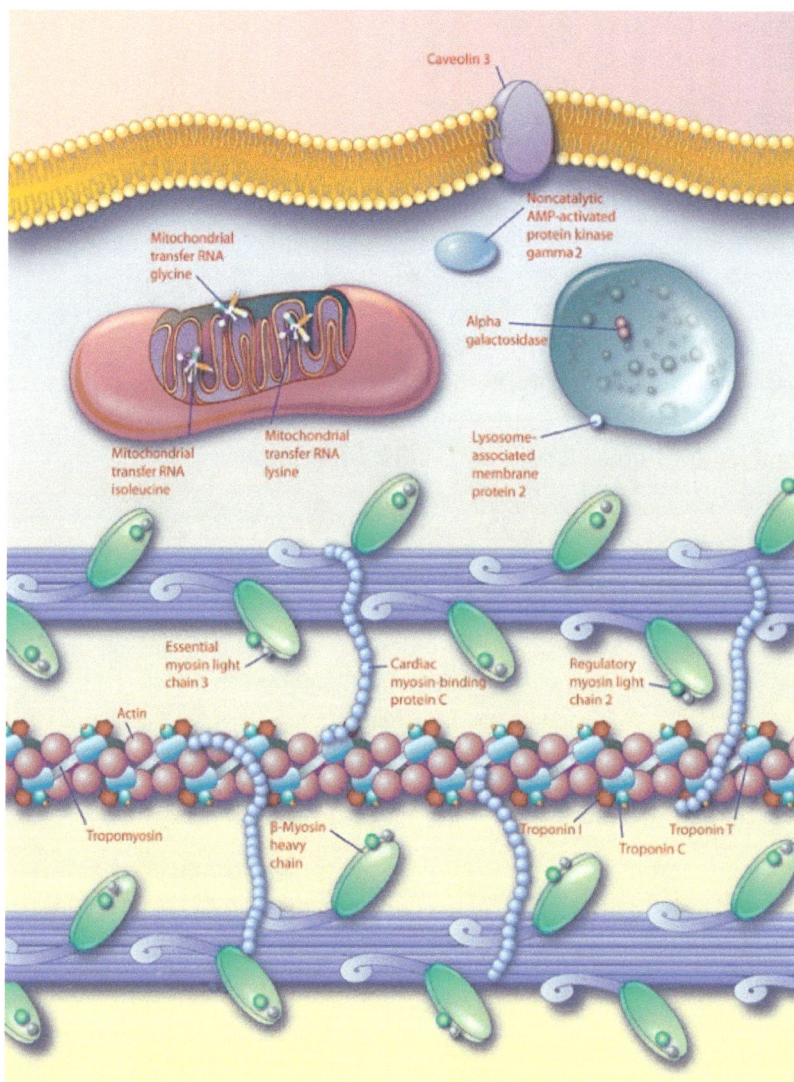

Figure 3: Cardiac sarcomere and proteins involved in HCM (Images courtesy of GeneDX (http://www.genedx.com/)

Most sarcomere mutations are believed to act in a dominant negative manner (i.e affecting the expression of the normal gene product). The exceptions to this dominant negative model for HCM are the loss-of-function variants resulting in insufficient protein for normal function and leading to haploinsufficiency; these variants occur less frequently but are prevalent in the *MYBPC3* gene (Andersen *et al.*, 2004).

Gene	Protein	HCM associated Mutations*	Location or Function**
ACTA1	actin, alpha 1	1	Sarcomere, skeletal muscle
ACTC1	actin, alpha, cardiac muscle 1	14	Sarcomere, cardiac muscle
ACTN2	actinin, alpha 2	4	Z-disk
ANKRD1	ankyrin repeat domain 1	3	Z-disk and nucleus (transcription factor)
BRAF	v-raf murine sarcoma viral oncogene homolog B1	1	Cytoplasmic serine/threonine kinase
COA5	cytochrome c oxidase assembly factor 5	1	Mitochondrial
CALM3	calmodulin 3 (phosphorylase kinase, delta)	1	Calcium sensor and signal transducer
CALR3	calreticulin 3	2	Endoplasmic reticulum chaperone
CASQ2	calsequestrin 2	1	Sarcoplasmic reticulum; calcium storage
CAV3	caveolin 3	1	Plasma membrane
COX15	cytochrome c oxidase assembly homolog 15	2	Mitochondrial respiratory chain
CSRP3	cysteine and glycine-rich protein 3	11	Z-disk
DES	Desmin	1	Intermediate filament
FHL1	four and a half LIM domains 1	3	Biomechanical stress sensor
FHOD3	formin homology 2 domain containing 3	1	Actin-organizing protein
FXN	Frataxin	1	Mitochondrial iron transport and respiration
GLA	galactosidase, alpha	1	Lysosome
JPH2	junctophilin 2	4	Junctional membrane complexes; calcium signaling
KLF10	Kruppel-like factor 10	6	Transcriptional repressor; inhibits cell growth
MAP2K1	mitogen-activated protein kinase kinase 1	1	MAP kinase kinase; signal transduction
MAP2K2	mitogen-activated protein kinase kinase 2	1	MAP kinase kinase; signal transduction
MRPL3	mitochondrial ribosomal protein L3	1	Mitochondrial Ribosomal Protein
MTO1	mitochondrial tRNA translation optimization 1	2	Mitochondrial tRNA modification
MYBPC3	myosin binding protein C, cardiac	373	Sarcomere
MYH6	alpha-myosin heavy chain	4	Sarcomere
MYH7	beta-myosin heavy chain	307	Sarcomere

MYL2	ventricular myosin regulatory light chain	14	Sarcomere
MYL3	myosin light chain 3	12	Sarcomere
MYLK2	myosin light chain kinase 2	2	Calcium/calmodulin dependent kinase
MYO6	myosin VI	1	Actin-based reverse-direction motor protein
MYOM1	myomesin 1	1	Sarcomere
MYOZ2	myozenin 2	2	Z-disk
MYPN	Myopalladin	7	Z-disk
NDUFAF1	NADH dehydrogenase (ubiquinone) complex I, assembly factor 1	2	Mitochondrial chaperone
NDUFV2	NADH dehydrogenase (ubiquinone) flavoprotein 2	1	Mitochondrial respiratory chain
NEXN	Nexilin	2	Z-disk
OBSCN	Obscurin	1	Sarcomere
PDLIM3	PDZ and LIM domain 3	1	Z-disk
PRKAG2	5'-AMP-activated protein kinase subunit gamma-2	7	Energy sensor protein kinase
PLN	Phospholamban	7	Sarcoplasmic reticulum; regulates Ca(2+)-ATPase
RAF1	v-raf-1 murine leukemia viral oncogene homolog 1	1	Serine/threonine-protein kinase; signal transduction
SLC25A3	solute carrier family 25, member 3	1	Phosphate carrier protein (cytosol to mitochondria)
SLC25A4	solute carrier family 25, member 4	2	Adenine nucleotide translocator (cytosol/mitochondria)
SOS1	son of sevenless homolog 1	2	Guanine nucleotide exchange factor for RAS proteins; signal transduction
SRI	Sorcin	1	Calcium-binding; modulates excitation-contraction coupling
TCAP	Telethonin	3	Z-disk
TNNC1	troponin C	7	Sarcomere
TNNI3	troponin I	45	Sarcomere
TNNT2	troponin T	50	Sarcomere
TPM1	alpha-tropomyosin	16	Sarcomere
TRIM63	tripartite motif-containing 63	3	Sarcomere; regulates protein degradation
TTN	Titin	3	Sarcomere
VCL	Vinculin	1	Sarcomere

Table 1: HCM associated genes, proteins, mutations and protein localization or function. * - Human Genome Mutation Database (http://www.hgmd.cf.ac.uk/ac/index.php); ** - National Center for Biotechnology Information (NCBI) (http://www.ncbi.nlm.nih.gov/)

These sarcomere protein abnormalities ultimately appear to converge on increased actin activated ATPase activity, disruption of actin-myosin interaction and force generation, and altered intracellular calcium signaling in cardiomyocytes as the major common paths leading to the anatomic (hypertrophy, myofiber disarray, and fibrosis) and functional features (pathological signaling and diastolic dysfunction) characteristic of HCM (Teekakirikul *et al.*, 2013; Fatkin D & Graham RM 2002; Sequeira *et al.*, 2013; Witjas-Paalberends *et al.*, 2013). More recently scientific data suggests that LVH can be caused by perturbations of transforming growth factor b and CaMKII Mef2 signaling pathways (Teekakirikul *et al.*, 2010).

Sarcomere gene mutations have been identified in up to 60% of familial HCM and in 40% of sporadic HCM (Ho, 2010). Most of HCM associated mutations/variants are private (within a family) and only a small number of variants are present at higher population frequencies, the most common of which, a 25-bp deletion in intron 32 of the *MYBPC3* gene, is present in 4% of the Southeast Asian Indian population and increases the risk for heart failure by >6 fold (Dhandapany *et al.*, 2009). In the Netherlands, for instance a single founding mutation also accounts for a substantial percentage of HCM (Alders *et al.*, 2003), while in the US, there is marked genetic heterogeneity and most HCM-patients have a unique pathogenic mutation (Alcalai *et al.*, 2008).

The marked genetic heterogeneity, the highly variable intra- and inter- family expressivity and the incomplete penetrance poses some problems in the establishment of complete genotype-phenotype correlations. Despite this, few exceptions has been attempted namely at the gene level. For example, some *TNNT2* mutations have been associated with an appreciable risk of arrhythmia and minor hypertrophy (Watkins *et al.*, 1995), *MYH7* variants lead to a significant LVH after the second decade of life and are thought to be associated with an increased risk of heart failure and SCD (Ho *et al.*, 2010a), and some pathogenic variants in *MYBPC3* are believed to be associated with a later onset (high prevalence of loss-of-function variants) (Niimura *et al.*, 2002) although others have also been identified in a significant proportion of HCM patients with childhood-onset LVH (usually missense variants; possible with more severe functional consequences) (Morita *et al.*, 2008). For a more detailed information regarding genes, mutations and clinical phenotype see table 2.

Causal genes for HCM	Encoded Protein	Frequency Familial (%)ᵛ	Frequency Sporadic (%)*	Clinical Features, associated phenotype	References
Sarcomere Thick filament					
MYH7	Beta-myosin heavy chain	30-40	25-35*	Moderate to severe hypertrophy, high disease penetrance and variable prognosis. Younger onset is typical. Severe LVH, Heart failure, SCD	Watkins et al 1992; Charron et al 1998; Marian et al 2001; Seidman & Seidman 2001; Fatkin, 2002; Erdmann et al 2003; Richard et al 2003; Ingles et al 2005; Van Driest et al 2005; Morita et al 2008; Ho et al 2010; Keren et al 2008; Lopes et al 2013; 2013b; Seidman & Seidman, 2011; 2013, 2013b; Teekakirikul et al 2013
MYBPC3	Myosin binding protein C, cardiac	30-40	20-30*	Usually milder disease. Although it can be severe; some older onset;	Watkins et al 1995b; Charron et al 1998, Marian et al 2001; Seidman & Seidman 2001; Fatkin 2002; Niimura et al 2002; Erdmann et al 2003; Richard et al 2003; Andersen et al 2004; Ingles et al 2005; Van Driest et al 2005; Keren et al 2008; Morita et al 2008; Ho et al 2010; Seidman & Seidman, 2011; Lopes et al 2013, 2013b; Teekakirikul et al 2013

TNNT2	Troponin T	10-20	3-5*	Mild LVH, SCD more common	Thierfelder et al 1994; Watkins et al 1995; ; Moolman et al 1997; Marian et al 2001; Seidman & Seidman 2001;Varnava et al 2001; Fatkin 2002; Erdmann et al 2003; Richard et al 2003; Ingles et al 2005; Van Driest et al 2005; Keren et al 2008; Morita et al 2008 Ho et al 2010; Lopes et al 2013, 2013b; Teekakirikul et al 2013
MYL2	Ventricular myosin regulatory light chain 2	Rare**	Rare**	Skeletal myopathy Midcavity obstruction Common in HCM families with a malignant prognosis.	Poetter et al 1996; Seidman & Seidman 2001; Fatkin 2002; Richard et al 2003; Ingles et al 2005; Van Driest et al 2005; Morita et al 2008, Lopes et al 2013, 2013b; Teekakirikul et al 2013
MYL3	Myosin light chain 3	Rare**	Rare**	Skeletal myopathy Midcavity obstruction	Poetter et al 1996; Seidman & Seidman 2001; Fatkin 2002; Richard et al 2003; Ingles et al 2005; Van Driest et al 2005; Morita et al 2008, Lopes et al 2013, 2013b; Teekakirikul et al 2013
MYH6	Alpha-myosin heavy chain	Rare**	Rare**	Late onset	Carniel et al 2005; Fatkin 2002; Lopes et al 2013, 2013b; Teekakirikul et al 2013
Sarcomere Thin filament					
TNNI3	Troponin I	2-5	?	Very heterogeneous disease expression. Sudden death with severe disease	Kimura et al 1997; Seidman & Seidman 2001; Fatkin 2002; Niimura et al 2002; Mogensen et al 2004; Van Driest et al 2005; Morita et al 2008; Ho et al 2010;Teekakirikul et al 2013
TPM1	Alpha-tropomyosin	2-5	?	Variable prognosis, sudden death	Thierfelder et al 1994; Watkins et al 1995; Fatkin 2002; Seidman & Seidman 2001; Erdmann et al 2003; Heller et al 2003; Chang et al 2005; Van Driest et al 2005; Morita et al 2008; Ho et al 2010; Karibe et al 2011; Teekakirikul et al 2013
TNNC1	Troponin C	Rare**	Rare**	Typical HCM	Seidman & Seidman 2001; Erdmann et al 2003; Fatkin 2002; Richard et al 2003; Teekakirikul et al 2013
TTN	Titin	Rare**	Rare**	Typical HCM	Satoh et al 1999; Bos et al 2006; Lopes et al 2013b; Teekakirikul et al 2013
ACTC1	Actin, alpha, cardiac muscle	Rare**	Rare**	Apical hypertrophy Midcavity obstruction Some late onset mutations.	Olson et al. 2000; Seidman & Seidman 2001; Wong et al 2001; Fatkin 2002; Niimura et al 2002; Richard et al 2003; Ingles et al 2005; Van Driest et al 2005, Vang et al 2005; Bookwalter et al 2006; Lopes et al 2013, 2013b; Teekakirikul et al, 2013
Z- Disk					
TCAP	Telethonin	Rare**	Rare**	Variable hypertrophy Typical HCM, variable penetrance	Hayashi et al 2004; Bos et al 2006; Teekakirikul et al 2013
CSRP3	Cysteine and glycine-rich	Rare**	Rare**	Variable hypertrophy and skeletal myopathy Late onset, variable	Fatkin 2002; Bos et al 2006; Teekakirikul et al 2013

	protein 3			penetrance	
MYOZ2	Myozenin 2	Rare**	Rare**	Early onset of symptoms, pronounced cardiac hypertrophy, and cardiac arrhythmias	Osio et al 2007; Posch et al 2008; Teekakirikul et al 2013
VCL	Vinculin	Rare**	Rare**	Obstructive midventricular Hypertrophy	Vasile et al 2006: Teekakirikul et al 2013
Ca^{2+}-handling protein					
PLN	Phospholamban	Rare**	?	Typical HCM, variable penetrance	Landstrom et al 2011; 2012; Teekakirikul et al 2013
CASQ2	Calsequestrin 2	Rare**	?	Typical HCM	Keren et al 2008; Landstrom et al 2012
JPH2	Junctophilin 2	Rare**	?	Typical HCM	Keren et al 2008; Landstrom et al 2012

Table 2: Hypertrophic cardiomyopathy: disease-causing genes and associated clinical features and phenotypes; ¥Hershberger et al 2009; *Keren et al 2008; **Rare - Means < 1 %; ? - Means unknown

For the last decades the management strategy for families living with HCM has been described in the literature and followed routinely by cardiologists over the world (Ho, 2010, O'Mahony *et al*., 2013). Serial screening in HCM families includes an echocardiogram, electrocardiogram and evaluation by a cardiologist (Maron *et al*., 2003, O'Mahony *et al*., 2013). This strategy is considered time consuming and an expensive process for families and medical community. In the last decade, major progresses have been achieved in the understanding of the genetic basis underlying HCM and genetic testing has been offer as a service (Ackerman *et al.,* 2011; Wang *et al*., 2010, Ho *et al.,* 2011). Clinical guidelines for HCM recommend comprehensive testing for at least five HCM genes (*MYBPC3*, *MYH7*, *TNNI3*, *TNNT2*, and *TPM1*) (Ackerman *et al.,* 2011, Ho *et al*., 2011). Genetic testing for HCM is primarily used to identify families with a detectable genetic cause of disease and to screen at-risk family members. Testing can also help rule out nongenetic conditions, such as athlete's heart, although only when a pathogenic variant is identified (Ho, 2010; Wheeler *et al*., 2009). Since the late 90s traditional genotyping strategies such as SSCP (Single Strand Conformation Polymorphism), DHPLC (Denaturing High Pressure Liquid Chromatography) and dideoxy sequencing of amplified protein encoding exons have been employed (Larsen *et al.,* 1999, Mogensen *et al*., 2003). Nevertheless, these technologies are considered low throughput, with high cost and has a low sensitivity. In 2003, genetic testing entered the mainstream of the healthcare system with automated DNA sequencing providing rapid, reliable, and comprehensive molecular diagnosis on a fee-for-service basis (Maron *et al*., 2012). Although current clinical guidelines recommend routine genetic testing in patients with HCM (Anderson *et al.,* 2004; Hershberger *et al*., 2009; Ho, 2010) its use in everyday clinical practice has been limited by the cost and complexity of conventional sequencing technologies. Advances in high throughput technologies have the potential to solve this problem by analyzing substantially larger genomic regions at a lower cost than conventional capillary Sanger sequencing (Geier *et al*., 2008). In the last years, high throughput technologies such as High Resolution Melting (Millat *et al*., 2010; Santos *et al*., 2012), resequencing DNA arrays (Fokstuen *et al.,* 2008), Next Generation Sequencing (NGS) (Lopes *et al*., 2012; Lopes *et al.*, 2013) and iPlex Mass Array (Santos *et al*., 2011) have emerged to detect HCM pathological mutations enabling the test of a large number of genes simultaneously with lower costs and more rapidly. Nevertheless, some of these new technologies also pose new challenges, in particular, NGS and HRM given their potential to identify a large number of variants of unclear clinical significance (VUS) (Lopes *et al.*, 2013; Santos *et al.*, 2012). Indeed, distinguishing pathogenic mutations from VUS or rare nonpathogenic variants regarding genetic testing interpretation is considered a new challenge. Notably, generally accepted guidelines for interpreting VUS are currently lacking, with estimated frequencies varying dramatically from 5% to 50% (Maron *et al.*, 2012), and being so, when a VUS is identified, its utility in confirming the diagnosis in a proband with suspected disease is limited and it cannot be used for predictive gene testing in at-risk relatives. Additionally, laboratory commercial testing strategies vary widely, employing from 3 to 7 descriptive pathogenicity classes to construct formal reports, thereby creating the distinct possibility that different interpretations of pathogenicity may emanate from different laboratories for the same mutation (Maron *et al.*, 2012). In this regard, it has become critical to carefully review the scientific evidence underlying a proclaimed disease gene. Genes with low detection rates (Table 2) usually have a limited number of studies and many studies infer disease association based on the absence from a small number of healthy control individuals and evolutionary conservation of the affected amino acid. Indeed, screening 300 chromosomes identifies only 80% of all rare benign variation and that more than 6000 chromosomes are necessary to identify the full spectrum (Ionita-Laza *et al.*, 2009). Additional genetic evidence, such as segregation with disease and functional data that would bring a stronger support, is rarely available (Teekakirikul *et al.*, 2013).

Taking all this into consideration the process of genetic testing involves more and more a close collaboration between molecular geneticists and genetic counselors at the testing laboratory and the referring health care provider and the family. Genetic test results often initiate a cascade of events, including familial segregation studies and iterative reevaluation of clinical and molecular evidence, to determine the clinical significance of novel variants. Although clinical sequencing of emerging disease genes is increasingly performed, it is important to realize that it can take years until the spectrum of pathogenic and benign variation has been characterized. Until then, testing often yields many VUSs, and these inconclusive results can be problematic for the patient (Aatre *et al.*, 2011). The rapidly increasing number of sequenced genomes is beginning to remedy this problem, as the spectrum of rare benign variation is better defined (Teekakirikul *et al.*, 2013). As this is a rapidly expanding field, recommendations for HCM genetic testing will be reinforced. Nevertheless, it should be noted that there is a positive impact of identifying a mutation in an individual since it often provides an explanation for why the disease has occurred and also allows for cascade testing of other affected and unaffected family members. Testing of affected family members is performed as a confirmation of their disease status and to exclude the possibility of a "phenocopy". This enables an accurate risk assessment to be given for their offspring. Asymptomatic family members can be offered a predictive genetic test to clarify whether they are at risk of developing clinical disease and to determine the inheritance risk to their children. As the decision of having a predictive genetic test is complex, it should be made in the context of a clinical genetics service offering pre- and post-test genetic counselling. Additionally, it should be noted that, in most cases, the presence of a mutation on a genetic test will not alter the clinical management of an individual who is already known to be affected. However, in cases where an unaffected individual receives a positive predictive gene test result, an ongoing surveillance programme should be recommended. Due to variable age of onset, surveillance should be started early, and may be determined by the natural history in the family. Genotype-phenotype correlations, if known, could be an important consideration in determining screening for asymptomatic mutation positive individuals (Teekakirikul *et al.*, 2013; Maron *et al.*, 2010). Indeed, in the clinical practice genotyping HCM-patients has proven to be useful for risk stratification, with particular regard to the SCD event (Elliot *et al.*, 2000, Spirito *et al.,* 2000, Marian, 2003, Frenneaux, 2004; Hershberger *et al.*, 2009). An accurate diagnostic molecular approach to establish meaningful relationships among individual gene mutations, phenotype, and outcome in HCM cohorts is therefore considered of utmost importance (Arad 2002, Frenneaux , 2004, Bos *et al.,* 2006, Santos *et al.,* 2012, Seidman & Seidman, 2011). The management of the clinical aspects of HCM, integrating the clinical, diagnostic, and therapeutic recommendations based on a synthesis of all data is particularly relevant with HCM because of the complexity of decision analysis for clinical interventions (eg, the assessment of outflow tract obstruction, and if present, selection of a treatment plan that may involve surgical or catheter-based interventions or a positive family history of SCD, may increase the threshold for preventive implantation of an automated implantable cardioverter defibrillator) (Teekakirikul *et al.*, 2013; Maron *et al.*, 2010; Hershberger *et al.*, 2009).This also poses several implications for the mutation-positive individuals since they should receive appropriate lifestyle modification advices as part of result follow-up.

Through large-scale gene sequencing, new data have emerged in HCM suggesting that double (or triple) or compound pathogenic mutations can be associated with more severe disease expression and adverse prognosis (e.g., advanced heart failure or SCD, even in the absence of conventional risk markers (Maron *et al.*, 2012). While it is possible that multiple mutations will prove to be prognostic markers or arbitrators of ambiguous risk profiles, current evidence is preliminary and prospective long-term studies in large populations are required (Arad 2002, Frenneaux , 2004, Bos *et al.*, 2006, Maron *et al.*, 2013, Santos *et al.,* 2012, Seidman & Seidman, 2011).

The benefits for establishing the molecular basis for HCM are not limited to researchers. Indeed, for clinicians, knowledge about the genetic causes of human HCM is of immediate and practical value. The practical information about genetic causes has considerable implications provides insights into prognosis, accurate diagnosis and screening strategies for at-risk familial members (Hershberger *et al.*, 2009).

Another important aspect is the use of genetic test results in guiding clinical management such as the case of enzyme replacement therapy for storage disorders that can present as isolated LVH (Rozenfeld & Neumann, 2011). In this regard, an emerging area is the use of genotype data to guide therapeutic decisions in preclinical individuals. Studies using animal model suggest that calcium channel blockers, such as diltiazem, may delay the clinical progression of disease (Semsarian *et al.*, 2002). Additionally, animal studies have also shown evidence of a connection between HCM and increased transforming growth factor b signaling. A combined therapy using an anti-transforming growth factor b antibody and losartan (an angiotensin II receptor type 1 antagonist) was shown to prevent cardiac fibrosis and hypertrophy in a sarcomere mutation positive mice (Teekakirikul *et al.*, 2010). All these studies may open additional therapeutic avenue for HCM.

4   HCM New Insights: Translating Transcriptomics into Diagnostic Markers

One of the major concerns regarding HCM is the phenotypic variability even in related patients carrying the same disease-causing mutation (Keren *et al.*, 2008). This has drawn several concerns in the establishment of complete genotype-phenotype correlations based only on their genetic analysis results and raises the fact that HCM phenotypic and genetic variability cannot be explained exclusively on the basis of the type of genetic defect or the gene that is altered per se (Fatkin *et al.*, 2002). Indeed, disease manifestation are likely to be influenced not only by genetic factors such as mutations, but also by modifier genes, and environmental factors such as lifestyle, degree of physical exercise and blood pressure (Fatkin *et al.*, 2002).

Despite significant advances in the relations between structure and function of the components of the contractile apparatus, there is limited knowledge of how a particular mutation can induce clinical HCM. Cardiac muscle development is characterized by the activation of contractile protein genes and subsequent modulation of expression by physiological and pathological stimuli (Clerk *et al.*, 2007; Kehat *et al.*, 2010). Structural remodeling, meaning changes in the size, shape and function of the heart, is a key determinant of whether cardiac hypertrophy is classified as pathological or physiological. Pathological hypertrophy is associated with structural rearrangement of components of the normal chamber wall that involves cardiac myocyte hypertrophy, cardiac fibroblast proliferation, fibrosis, and cell death (apoptotic and necrotic) (Manabe *et al.*, 2002). During the HCM development, cardiomyocytes undergo a remodeling process that, while initially compensatory, ultimately accelerates functional deterioration namely caused by cardiomyocyte disarray and tissue fibrosis responsible for the onset of cardiac failure (Maron *et al.*, 1987; Klues *et al.*, 1995; Nimura *et al.*, 1998; Marian *et al.*, 2000; Olivotto *et al.*, 2001; Varnava *et al.*, 2001; Maron *et al.*, 2004). In this regard, the understanding of the molecular changes within the myocardial tissue that for instances occur in response to HCM causal mutations may advance mechanistic insights that account for disease. This important issue could be tackled by characterizing the key players in cardiac tissues during HCM induced sarcomere remodeling. In this context the transcriptional profile involved in the contractile function and HCM progression, may represent valuable candidates for recognition of HCM (Watkins *et al.*, 1996; Cooper *et al.*, 2005; Lawler *et al.*, 2007; Theis *et al.*, 2009). Gene expression during HCM remodelling in myocardial tissue – ventricle and auricle was performed by our group (our results not published; Santos *et al.*, 2009 and Santos *et al.*, 2010 both oral presentation in international meetings; Santos *et al.*, 2012; Fernandes *et al.*, 2013 both poster presentation in international meetings). In an expression study in human HCM tissue an increased myofilamet proteins level in patients with either MYBPC3- or MYH7- mediated HCM suggest a dominant negative mechanism (Theis *et al.*, 2009). Our results point out to the hypothesis that transcriptional variants may correlated with the clinical and genetic profile (Santos *et al.*, 2009 and Santos *et al.*, 2010 both oral presentation in congress; Santos *et al.*, 2012; Fernandes *et al.*, 2013 both poster presentation in congress). The extraordinary degree of analytical power of the current high-throughput technologies provides opportunities to gain novel insights into cell biology and associated pathophysiological processes. Cardiac molecular changes that prompt cardiac remodeling could be evaluated by comprehensive transcriptional analyses that quantify key molecules as myocardial mRNAs and microRNAs (miRNAs) within HCM heart tissues. High throughput transcriptomic analyses of mRNAs enable scientists to gain a comprehensive view of transcriptional changes within tissue. Heart tissue mRNAs could be systematically studied using different and complementary methods, namely RNA sequencing (RNA-Seq), Quantitative Real Time gene expression (qRT-PCR), Deep Serial Analysis Gene Expression (DSAGE). These approaches allow quantifying mRNA and defining gene splice variation. Also, custom or commercially available cDNA microarrays can simultaneously examine the expression of thousands of transcripts from several biological specimens. Most important, the correlation of genomic and transcriptomic strategies allow characterizing transcriptional responses related to HCM mutations, and as so to gain fundamental mechanistic insights that could explain the range of clinical manifestations and symptoms associated with HCM (Watkins *et al.*, 1996; Cooper *et al.*, 2005; Margulies & Matiwala, chapter 36; Lawler *et al.*, 2007; Theis *et al.*, 2009).

For the transcriptional profiling of HCM in human cardiac tissue a range of logistical and technical factors tend to undermine the settlements that could be acquired by this approach. Foremost, all studies obtain failing human ventricular myocardium at the time of myectomy or cardiac transplantation (Margulies & Matiwala, chapter 36). This sampling approach excludes some of the information that could be obtained by a time sampling strategy to enquire about disease progression. If possible, gene expression analysis should be conducted at multiple time points of sampling that has proved to be informative in animal models studies. Also, myocardial profiling from failing hearts is focused in end state of the disease and probably the inherent transcriptional changes correspond to an adaptive cellular and molecular mechanisms rather than the cause of the pathology. Moreover, the time of onset, etiology and therapeutics associated to each individual can confound the true significance of the obtained data. Another logistical issue concerns with the complicated issue to obtain an appropriate healthy human myocardial control tissue. Because of rapid mRNA degradation, samples obtained at necropsy are not suitable.

Despite the above considerations, the use of gene expression analysis does provide an opportunity to take aware of the transcriptional portrait of cardiomyopathies by simultaneous analysis of several genes from diverse pathways. Studies regarding the profiling of transcription patterns in myocardial tissues have already produced novel evidences that contribute to the understanding of cardiomyopathies cardiac remodeling (Lee *et al.*, 2000; Lim *et al.,* 2001; Hawng *et al.*, 2002). An example is related with the molecular distinction between HCM and DCM being these data obtained from transcriptional profiling data (Hwang *et al.*, 2002). In most cases, familial HCM is caused by mutation in one of sarcomeric proteins, while cytoskeletal mutations can lead to a DCM (Fatkin *et al.*, 2002). Hwang *et al.* demonstrated sets of genes that were differentially expressed among the patients with DCM and HCM, despite the common endpoint of severe heart failure (Hwang *et al.*, 2002). Among upregulated genes, the ones related to immune responses were more mostly identified in DCM, while the genes related to protein synthesis were more distinguished in HCM. On the other hand, the genes related to metabolism were more downregulated in DCM than in HCM. Genes related to cell signaling and cell structure tended to be further reduced in HCM compare to DCM (Hwang *et al.*, 2002). In this example the obtained data of transcriptional profiling supports the concept that distinct etiologies of cardiomyopathies, progress through different patterns of cardiac remodeling, involving distinct molecular dynamics. Another example, is regarded the end-stage DCM in which Barrans and collaborators (Barrans *et al.*, 2002) identified a significant transcriptional convergence. These author compared DCM and healthy cardiac tissues and observed the deregulation of more than 100 genes in the failing hearts. In addition it was identified an upregulation of classic markers of hypertrophy, such as sarcomeric and cytoskeletal proteins, transcriptional factors and genes involved with energy metabolism (Barrans *et al.*, 2002).

It is well documented that the cellular responses characteristic of cardiac hypertrophy include an increase in cell size due to accelerated synthesis of sarcomeric and structural proteins, and reprogramming of the fetal cardiac genes (Komuro *et al.*, 1993; Sadoshima *et al.*, 1997). Some of the contractile proteins, ion channels and metabolic enzymes have both fetal and adult isoforms, which have similar, but not identical, functions. Studies regarding gene expression reported that the transcriptional control during cardiac hypertrophy involves switching of gene expression from normally expressed adult isoforms to fetal isoforms (Komuro *et al.*, 1993; Sadoshima *et al.,* 1997; Friddle *et al.*, 2000).

Tan and collaborators (Tan *et al.*, 2002) reported an accentuated transcriptional convergence among the different diseased hearts. Interestingly, many of the deregulated genes in end-stage failing human hearts include the genes also expressed during fetal development. This data supports the evidence that many of the transcriptional changes observed in severely failing human hearts obtained at the time of transplantation are responses to, rather than causes of, sustained myocardial stress and overall the heart failure phenotype (Vikstrom *et al.*, 1998).

Marston *et al* (2009) studied the cellular mechanisms responsible for sarcomere stoichiometric alteration in HCM using human myectomy samples, and were able to demonstrate that mutations in cardiac myosin-binding protein-C (MyBP-C), cause HCM through a mechanism of haploinsufficiency. Most of sarcomere gene mutations that cause HCM are missense alleles that encode dominant negative proteins. MyBP-C mutations are considered an exception as frequently encode truncated proteins. The authors compared ventricular muscle from patients undergoing surgical myectomy with samples from donor hearts (Marston *et al.*, 2009). MyBP-C protein and mRNA levels were quantified from cardiac tissues using immunoblotting and RT-PCR. The absence of any detectable truncated MyBP-C argues against its incorporation in the myofiber and any dominant negative effect. In contrast, the lowered relative level of full length protein in both truncation and missense *MYBPC3* mutations argues strongly that haploinsufficiency is sufficient to cause the disease (Marston *et al.*, 2009).

In addition, recent data have demonstrated that using PMAGE (for "polony multiplex analysis of gene expression") is possible to identify early transcriptional changes that preceded pathological manifestations of HCM in mice carrying a disease-causing mutation (Kim *et al.*, 2007). The authors describe a sensitive mRNA profiling technology that provided a comprehensive profile of cardiac mRNAs, including low-abundance mRNAs encoding signaling molecules and transcription factors that are likely to participate in disease pathogenesis.

In recent years, it has become increasingly apparent that therapeutic interventions have effects on transcriptional profiles in failing hearts prompting the ability to induce regression of the pathological phenotype (Margulies & Matiwala, chapter 36). In both animal models and clinical settings, this phenomenon of so-called 'reverse remodeling' has been observed via both medical interventions and surgical interventions. The cellular and organ level mechanisms that drive the process of myocardial recovery and reverse remodeling are still under enquire in a way similar to the processes that drive the progression of cardiomyopathy in diseased hearts. As so the use of transcriptional profiling may provide new insights into the molecular biology of myocardial reverse remodeling. Interestingly, in what concerns DCM therapeutics and the intrinsic targets, Yasumura and collaborators (2003) identified an increase in SERCA and phospholamban abundance and a decrease in β myosin heavy chain (β -MHC) and sodium-calcium exchanger. Gene expression of right ventricular endomyocardium was assessed by qRT-PCR (Yasamura *et al.*, 2003). These results provide further evidence that β-blocker treatment affects expression of sarcomeric proteins and calcium regulatory proteins (Yasamura *et al.,* 2003). The authors reported that ventricular functional recovery by β-blocker therapy is attributed to time-dependent biologic effects on cardiomyocyte (Yasamura *et al.*, 2003). The obtained data indicate that transcriptional profiling may provide clues of the mechanisms of myocardial adaptations observed during pharmacological therapies. Commonly prescribed therapeutic agents for cardiovascular disease exert pleiotropic effects on cardiomyocytes and cardiac fibroblasts having beneficial outcomes on the remodeling heart. These include drugs for reducing hypertension, as ACE inhibitors, angiotensin receptor blockers, beta-blockers, for cholesterol levels as statins, fibrates and for insulin resistance as thiazolidinediones (Porter *et al.,* 2009).

The above transcriptional profiling studies using human myocardial specimens with cardiomyopathies, and HCM could reveal the mechanisms how gene mutations trigger a variety of transcriptional adaptations. These studies further demonstrate that transcriptional regulation of severe hypertrophy or dysfunction, are more likely to represent model-specific changes rather than non-specific responses to the development of heart failure and myocardial stress or injury (Margulies & Matiwala, chapter 36). Nevertheless, a more accurate evaluation of transcriptional profiling must be complemented with assessments of protein abundance and post-translational modifications.

In parallel with mRNA evaluation, microRNAs (miRNAs), non-protein-coding small RNAs of 20-23 nucleotides, have emerged as one of the central players of gene expression regulation (Thum, 2011). miRNAs act as negative regulators of gene expression by inhibiting the translation or promoting the degradation of target mRNAs (Thum, 2011). Recent studies have uncovered important roles for miRNAs, in the control of diverse aspects of cardiac function (including cardiomyocyte growth, integrity of the ventricular wall and contractility) and of the pathological heart (Olson & Rooj, 2007; Cheng *et al.*, 2007; da Costa Martins *et al.*, 2008; Thum *et al.*, 2008; Wang & Yang, 2012). Specific miRNAs are misexpressed in diseased heart, and gain- and loss-of-function experiments in mice have shown the importance of these miRNAs as necessary and sufficient to evoke cardiac hypertrophy and heart failure (Olson & Rooj, 2007; Divakaran *et al.*, 2008). Microarray and qRT-PCR analyses also have demonstrated a collection of miRNAs that are up/downregulated during pathological cardiac remodeling in hypertrophic and failing hearts (Olson & Rooj 2007; Cheng *et al.*, 2007; da Costa Martins *et al.*, 2008; Thum *et al.*, 2008; Wang & Yang, 2012). *In vitro* experiments using either overexpression or knockdown of miRNAs in cultured cardiomyocytes indicate that a subset of miRNAs are indeed actively involved in cardiomyocyte hypertrophy. However, a major challenge remains in to identify the mRNA targets of the miRNAs that participate in cardiac remodeling and to understand the functions of their target mRNAs. Indeed each miRNA could repress up to hundreds of transcripts, and it is thus hypothesized that miRNAs form large-scale regulatory networks across the transcriptome through miRNA response elements (MREs) (Cheng *et al.*, 2007).

In our research we have been tackling some of the pathways involved in HCM remodeling through an integrated evaluation of the transcriptional profile in human HCM cardiac tissue not only at the level of sarcomere genes expression levels but also miRNA profiling (our unpublished results; Fernandes *et al.*, 2013; Santos *et al.*, 2013 - poster presentations in international meetings). These miRNA expression profiling studies are important for revealing novel miRNA-based pathways underlying the cardiac remodeling and therefore to inquire the potential role for miRNAs in regulating the changes in gene expression that occur during cardiac hypertrophy. As so, the use of specific miRNA for targeting deregulated mRNA could be an opportunity for potential therapeutic of heart diseases, namely in controlling cardiac remodeling typical of HCM, and so specific miRNAs may themselves become therapeutic targets in HCM.

To date, several tools are available to selectively target miRNA pathways. Chemically engineered oligonucleotides, termed "mimic" and "antagomirs", and adenovirus that expresses specific sense or antisense miRNAs, have been developed and evaluated for their therapeutic effect on cardiac diseases (Wang & Yang, 2012). It is possible to use chemically modified oligonucleotide to target specific miRNAs and/or to disrupt the binding between a specific miRNA and a specific mRNA target. Dysregulation of cardiomyocyte miRNAs disturbs cardiac homeostasis by disrupting the cellular responses of cardiomyocytes to various signaling pathways. Recent studies have demonstrated that re-expression of downregulated anti-hypertrophic miRNAs or knockdown of upregulated pro-hypertrophic miRNAs is able to modulate cardiac remodeling, and serve as a promising therapeutic approach (Wang & Yang, 2012).

As tools for diagnosis and clinical evaluation of HCM improve, the lack of rationale therapies for this condition remains a major obstacle in care and management of HCM patients and families. However, genomics and transcriptomics inherent knowledge allow the development of new therapies to slow or prevent disease development. The identification of disease genes in several inherited cardiac diseases has raised expectations for new forms of treatment for some inherited cardiomyopathies there are realistic prospects that molecular insights will soon lead to novel treatments (Watkins *et al.*, 2011). Despite these promising advances, further research continues to determine how the binding of multiple miRNAs affects the expression of individual targeted mRNAs. Also, it is important to understand how multiple miRNA targets are interlinked to affect the various pathways and cardiac remodeling. A new concept- "competing endogenous RNA (ceRNA)" has emerged trying to explain how different types of RNAs interact to each other using MREs (Cheng *et al.*, 2007).

The high frequency of novel genetic alterations, for instance in new genes, identified in genome of HCM patients trough the new sequencing technologies illustrate the difficulties in translating genetics complexity into the clinical framework. Also gene expression evaluation using transcriptomic arrays of mRNA and miRNA still fail to be informative at a diagnostic level. Genetic and transcriptional datasets correlated with clinical datasets will be important to understand how different HCM causal mutations produce HCM clinical manifestations (variable hypertrophy, fibrosis, diastolic dysfunction, arrhythmias and heart failure). Importantly, the knowledge obtained from the data integration of these datasets will be useful in the assessment of genotype–phenotype correlations by identifying low penetrance cases with important clinical implications on HCM therapeutic and prevention. Informatics tools are currently being used to store, integrate and analyse biological, genetic and clinical data.

5   Translational Bioinformatics Approaches in HCM Research

HCM is, as previously demonstrated, a complex disease whose study requires the effective integration and analysis of a number of heterogeneous features that originate from genotypic, phenotypic, and environmental sources. Computational approaches that take into account heterogeneous features, to improve clinical guidelines on treatments and disease prevention, are being developed in a very promising area of research named translational bioinformatics (Drolet & Lourenzi. 2011; Roque *et al.*, 2011). This emerging research field is a discipline that was built on the successes of bioinformatics and health informatics for the study of complex diseases. The American Medical Informatics Association (AMIA), which considers the new field as a third major domain of informatics, defined translational bioinformatics as "... the development of storage, analytic, and interpretive methods to optimize the transformation of increasingly voluminous biomedical data into proactive, predictive, preventative, and participatory health." (Butte, 2009).

In this section we describe how computational approaches, that take advantages of Semantic Web technologies (Berners-Lee *et al.*, 2001), are being developed to model, integrate and analyse large volumes of heterogeneous data, in order to provide new insights for the diagnosis and prognosis of complex diseases like HCM.

Semantic Web and Linked Open Data technologies are being adopted in science and business to overcome the limitations of the conventional data integration approaches and make data as open as possible (see, http://www.w3.org/). During the last decade, several approaches have been put into practice to integrate heterogeneous data sources for the domains of biomedicine, medicine and bioinformatics (Chen *et al.*, 2013; Goble & Stevens, 2008; Antezana *et al.*, 2009a; Agorastos *et al.*, 2009). These new technologies open a new dimension to data integration, a big current challenge in biological and biomedical knowledge management (Attwood *et al.*, 2009; Antezana *et al.*, 2009b). The first approaches that have been developed, using Semantic Web technologies, aimed only to browse, visualize and search RDF data (RDF Primer http://www.w3.org/TR/2004/REC-rdf-primer-20040210/). Now, new developments already include more powerful tools such as the ones required to perform hypothesis testing.

Decision support based on translational bioinformatics means better information and workflow management, efficient literature and resource retrieval, and communication improvement. As new high-throughput typing and sequencing technologies gain popularity and provide unprecedented opportunities to characterize individual genomic landscapes and identify mutations relevant for diagnosis and therapy, data analysis poses significant challenges that led to the development of a large number of tools supporting specific parts of the analysis workflow or providing a complete solution. A typical computational workflow in this context encompasses four stages: (1) Data capture; (2) Data integration; (3) Data Analysis; and (4) Data visualization and reporting.

Acquisition and dissemination of genotypic, phenotypic and clinical data requires the availability and cross compatibility of simple and cost-effective information management systems, to enable more rapid adoption of data collection standards and broader use of comprehensive data and metadata tracking. In a recently proposed translational bioinformatics approach for HCM, the authors focused on the identification of associations between clinical and genotypic data with the objective of helping physicians predict the likely outcome of the disease, for every individual patient, with respect to the occurrence of a sudden cardiac death event (Machado *et al.*, 2012). The proposed framework integrates clinical and genetic data mediated by a semantic data model representing the disease and explores data mining models depicting the clinical-genetic associations.

Still in the context of cardiovascular diseases, another work reasoned that an integrative genomics-phenomics approach could expedite disease candidate gene identification and prioritization. To approach the problem of inferring likely causality roles, the authors generated Semantic Web methods-based network data structures and performed centrality analyses to rank genes according to model-driven semantic relationships (Gudivada *et al.,* 2008). In a different direction, methods have also been proposed to exploit bio-ontologies for guiding data selection within the preparation step of the Knowledge Discovery in Databases (KDD) process. For familial hypercholesterolemia dataset, three scenarios have been proposed in which domain knowledge and ontology elements such as properties and class descriptions have been taken into account for data selection, before the data mining step (Coulet *et al.*, 2008). In the context of cerebrovascular diseases, the Neuroweb European Project (Colombo *et al.,* 2010) was created to support genetic association studies, through the integration of clinical and genetic databases from four clinical institutions. The data is maintained in relational format and at its original location, thus in accordance with a database federation approach. All these systems envisage supporting the development of an open network of data, improving interoperability.

Regarding data integration, it does not only provide better data access, but also improves knowledge representation. Ontologies and controlled vocabularies play an important role at this stage since they provide a standard way of representing knowledge. Usually, these vocabularies are references accepted by a specific user community, such as the Gene Ontology (Ashburner *et al.*, 2000) and the Systematized Nomenclature of Medicine-Clinical Terms (SNOMED-CT) (http://www.ihtsdo.org/snomed-ct/). Strategies based on multiple vocabularies have also been developed, namely in pharmacogenomics considering the Human Disease Ontology and the Pharmacogenomics Knowledge Base (Hoehndorf *et al.*, 2012). New efforts like the Cardiovascular Gene Ontology Annotation Initiative encourage the creation of an information-rich resource for the cardiovascular-research community, enabling researchers to rapidly evaluate and interpret existing data (http://www.ucl.ac.uk/cardiovasculargeneontology).

Most of the times the data integration stage starts with the creation of a semantic model for the domain under study, however one of the important features of using semantic web technologies is that they enable linking the data in a way that the structure that represents the knowledge emerges from the data. This means that the semantic model can emerge from the links between the data.

Usually, building a semantic model for a given disease includes collecting its domain knowledge, e.g. clinical and genetic, in the form of keywords and scientific publications directly from the biomedical experts. This domain knowledge is used to identify relevant biomedical ontologies, to which modularization techniques can be applied in order to extract the modules that contain the concepts of interest. Previous work on semantic modelling on HCM (Machado *et al.*, 2012), has shown that the semantic data model provides a useful framework for the integration of data not only from two heterogeneous domains of knowledge, clinics and genetics, but also from different medical institutions and research groups. In this work the authors propose a semantic model with three modules: 1) *Genotype Analysis* (with 19 concepts and approximately 39 properties), containing concepts associated with the genetic testing of biological samples; 2) *Medical Classifications* (with two high-level concepts: Angina Classification and Heart Failure Classification), containing medical standards used in the characterization of clinical elements such as patient symptoms; and 3) *Clinical Evaluation* (with a total of 63 concepts and approximately 60 object and data properties), that is the main module and that imports the other two. This last module additionally contains administrative concepts and clinical data elements that play an important role in the diagnosis and the prognosis of HCM patients. All the concepts have also been mapped to external controlled vocabularies, such as ontologies, to facilitate the interaction with other systems. Controlled vocabularies like SNOMED CT (version 2010 01 31), the National Cancer Institute Thesaurus (NCIt) (version 10.03), the Gene Regulation Ontology (version 0.5, released on 04 20 2010) and to the Sequence Ontology (released on 11 22 2011) have been considered. The concepts modelled in this work have also been identified and defined with the help of physicians, geneticists and molecular biologists based on the data elements collected during their activities. The model was populated with data from four medical institutions and two research centers. In opposition to ontology modularization state-of-the-art approaches, the work presented by Machado et al. (Machado *et al.*, 2012) did not rely on the exploitation of a single biomedical ontology (Wennerberg *et al.*, 2011), since clinical and genetic conceptualizations have been collected from multiple ontologies. In these scenarios, methods like local evidence content (Couto *et al.*, 2005), ontology matching (Pesquita *et al.*, 2011) and disjunctive common ancestors identification (Couto *et al.*, 2011), can be used to retrieve concepts and keywords from different places. Although these techniques can help in building a semantic model from scratch, it is very important and useful if semantic models can be reused from other diseases or if manually developed models, validated by experts, are made available (Machado *et al.*, 2010). For data storage and access purposes, this framework makes use of the sdlink system (http:/kdbio.inesc-id.pt/sdlink/), which allows the input of the data according to a semantic model or ontology. This system was developed based on Semantic Web technologies (Francisco *et al.*, 2012), and its utilization as a clinical decision support system is under evaluation by physicians and biomedical experts.

Many workflows do not consider data integration and analysis as being part of two different stages, since data-mining techniques can be used both for knowledge extraction to support data representation and to obtain correlations between heterogeneous data sources that will help on the clinical diagnosis. In this context we are considering that upon completion of the data integration stage, the data is analysed by using data mining techniques in order to infer genotype-phenotype correlations, or, more specifically, to develop models for the association between the presence of certain mutations and the resulting physical traits.

In the case of HCM data analysis, the data elements that usually need to be integrated correspond to the presence/absence of each mutation in the genome of the patients (genotypic data) and to the clinical elements upon which the clinicians rely to provide a diagnose (phenotypic and clinical data). The latter normally include the results from physical examinations (e.g. electrocardiogram, echocardiogram), as well as the clinical history of the individual (e.g. age at diagnosis, sudden deaths in the family). Since there is a dynamic aspect associated with this type of disease, an object *date* was included in the top concepts (Person, Procedure, Clinical Finding, Health Care Site and Observable Entity) of the *Clinical Evaluation* module. By detailing a date to every Clinical Finding, that describes a specific stage of the disease, and to the Procedure or Observable entity, which can be a physical examination or a cardiovascular measurement, respectively, it is possible to analyse the evolution of the clinical scenario for each patient.

Although a large number of studies have been conducted on the linkage between specific mutations and the risk of specific illnesses (Roque *et al.*, 2011; Aslam *et al.*, 2011), models for the more general case of genotype to phenotype association in the presence of high disease complexity, both genetic and clinical, remain largely unexplored. Supervised machine learning techniques, such as decision trees and support vector machines, offer the potential to identify more complex relationships than those identified using simple correlation analysis, the standard practice in genotype-phenotype association models. Standard statistical analysis may identify correlations between one or a small set of specific mutations, but in more complex cases these correlations will not be significant enough to lead to concrete diagnosis methods. The models obtained using data mining techniques are expected to be of great interest both in terms of their predictive ability and their practical usability for physicians.

The exponential growth of genomic and also transcriptomic data, along with parallel achievements in acquiring and analyzing clinical data position the biomedical research enterprise to deliver on the promise of personalize medicine. Presently, data generated by new tests overwhelms current information technology systems and human interpretation capabilities. The need for sophisticated data analysis tools is leading the genetics industry to a fundamental shift from a clinical science focus to a translational bioinformatics focus.

6   Key Points and Concluding Remarks

HCM pathogenic mutations remain elusive in 30% to 40% of investigated HCM patients. This may be explained by the limitations of genotyping strategies with respect to yet-to-be discovered genes. Although cardiac hypertrophy is initially compensatory and beneficial, prolongation of this process leads to deleterious outcomes such as heart failure, arrhythmia, and in last instance SCD. Cellular and molecular studies to enquire about cardiac process of adaptation suggest that the genetic mutations cause functional defects that activate signaling molecules that ultimately prompts for cardiac remodeling adaptation. One fundamental issue in HCM has been whether cardiac remodeling encompassing cardiac hypertrophy and fibrosis, once established, can be reversed or prevented. Accordingly, the elucidation of molecular mechanisms underlying key processes generating cardiac hypertrophy is an important subject of intense research from a clinical point of view. The identification of key molecules that contribute to explain HCM phenotypic heterogeneity may provide important clues about the mechanisms by which HCM causes heart cellular remodeling. The knowledge about specific mRNA, miRNAs and their regulated networks will allow using these molecules as key molecular biomarkers related with their function in HCM and the molecular mechanism underlying cardiac hypertrophy and heart failure. Biological heterogeneity has considerable impact on the translation of basic discoveries into clinical ascertainment of genetic cause of human cardiomyopathies. Computational approaches that take into account heterogeneous features for better providing clinical guidelines on treatments and disease prevention are being developed in a very promising area of research named translational bioinformatics. By using new semantic web based knowledge systems it is possible to have an integrated environment for querying, retrieving and analysing linked data and integrate heterogeneous data resources. In the case of HCM data analysis, the data elements that usually need to be integrated correspond to the presence/absence of each mutation in the genome of the patients (genotypic data), transcriptomic data (at the level of mRNA and miRNA) and to the clinical elements upon which the clinicians rely to provide a diagnose (phenotypic and clinical data). Several factors can impact on the availability and utility of genetic testing, such as access to testing, cost of testing and the mutation detection rate. These factors vary greatly depending on the disease and the technology used, nevertheless, genetic testing for HCM is available now at a much lower cost and timeframe and has a relatively high probability (up to 75%) of finding a mutation in a proband (Teekakirikul *et al.*, 2013). Incumbent on the professional ordering genetic testing for HCM is the need to be skilled in interpreting the genetic test results and the consequent counseling based on the integration of the results (positive or negative), the family history, the clinical data of the patient, and any other known affected or unaffected family members. Ideally, the practitioner will also be skilled in the management of the clinical aspects of HCM, integrating the clinical, diagnostic, and therapeutic recommendations based on a synthesis of all data.

Genetic testing for HCM has seen major advancements in recent years with the introduction of new technologies for mutation detection, such as genome-wide sequencing which promises to rapidly increase the rate of variant detection and should enable more families to acquire genotype results. However, this has brought also new challenges for sequence variant interpretation and many variants of uncertain significance are likely to be found. Nevertheles, the positive identification of a mutation or a negative result in a family member can bring great benefits to management of HCM due to a better surveillance programme in the first case and less frequent intervals for clinical screening due to the reduced evidence of genetic risk.The understanding of HCM clinical and genetic heterogeneity and the development of new targeted therapies and accurate genetic diagnosis depends of a multidisciplinary approach that integrates experts in the fields of basic research, pathology, cardiology, medical geneticists and bioinformaticians working closely to bring cutting-edge research advances to manage and improve HCM patient care.

Acknowledgement

Isabel Carreira, Manuel Antunes, Carolino Monteiro, Nuno Cardim, Isabel Gaspar, Cátia Machado and Francisco Couto for their contribution to our work.

References

Aatre, R.D., Day, S.M. (2011). Psychological issues in genetic testing for inherited cardiovascular diseases. Circ Cardiovasc Genet (4):81-90.

Ackerman, M.J., Priori, S.G., Willems, S., Berul, C., Brugada, R., Calkins, H., Camm, A.J., Ellinor, P.T., Gollob, M., Hamilton, R., Hershberger, R.E., Judge, D.P., Le Marec, H., McKenna, W.J., Schulze-Bahr, E., Semsarian, C., Towbin, J.A., Watkins, H., Wilde, A., Wolpert, C., Zipes, D.P. (2011). HRS/EHRA expert consensus statement on the state of genetic testing for the channelopathies and cardiomyopathies this document was developed as a partnership between the Heart Rhythm Society (HRS) and the European Heart Rhythm Association (EHRA). Heart Rhythm (8):1308-1339.

Agorastos, T., Koutkias, V., Falelakis, M., Lekka, I., Mikos, T., Delopoulos, A., Mitkas, P.A., Tantsis, A., Weyers, S., Coorevits, P., Kaufmann, A.M., Kurzeja, R. & Maglaveras, N. (2009). Semantic Integration of Cervical Cancer Data Repositories to Facilitate Multicenter Association Studies: the ASSIST Approach. Cancer Informatics. (8): 31-44.

Alcalai, R., Seidman, J.G., Seidman, C.E. (2008). Genetic basis of hypertrophic cardiomyopathy: From bench to the clinics. J Cardiovasc Electrophysiol (19):104-110.

Alders, M., Jongbloed, R., Deelen, W., van den Wijngaard, A., Doevendans, P., Ten Cate, F., Regitz-Zagrosek, V., Vosberg, H.P., van Langen, I., Wilde, A., et al (2003). The 2373insG mutation in the MYBPC3 gene is a founder mutation, which accounts for nearly one-fourth of the HCM cases in the Netherlands. Eur Heart J (24):1848-1853.

Ahmad F., Seidman J.G., Seidman C.E. (2005). The genetic basis for cardiac remodeling. Annu Rev Genomics Hum Genet (6):185-216.

Andersen, P.S., Havndrup, O., Bundgaard, H., Larsen, L.A., Vuust, J., Pedersen, A.K., Kjeldsenm K., Christiansen, M. (2004). Genetic and phenotypic characterization of mutations in myosin-binding protein C (MYBPC3) in 81 families with familial hypertrophic cardiomyopathy: total or partial haploinsufficiency. Eur J Hum Genet (12):673-677.

Antezana, E., Blond, W., Egaa, M., Rutherford, A., Stevens, R., De Baets, B., Mironov, V., & Kuiper, M. (2009a). BioGateway: a semantic systems biology tool for the life sciences. BMC Bioinformatics, (10):S11

Antezana, E., Kuiper, M., & Mironov, V. (2009b). Biological knowledge management: the emerging role of the Semantic Web technologies Briefings on Bioinformatics (10): 392-407

Arad, M., Maron, B.J., Gorham, J.M., Johnson, W.H. Jr, Saul, J.P., Perez-Atayde, A.R., Spirito, P., Wright, G.B., Kanter, R.J., Seidman, C.E., Seidman, J.G. (2005). Glycogen storage diseases presenting as hypertrophic cardiomyopathy. N Engl J Med (352):362-37214.

Ashburner, M., Ball, C.A., Blake, J.A., Botstein, D., Butler, H., Cherry, J.M., Davis, A.P., Dolinski, K., Dwight, S.S., Eppig, J.T., Harris, M.A., Hill, D.P., Issel- Tarver, L., Kasarskis, A., Lewis, S., Matese, J.C., Richardson, J.E., Ringwald, M., Rubin, G.M. & Sherlock, G. (2000). Gene Ontology: Tool for the Unification of Biology. Nature Genetics (25): 25-29.

Attwood, T.K., Kell, D.B., McDermott, P., Marsh, J., Pettifer, S.R., & Thorne, D. (2009). Calling International Rescue: knowledge lost in literature and data landslide! Biochemical Journal (424): 317-333.

Barrans, J.D., Allen, P.D, Stamatiou, D., Dzau, V.J. Liew C.C. (2002). Global Gene Expression Profiling of End-Stage Dilated Cardiomyopathy Using a Human Cardiovascular-Based cDNA Microarray. Am J Pathol. (160):2035-4.

Basso, C., Thiene, G., Corrado, D., Buja, G., Melacini, P., Nava A. (2000). Hypertrophic cardiomyopathy and sudden death in the young: pathologic evidence of myocardial ischemia. Human pathology.(31):988–998.

Berners-Lee, T., Hendler, J. & Lassila, O. (2001). The SemanticWeb. Scientific American, 29-37.

Biagini, E., Coccolo, F., Ferlito, M., Perugini, E., Rocchi, G., Bacchi-Reggiani, L., Lofiego, C., Boriani, G., Prandstraller, D., Picchio, F.M., Branzi, A.,Rapezzi, C. (2005) Dilated-hypokinetic evolution of hypertrophic cardiomyopathy: prevalence, incidence, risk factors, and prognostic implications in pediatric and adult patients. J Am Coll Cardiol (46): 1543-1550

Butte, AJ. (2009). Translational bioinformatics applications in genome medicine. Genome Medicine (1):64

Bookwalter, C.S., Trybus, K.M. (2006). Functional consequences of a mutation in an expressed human a-cardiac actin at a site implicated in familial hypertrophic cardiomyopathy. J Biol Chem (281):16777–16784.

Bos, J.M., Poley, R.N., Ny, M., Tester, D.J., Xu, X., Vatta, M., Towbin, J.A., Gersh, B.J, Ommen, S.R, Ackerman, M.J. (2006). Genotype phenotype relationships involving hypertrophic cardiomyopathyassociated mutations in titin, muscle LIM protein, and telethonin. Mol Genet Metab (88):78–85.

Carniel, E., Taylor, M.R., Sinagra, G., Di Lenarda, A., Ku, L., Fain, P.R., Boucek, M.M., Cavanaugh, J., Miocic, S., Slavov, D., Graw, S.L., Feiger, J., Zhu, X.Z., Dao, D., Ferguson, D.A., Bristow M,R., Mestroni, L. (2005). Alpha-

myosin heavy chain: a sarcomeric gene associated with dilated and hypertrophic phenotypes of cardiomyopathy. Circulation. (5);112(1):54-9.

Chang, A.N., Harada, K., Ackerman, M.J., Potter, J.D. (2005). *Functional consequences of hypertrophic and dilated cardiomyopathy-causing mutations in alfa-tropomyosin. J Biol Chem (280):34343–34349.*

Charron, P. , Dubourg, O., Desnos, M., Isnard, R., Hagege, A., Bonne, G., Carrier, L., Tesson, F., Bouhour, J.B., Buzzi, J.C., Feingold, J., Schwartz, K., Komajda, M. (1998) *Genotype–phenotype correlations in familial hypertrophic cardiomyopathy: a comparison between mutations in the cardiac protein-C and the β-myosin heavy chain genes. Eur Heart J (19): 139–145*

Chen, H., Yu, T., & Chen, J.Y. (2013). *Semantic Web meets Integrative Biology: a survey Briefings on Bioinformatics (14): 109-125.*

Cheng, Y., Ji, R., Yue, J., Yang, J., Liu, X., Chen, H., Dean, D.B., Zhang C. (2007). *MicroRNAs are aberrantly expressed in hypertrophic heart: do they play a role in cardiac hypertrophy? Am. J. Pathol. (170):1831-40.*

Cirino, A.L., & Ho, C.Y. (2011). *Familial Hypertrophic Cardiomyopathy Overview. GeneReviews™ Pagon RA, Adam MP, Bird TD, editors. Seattle, University of Washington.*

Clerk, A., Cullingford, T.E., Fuller, S.J., Giraldo, A., Markou, T., Pikkarainen, S., Sugden, P.H.. (2007). *Signaling pathways mediating cardiac myocyte gene expression in physiological and stress responses. J Cell Physiol. (212):311-22.*

Colombo, G., Merico, D., Boncoraglio, G., Paoli, F.D., Ellul, J., Frisoni, G., Nagy, Z., van der Lugt, A., Vassanyi, I. & Antoniotti, M. (2010). *An Ontological Modeling Approach to Cerebrovascular Disease Studies: the NEUROWEB Case. Journal Biomedical Informatics (43): 469-484*

Cooper, T.A. (2005). *Alternative Splicing Regulation Impacts Heart Development. Cell. (120):1-2.*

Coulet, A., Smail-Tabbone, M., Benlian, P., Napoli, A., & Devignes, M., (2008). *Ontology-guided data preparation for discovering genotype-phenotype relationships. BMC Bioinformatics (9): S3*

Couto, F.M., Silva, M.J. & Coutinho, P.M. (2005). *Finding genomic ontology terms in text using evidence content. BMC Bioinformatics (6): S21*

Dhandapany, P.S., Sadayappan, S., Xue, Y., Powell, G.T., Rani, D.S., Nallari, P., Rai, T.S., Khullar, M., Soares, P., Bahl, A., et al (2009). *A common MYBPC3 (cardiac myosin binding protein C) variant associated with cardiomyopathies in South Asia. Nat Genet (41):187-191.*

Divakaran, V. & Mann, D.L. (2008).*The Emerging Role of MicroRNAs in Cardiac Remodeling and Heart Failure. Circulation Research.(103): 1072-1083.*

Drolet, BC. & Lorenzi, NM. (2011). *Translational research: understanding the continuum from bench to bedside, Translational Research (157): 1-5.*

Erdmann, J., Daehmlow, S., Wischke, S., Senyuva, Mm, Werner, U., Raible, J., Tanis, N., Dyachenko, S., Hummel, M., Hetzer, R., Regitz-Zagrosek, V. (2003). *Mutation spectrum in a large cohort of unrelated consecutive patients with hypertrophic cardiomyopathy. Clin Genet. (64): 339-349.*

Fatkin, D, Graham, R.M. (2002). *Molecular Mechanisms of Inherited Cardiomyopathies. Physiol Rev (82): 945–980.*

Fernandes, A.R., Marques, V., Nunes, A.C., Freitas, A.T., Gouveia, M.R., Antunes, M., Carreira, I.M., Gaspar, I.M., Monteiro, C., Santos S. (2013). *microRNA Transcriptional Evaluation in Obstructive Hypertrophic Cardiomyopathy: a preliminary study using human myectomy samples. Cardiac Remodeling, Signaling Matrix and Heart function. Flash Presentation. Keystone Symposia 2013.*

Francisco A., Reis P.M., Abdulrehman D., Vaz C., Santos M., & Freitas A.T. (2012). *sdlink: An Integrated System for Linking Biological and Biomedical Semantic Data. Conference on Semantics in Healthcare and Life Sciences (CSHALS).*

Friddle, C.J., Koga, T., Rubin, E.M., Bristow, J. (2000). *Expression profiling reveals distinct sets of genes altered during induction and regression of cardiac hypertrophy. Proc Natl Acad Sci U S A. (97):6745–50.*

Geier, C., Gehmlich, K., Ehler, E., Hassfeld, S., Perrot, A., Hayess, K., Cardim, N., Wenzel, K., Erdmann, B., Krackhardt, F., Posch, M.G., Osterziel, K.J., Bublak, A., Nagele, H., Scheffold, T., Dietz, R., Chien, K.R., Spuler, S., Furst, D.O., Nurnberg, P., Ozcelik, C. (2008). Beyond the sarcomere: cSRP3 mutations cause hypertrophic cardiomyopathy. Hum Mol Genet (17):2753-2765.

Gersh, B.J., Maron, B.J., Bonow, R.O., Dearani, J.A., Fifer, M.A., Link, M.S., Naidu, S.S., Nishimura, R.A., Ommen, S.R., Rakowski, H., Seidman, C.E., Towbin, J.A., Udelson, J.E., Yancy, C.W. (2011). ACCF/AHA guideline for the diagnosis and treatment of hypertrophic cardiomyopathy: executive summary: A report of the American College of Cardiology Foundation/American Heart Association Task Force on Practice Guidelines. Circulation (124): 2761–2796.

Girolami, F. Olivotto, I. Passerini,. I. , Zachara, E., Nistri, S., Re, F., Fantini, S., Baldini, K., Torricelli, F., Cecchi, F.(2006). A molecular screening strategy based on beta-myosin heavy chain, cardiac myosin binding protein C and troponin T genes in Italian patients with hypertrophic cardiomyopathy. J Cardiovasc Med (Hagerstown). (7:)601-607

Goble, C. & Stevens R. (2008). State of the nation in data integration for bioinformatics. Journal of Biomedical Informatics (41): 687-693.

Gudivada, R.C., Qu, X.A., Chen, J., Jegga, A.G., Neumann, E.K. & Aronow, B.J. (2008). Identifying Disease-Causal Genes Using Semantic Web-based Representation of Integrated Genomic and Phenomic Knowledge. Journal Biomedical Informatics (41): 717-729.

Harris, K.M., Spirito, P., Maron, M.S., Zenovich, A.G., Formisano, F., Lesser, J.R., Mackey-Bojack, S., Manning, W.J., Udelson, J.E., Maron, B.J. (2006). Prevalence, clinical profile, and significance of left ventricular remodeling in the end-stage phase of hypertrophic cardiomyopathy. Circulation (114): 216-225.

Harvey, P.A. & Leinwand, L.A. (2011). Cellular mechanisms of cardiomyopathy. J. Cell Biol. (194):355–365.

Hayashi, T., Arimura, T., Itoh-Satoh, M., Ueda, K., Hohda, S., Inagaki, N., Takahashi, M., Hori, H., Yasunami, M., Nishi, H., Koga, Y., Nakamura, H., Matsuzaki, M., Choi, B.Y., Bae, S.W., You, C.W., Han, K.H., Park, J.E., Knöll, R., Hoshijima, M., Chien, K.R., Kimura, A. (2004). Tcap gene mutations in hypertrophic cardiomyopathy and dilated cardiomyopathy. J Am Coll Cardiol (44):2192–2201.

Heller, M.J., Nili, M., Homsher, E., Tobacman, L.S. (2003). Cardiomyopathic tropomyosin mutations that increase thin filament Ca2þ sensitivity and tropomyosin N-domain flexibility. J Biol Chem (278):41742–41748.

Hershberger, R.E., Lindenfeld, J., Mestroni, L.,Seidman, C.E. Taylor, M.R.G., Towbin, J.A. (2009). Genetic Evaluation of Cardiomyopathy - A Heart Failure Society of America Practice Guideline. Journal of Cardiac Failure (15): 83-97.

Ho, C.Y. (2010). Genetics and clinical destiny: improving care in hypertrophic cardiomyopathy. Circulation (122):2430-2440.

Ho, C.Y. (2010a). Hypertrophic cardiomyopathy. Heart Fail Clin (6):141-159.

Hoehndorf, R., Dumontier, M. & Gkoutos, G. (2012). Identifying aberrant pathways through integrated analysis of knowledge in pharmacogenomics. Bioinformatics, (28) :2169-2175.

Hwang, J.J, Allen, P.D., Tseng, G.C, Lam, C.W, Fananapazir, L., Dzaul, V.J., Liew, C.C. (2002). Microarray gene expression profiles in dilated and hypertrophic cardiomyopathic end-stage heart failure. Physiol Genomics. (10): 31–44.

Ingles, J., Doolan, A., Chiu, C., Seidman, J., Seidman, C., Semsarian, C. (2005). Compound and double mutations in patients with hypertrophic cardiomyopathy: implications for genetic testing and counselling. J Med Genet. (42):10,e59.

Ionita-Laza, I., Lange, C., Laird, M.N. (2009). Estimating the number of unseen variants in the human genome. Proc Natl Acad Sci USA (106):5008-5013.

Karibe, A., Tobacman, L.S., Strand, J., Butters, C., Back, N., Bachinski, L.L., Arai, A.E., Ortiz, A., Roberts, R., Homsher, E., Fananapazir, L. (2001). Hypertrophic cardiomyopathy caused by a novel alpha-tropomyosin mutation (V95A) is associated with mild cardiac phenotype, abnormal calcium binding to troponin, abnormal myosin cycling, and poor prognosis.Circulation (103):65–71.

Keren, A., Syrris, P, McKenna, W.J. (2008). Hypertrophic cardiomyopathy: the genetic determinants of clinical disease expression. Nat Clin Pract Cardiovasc Med. (3):158-68.

Kehat, I., Molkentin, J.D. (2010). Molecular Pathways Underlying Cardiac Remodeling During Pathophysiological Stimulation. Circulation (122): 2727-2735.

Kim, J.B., Porreca, G.J., Song, L., Greenway, S.C., Gorham, J.M., Church G.M., Seidman,   C.E., Seidman, J.G.   (2007). Polony multiplex analysis of gene expression (PMAGE) in mouse hypertrophic cardiomyopathy. Science (316):1481–1484

Kimura A, Harada H, Park JE, Nishi H, Satoh M, Takahashi M et al. Mutations in the cardiac troponin I gene associated with hypertrophic cardiomyopathy. Nat Genet 1997;16:379–382.

Klues, H.G., Schiffers, A. Maron, B.J. (1995) Phenotypic spectrum and patterns of left ventricular hypertrophy in hypertrophic cardiomyopathy: morphologic observations and significance as assessed by two-dimensional echocardiography in 600 patients. J. Am. Coll. Cardiol. (26):1699-1708.

Komuro, I., Yazak,i Y. (1993). Control of cardiac gene expression by mechanical stress. Annu Rev Physiol. (55): 55–75.

Landstrom, A.P., Adekola, B.A., Bos. J.M., Ommen, S.R, Ackerman, M.. (2011). PLN-encoded phospholamban mutation in a large cohort of hypertrophic cardiomyopathy cases: summary of the literature and implications for genetic testing. J Am Heart J.161(1):165-71

Landstrom, A.P., Ackerman, M.J. (2012). Beyond the cardiac myofilament: hypertrophic cardiomyopathy- associated mutations in genes that encode calcium-handling proteins. Curr Mol Med.12(5):507-18.

Lawler, P.R., Yongzhong, W., Steinbrüchel D., Blagoja, D., Paulsson-Berne, G., Kastrup, J., Hansson, G.K. (2007). Gene expression signals involved in ischemic injury, extracellular matrix composition and fibrosis defined by global mRNA profiling of the human left ventricular myocardium. Journal of Molecular and Cellular Cardiology. (42): 870–883

Lee, M.L., Kuo, F.C., Whitmore, G.A., Sklar, J. (2000) Importance of replication in microarray gene expression studies: statistical methods and evidence from repetitive cDNA hybridizations.Proc Natl Acad Sci USA (97): 9834–9839.

Lim, D.S., Roberts, R., Marian, A.J. (2001). Expression profiling of cardiac genes in human hypertrophic cardiomyopathy: insight into the pathogenesis of phenotypes. J Am Coll Cardiol (38):1175–1180.

Lopes, L.R., Rahman, M.S., Elliott, P.M. (2013). A systematic review and meta-analysis of genotype–phenotype associations in patients with hypertrophic cardiomyopathy caused by sarcomeric protein mutations. Heart doi:10.1136/heartjnl-2013-303939.

Lopes, L.R., Zekavati, A., Syrris, P., Hubank, M., Giambartolomei, C., Dalageorgou, C., Jenkins, S., McKenna, W., Elliott, P.M.. (2013b). Genetic complexity in hypertrophic cardiomyopathy revealed by high-throughput sequencing. J Med Genet.;50(4):228-39.

Manabe, I., Shindo, T., Nagai, R. (2002). Gene expression in fibroblasts and fibrosis: involvement in cardiac hypertrophy. Circ Res. (91):1103–13

Machado, C., Couto, F.M., Fernandes, A.R., Santos, S., & Freitas, A.T. (2012). Toward a Translational Medicine Approach for Hypertrophic Cardiomyopathy. 3rd International Conference on Information Technology in Bio- and Medical Informatics, LNCS (7451): 151-165.

Machado. C., Couto, F.M., Fernandes, A.R., Santos, S., Cardim, N., & Freitas, A.T. (2010). Semantic characterization of hypertrophic cardiomyopathy disease. First Workshop on Knowledge Engineering, Discovery and Dissemination in Health (KEDDH).

Margulies, K.B & Matiwala, S. (2005). Molecular Mechanisms Of Cardiac Hypertrophy And Failure. Taylor and Francis. Edited by Richard A Walsh. Chapter 36: 797-816.

Marian, A.J. (2000). Pathogenesis of diverse clinical and pathological phenotypes in hypertrophic cardiomyopathy. Lancet (355):58-60.

Marian, A.J., Roberts, R. (2001). The molecular genetic basis for hypertrophic cardiomyopathy. J Mol Cell Cardiol (33):655.

Maron, B.J., Bonow, R.O., Cannon, R.O., Leon, M.B., Epstein, S.E. (1987). Hypertrophic cardiomyopathy: interrelations of clinical manifestations, pathophysiology, and therapy. N Engl J Med. (316):780-9.

Maron, B.J., Casey, S.A., Hauser, R.G., Aeppli, D.M. (2003). Clinical course of hypertrophic cardiomyopathy with survival to advanced age. J Am. Coll Cardiol (42):882-888.

Maron, B.J., Gardin, J.M., Flack, J.M., Gidding, S.S., Kurosaki, T.T., Bild, D.E. (1995). Prevalence of hypertrophic cardiomyopathy in a general population of young adults. Echocardiographic analysis of 4111 subjects in the CARDIA Study. Coronary Artery Risk Development in (Young) Adults. Circulation. (92):785–789.

Maron, M.S., Olivotto, I., Betocchi, S., Casey, S.A., Lesser, J.R., Losi, M.A., Cecchi, F., Maron, B.J.(2003). Effect of left ventricular outflow tract obstruction on clinical outcome in hypertrophic cardiomyopathy. N Engl J Med. (348):295-303.

Maron, M.S., Olivotto, I., Zenovich, A.G., Link, M.S., Pandian, N.G., Kuvin, J.T., Nistri, S., Cecchi, F., Udelson, J.E., Maron, B.J. (2006). Hypertrophic cardiomyopathy is predominantly a disease of left ventricular outflow tract obstruction. Circulation (114): 2232–2239.

Maron, B.J., Seidman, J.G., Seidman, C.E. (2004). Proposal for contemporary screening strategies in families with hypertrophic cardiomyopathy. J Am Coll Cardiol. (44): 2125–2132.

Maron BJ, Semsarian C. (2010). Emergence of gene mutation carriers and the expanding disease spectrum of hypertrophic cardiomyopathy. Eur Heart J. (31): 1551-3

Marston, S., Copeland, O., Jacques, A., Livesey, K., Tsang, V., McKenna, W.J., Jalilzadeh, S., Carballo, S., Redwood,, C., Watkins, H. (2009). Evidence from human myectomy samples that MYBPC3 mutations cause hypertrophic cardiomyopathy through haploinsufficiency. Circ Res. (105):219-22.

Millat, G., Chanavat, V., Crehalet, H., Rousson, R. (2010). Development of a high resolution melting method for the detection of genetic variations in hypertrophic cardiomyopathy. Clin Chim Acta Int J Clin Chem (411):1983-1991.

Miller, S.W. (2009). Cardiac Imaging: The Requisites. By Stephen W. Miller, Suhny Abbara, Lawrence Boxt, Mosby Elsevier, Philadelphia.

Mogensen, J., Murphy, R.T., Kubo, T., Bahl, A., Moon, J.C., Klausen, I.C., Elliott, P.M., McKenna, W.J. (2004). Frequency and clinical expression of cardiac troponin I mutations in 748 consecutive families with hypertrophic cardiomyopathy. J Am Coll Cardiol (44):2315–2531.

Moolman, J.C., Corfield, V.A., Posen, B., Ngumbela, K., Seidman, C., Brink, P.A., Watkins, H. (1997). Sudden death due to troponin T mutations. J Am Coll Cardiol (29): 549–555 32.

Moon, J.C., McKenna, W.J., McCrohon, J.A., Elliott, P.M., Smith, G.C., Pennell, D.J. (2003). Toward clinical risk assessment in hypertrophic cardiomyopathy with gadolinium cardiovascular magnetic resonance. J Am Coll Cardiol. (41):1561-7.

Morita, H., Rehm, H.L., Menesses, A., McDonough, B., Roberts, A.E., Kucherlapati, R., Towbin, J.A., Seidman, J.G., Seidman, C.E. (2008). Shared genetic causes of cardiac hypertrophy in children and adults. N Engl J Med (358):1899-1908.

Niimura, H., Bachinski, L.L., Sangwatanaroj, S., Watkins, H., Chudley, A.E., McKenna, W., Kristinsson, A., Roberts, R., Sole, M., Maron, B.J.,Seidman, J.G., Seidman, C.E. (1998). Mutations in the gene for cardiac myosin-binding protein C and late- onset familial hypertrophic cardiomyopathy. N Engl J Med. 338:1248–1257.

Niimura, H., Patton, K.K., McKenna, W.J., Soults, J., Maron, B.J., Seidman, J.G., Seidman, C.E. (2002). Sarcomere protein gene mutations in hypertrophic cardiomyopathy of the elderly. Circulation (105):446-451.

Nishikawa, T., Ishiyama, S., Shimojo, T., Takeda, K., Kasajima, T., Momma, K. (1996). Hypertrophic cardiomyopathy in Noonan syndrome. Acta Paediatr Jpn (38):91-98.

Olivotto, I., Cecchi, F., Casey, S.A., Dolara, A., Traverse, J.H, Maron, B.J. (2001). Impact of atrial fibrillation on the clinical course of Hypertrophic Cardiomyopathy. Circulation. (104):2517-24.

Olson, T.M., Doan, T.P., Kishimoto, N.Y, Whitby, F.G., Ackerman, M.J., Fananapazir, L. (2000). Inherited and de novo mutations in the cardiac actin gene cause hypertrophic cardiomyopathy. J Mol Cell Cardiol (32):1687–94.

Osio, A., Tan, L., Chen, S.N., Lombardi, R., Nagueh, S.F., Shete, S., Roberts, R., Willerson, J.T., Marian, A.J. (2007). Myozenin 2 is a novel gene for human hypertrophic cardiomyopathy. Circ Res (100):766–768.

Osterziel, K.J., Bit-Avragim, N., Bunse, M. (2002). Cardiac hypertrophy in Friedreich's ataxia. Cardiovasc Res (54):694.

Poetter, K., Jiang, H., Hassanzadeh, S., Master, S.R., Chang, A., Dalakas, M.C., Rayment, I., Sellers, J.R., Fananapazir, L., Epstein, N.D. (1996). Mutations in either the essential or regulatory light chains of myosin are associated with a rare myopathy in human heart and skeletal muscle. Nat Genet (13):63–69.

Porter, K.E., Turner, N.A. (2009). Cardiac fibroblasts: at the heart of myocardial remodeling . Pharmacol Ther. (123):255-78.

Posch,, M.G., Thiemann, L., Tomasov, P., Veselka,J., Cardim, N., Garcia-Castro, M., Coto, E., Perrot, A., Geier, C., Dietz, R., Haverkamp, W., Ozcelik, C. (2008). Sequence analysis of myozenin 2 in 438 european patients with familial hypertrophic cardiomyopathy. Med Sci Monit. (14): CR372-CR374.

Richard, P., Charron, P., Carrier, L., Ledeuil, C., Cheav, T., Pichereau, C., Benaiche, A., Isnard, R., Dubourg, O., Burban, M., Gueffet, J.P., Millaire, A., Desnos, M., Schwartz, K., Hainque, B., Komajda, M.; EUROGENE Heart Failure Project. (2003). Hypertrophic cardiomyopathy: distribution of disease genes, spectrum of mutations, and implications for a molecular diagnosis strategy. Circulation (107):2227-2232.

Rooij, E. & Olson, E.N. (2007). MicroRNAs: powerful new regulators of heart disease and provocative therapeutic targets. J Clin Invest (117):2369–2376.

Roque, F.S., Jensen, P.B., Schmock, H., Dalgaard. M., Andreatta. M., et al. (2011) Using Electronic Patient Records to Discover Disease Correlations and Stratify Patient Cohorts. PLoS Computational Biology (7): e1002141.

Rozenfeld, P., Neumann, P.M. (2011). Treatment of fabry disease: current and emerging strategies. Curr Pharm Biotechnol (12):916-922.

Sachdev, B., Takenaka, T., Teraguchi, H., Tei, C., Lee, P., McKenna, W.J., Elliott, P.M. (2002). Prevalence of Anderson-Fabry disease in male patients with late onset hypertrophic cardiomyopathy. Circulation (105): 1407-1411.

Sadoshima, J., Izumo, S. (1997). The cellular and molecular response of cardiac myocytes to mechanical stress. Annu Rev Physiol. (59):551–71.

Santos, S., Cavaco, D., Adragão, P., Sá, I.; Carreira, I.; Antunes, M., Cardim, N., Monteiro, C. (2009). Familial mutation screening and gene expression evaluation in hypertrophic cardiomyopathy profiling: implications for a molecular diagnosis strategy. Oral presentation. 28th Annual Scientific Meeting of the Belgian Society of Cardiology.

Santos, S., Fernandes, A.R., Freitas, A.T., Machado, C.M, Branco, P., Silveira, L., Carreira, I., Antunes, M., Monteiro, C. (2010). HCM sarcomere gene expression analysis: a machine learning approach". Key Note Speaker. Advances in qPCR European Conference, Select Biosciences. Dublin, Ireland.

Santos, S, Lança, V., Oliveira, H., Branco, P., Silveira, L., Marques, V., Brito, D., Madeira, H., Bicho, M., Fernandes, A.R. (2011). "Genetic diagnostic of hypertrophic cardiomyopathy using Mass Spectrometry and High Resolution Melting". Rev Port Cardiol. (30):7-18.

Santos, S., Marques, V., Pires, M., Nunes, A.C., Freitas, A.T., Gouveia, R., Antunes, M., Carreira, I., Gaspar, I.M., Monteiro, C., Fernandes, A.R. (2013). Novel insights in Hypertrophic Cardiomyopathy (HCM) evaluation: miRs as biomarkers of HCM cardiac remodeling. Flash Presentation. Heart Failure Congress. European Society of Cardiology.

Santos, S., Marques, V., Pires, M., Silveira, L., Oliveira, H., Lança, V., Brito, D., Madeira, H., Carreira, I.M., Gaspar, I.M., Monteiro, C., Fernandes, A.R. (2012). "High resolution melting: improvements in the genetic diagnosis of Hypertrophic Cardiomyopathy in a Portuguese cohort". BMC Medical Genetics (13):13-17.

Satoh, M., Takahashi, M., Sakamoto, T., Hiroe, M., Marumo, F., Kimura, A. (1999). Structural analysis of the titin gene in hypertrophic cardiomyopathy: identification of a novel disease gene. Biochem Biophys Res Commun (262):411–417.

Seidman, J.G. & Seidman, C. (2001). The genetic basis for cardiomyopathy: from mutation identification to mechanistic paradigms. Cell. Feb 23;104(4):557-67

Seidman, C.E. & Seidman, J.G. (2011). Identifying sarcomere gene mutations in hypertrophic cardiomyopathy: a personal history. Circ Res (108):743-750.

Sequeira, V., Wijnker, P.J.M., Nijenkamp, L.L.A.M., Kuster, D.W.D., Najafi, A., Witjas-Paalberends, E.R., Regan, J.A., Boontje, N., ten Cate, F.J., Germans, T., Carrier, L., Sadayappan, S., van Slegtenhorst, M.A., Zaremba, R., Foster, D.B., Murphy, A.M., Poggesi, C., dos Remedios, C., Stienen, G.J.M., Ho, C.Y., Michels, M. & van der Velden, J. (2013). Perturbed Length-Dependent Activation in Human Hypertrophic Cardiomyopathy With Missense Sarcomeric Gene Mutations Novelty and Significance. Circ Res. (112):1491-1505.

Semsarian, C., Ahmad, I., Giewat, M., Georgakopoulos, D., Schmitt, J.P., McConnell, B.K., Reiken, S., Mende, U., Marks, A.R., Kass, D.A., Seidman, C.E., Seidman, J.G. (2002). The L-type calcium channel inhibitor diltiazem prevents cardiomyopathy in a mouse model. J Clin Invest (109):1013-1020.

Tan, F.L., Moravec, C.S., Li, J., Apperson-Hansen, C, McCarthy, P.M., Young J.B.,, Bond, M. (2002). The gene expression fingerprint of human heart failure. Proc Natl Acad Sci USA. (99):11387–92.

Teekakirikul, P., Eminaga, S., Toka, O., Alcalai, R., Wang, L., Wakimoto, H., Nayor, M., Konno, T., Gorham, J.M., Wolf, C.M., Kim, J.B., Schmitt. J.P., Molkentin, J.D., Norris, R.A., Tager, A.M., Hoffman, S.R., Markwald, R.R., Seidman, C.E., Seidman, J.G. (2010). Cardiac fibrosis in mice with hypertrophic cardiomyopathy is mediated by non-myocyte proliferation and requires Tgf-b. J Clin Invest (120):3520-3529.

Teekakirikul, P, Kelly, M.A., Rehm, H.L., Lakdawala, N.K., & Funke, B.H. (2013).Inherited Cardiomyopathies Molecular Genetics and Clinical Genetic Testing in the Postgenomic Era. The Journal of Molecular Diagnostics (15):158-170.

Tian T., Liu Y., Zhou X. & Song L. (2013). Progress in the Molecular Genetics of Hypertrophic Cardiomyopathy: A Mini-Review. Gerontology (59):199–205.

Theis, J.L., Bos, J.M., Theis, J.D., Miller, D.V., Dearani, J.A., Schaff, H.V., Gersh, B.J., Ommen, S.R., Moss, R.L., Ackerman, M.J. (2009). Expression Patterns of Cardiac Myofilament Proteins - Genomic and Protein Analysis of Surgical Myectomy Tissue from Patients with Obstructive Hypertrophic Cardiomyopathy. Circ Heart Fail. (2):325-33.

Thierfelder, L., Watkins, H., MacRae, C., Lamas, R., McKenna, W., Vosberg, H.P., Seidman, J.G., Seidman, C. (1994). Alpha-tropomyosin and cardiac troponin T mutations cause familial hypertrophic cardiomyopathy: a disease of the sarcomere. Cell (77):701–12.

Thum, T. (2011). MicroRNA therapeuthics in cardiovascular Medicine. EMBO Mol Med (4): 3-14.

Thum, T, Catalucci, D., Bauersachs, J. (2008). MicroRNAs: novel regulators in cardiac development and disease. Cardiovascular Research. (79), 562–570.

Van Driest ,S.L., Ommen, S.R., Tajik, A.J., Gersh, B.J., Ackerman, M.J. (2005). Sarcomeric genotyping in hypertrophic cardiomyopathy. Mayo Clin Proc. (80):463-469.

Varnava, A.M., Elliott, P.M., Baboonian, C., Davison, F., Davies, M.J., McKenna, W.J. (2001). Hypertrophic cardiomyopathy: histopathological features of sudden death in cardiac troponin T disease. Circulation (104):1380–1384

Varnava, A.M., Elliott, P.M., Mahon, N., Davies, M.J., McKenna, W.J. (2001). Relation between myocyte disarray and outcome in hypertrophic cardiomyopathy. The American journal of cardiology. (88):275–279

Vang, S., Corydon, T.J., Borglum, A.D., Scott, M.D., Frydman, J., Mogensen, J., Gregersen, N., Bross, P. (2005). Actin mutations in hypertrophic and dilated cardiomyopathy cause inefficient protein folding and perturbed filament formation. Febs J (272):2037–2049.´

Vasile, V.C., Will, M.L., Ommen, S.R., Edwards, W.D., Olson, T.M., Ackerman, M.J. (2006). Identification of a metavinculin missense mutation, R975W, associated with both hypertrophic and dilated cardiomyopathy. Mol Genet Metab. (87):169-174.

Vikstrom, K.L., Bohlmeyer, T., Factor, S.M., Leinwand, L.A. (1998). Hypertrophy, pathology, and molecular markers of cardiac pathogenesis. Circ Res. (82):773–8.

Villard E, Perret C, Gary F, Proust C, Dilanian G, Hengstenberg C, Ruppert V, Arbustini E, Wichter T, Germain M, Dubourg O, Tavazzi L, Aumont MC, DeGroote P, Fauchier L, Trochu JN, Gibelin P, Aupetit JF, Stark K, Erdmann J, Hetzer R, Roberts AM, Barton PJ, Regitz-Zagrosek V; Cardiogenics Consortium, Aslam U, Duboscq-Bidot L, Meyborg M, Maisch B, Madeira H, Waldenström A, Galve E, Cleland JG, Dorent R, Roizes G, Zeller T, Blankenberg S, Goodall AH, Cook S, Tregouet DA, Tiret L, Isnard R, Komajda M, Charron P, Cambien F. A genome-wide association study identifies two loci associated with heart failure due to dilated cardiomyopathy. (2011). European Heart Journal, (32): 1065-1076.

Wang, L., Seidman, J.G., Seidman, C.E. (2010). Narrative review: harnessing molecular genetics for the diagnosis and management of hypertrophic cardiomyopathy. Ann. Intern. Med. (152):513–520: W181.

Wang, J. & Yang, X. (2012). The function of miRNA in cardiac hypertrophy. Cell Mol Life Sci.(69): 3561–3570.

Watkins, H., Rosenzweig, A., Hwang, D.S., Levi, T., McKenna, W., Seidman, C.E., Seidman, J.G. (1992). Characteristics and prognostic implications of myosin missense mutations in familial hypertrophic cardiomyopathy. N Engl J Med (326):1108–14.

Watkins, H., McKenna, W.J., Thierfelder, L., Suk, H.J., Anan, R., O'Donoghue, A., Spirito, P., Matsumori, A., Moravec, C.S., Seidman, J.G., Seidman, C.E. (1995). Mutations in the genes for cardiac troponin T and alpha-tropomyosin in hypertrophic cardiomyopathy. N Engl J Med (332):1058-1064.

Watkins, H., Conner, D., Thierfelder, L., Jarcho, J.A., MacRae, C., McKenna, W.J., Maron, B.J., Seidman, J.G., Seidman, C.E. (1995b). Mutations in the cardiac myosin binding protein-C gene on chromosome 11 cause familial hypertrophic cardiomyopathy. Nat Genet (11):434–7.

Watkins, H., Ashrafian, H., Redwood, C. (2011). Inherited Cardiomyopathies. N Engl J Med. (364):1643-56

Wennerberg, P., Schulz, K., & Buitelaar, P. (2011). Ontology modularization to improve semantic medical image annotation. Journal Biomedical Informatics (44): 155-162.

Wheeler, M., Pavlovic, A., DeGoma, E., Salisbury, H., Brown, C., Ashley, E.A. (2009). A new era in clinical genetic testing for hypertrophic cardiomyopathy. J Cardiovasc Transl Res (2):381-391.

Witjas-Paalberends, E.R. Piroddi, N., Stam, K., van Dijk, S.J., Sequeira, V., Ferrara, C., Scellini, B., Hazebroek, M., ten Cate, F.J., van Slegtenhorst, M., dos Remedios, C., Niessen, H.W.M., Tesi, C., Stienen, G.J.M., Heymans, S., Michels, M., Poggesi, C., & van der Velden, J. (2013). Mutations in MYH7 reduce the force generating capacity of sarcomeres in human familial hypertrophic cardiomyopathy. Cardiovascular Research doi: 10.1093/cvr/cvt119.

Wong, W.W., Doyle, T.C., Cheung, P., Olson, T.M., Reisler, E. (2001). Functional studies of yeast actin mutants corresponding to human cardiomyopathy mutations. J Muscle Res Cell Motil (22):665–674

Yasumura, Y, Takemura, K, Sakamoto, A, Kitakaze, M, Miyatake, K. (2003). ,Journal of Cardiac Failure. Changes in myocardial gene expression associated with β-blocker therapy in patients with chronic heart failure. J Card Fail. (9):469-74.

Glia and Blood-retinal Barrier: Effects of Ocular Hypertension

José M. Ramírez, Blanca Rojas, Beatriz I. Gallego
Elena S. García-Martín, Alberto Triviño
Instituto de Investigaciones Oftalmológicas Ramón Castroviejo
Facultad de Medicina
Universidad Complutense de Madrid, Spain

Ana I. Ramírez, Juan J. Salazar, Rosa de Hoz
Instituto de Investigaciones Oftalmológicas Ramón Castroviejo
Facultad de Óptica y Optometría
Universidad Complutense de Madrid, Spain

1   Introduction

Glaucoma, the second leading cause of blindness in the world, is a multifactorial neurodegenerative disease characterized by an irreversible decrease of retinal-ganglion cells (RCG) of the retina and their axons, the functional impact of which leads to a visual-field loss (Kerrigan-Baumrind, Quigley, Pease, Kerrigan, & Mitchell, 2000; Nork *et al.*, 2000; Quigley, Dunkelberger, & Green, 1989; Quigley, 2001).

Many of the proposed mechanisms in the development and progression of this pathology are linked to increased intraocular pressure (IOP). Although IOP was previously considered a major factor responsible for the glaucomatous neuropathy, today multiple factors are considered to act as the initial insult in glaucomatous atrophy. This initial damage leads to a retinal-ganglion-cell injury. Secondary insults such as glutamate excitotoxicity and oxidative stress exacerbates the dysfunction, leading to the death of RGCs (Kaushik, Pandav, & Ram, 2003). Growing evidence in clinical and experimental studies strongly suggests the involvement of the immune system in glaucoma, supporting the idea that both innate and adaptive immune responses accompany glaucomatous neurodegeneration (Tezel *et al.*, 2007; Tezel & Wax, 2007; Tezel, 2013; Wax & Tezel, 2002; Yang *et al.*, 2001).

It is generally accepted that glaucomatous damage is a consequence of axonal degeneration that ends with the death of ganglion cells, recent studies have shown the importance of glia in the pathogenic mechanism of the disease (Hernandez *et al.*, 2008; Johnson *et al.*, 2009; Newman, 2004; Prasanna *et al.*, Krishnamoorthy, & Yorio, 2011; Tezel & the Fourth ARVO/Pfizer Ophthalmics Research Institute Conference,Working Group, 2009) .

Under normal conditions, astrocytes and Müller glia in the retina and in the optic nerve make contact with retinal neurons, providing stability to the neural tissue (Ramírez *et al.*, 1996). Physiological studies have demonstrated that both cell populations perform equivalent functions, including: neurovascular coupling, storing glycogen, providing glucose to neurons, regulating the levels of extracellular potassium, playing a major role in the regulation and metabolism of neurotransmitters such as GABA, helping to remove CO_2 from the retina, and helping to the maintenance of water homeostasis in the retina (Bringmann *et al.*, 2006; Kimelberg & Nedergaard, 2010; Kumpulainen, *et al.*, 1983; Nag, 2011; Newman, 2004; Sofroniew & Vinters, 2010). Furthermore, astrocytes as well as Müller cells can induce and maintain blood-retinal barrier (BRB) properties within the vascular endothelial cells (Tout *et al.*, 1993).

Microglial cells are considered the resident macrophages of the central nervous system (CNS) and are involved in defence mechanisms against the destructive environment in addition to being able to facilitate regenerative processes. Microglia cells are responsible for the phagocytosis of cell debris resulting from apoptosis and normal death and have the capacity to surround damaged neurons and participate in synaptic stripping. In addition, these cells could provide trophic support to neurons and release anti-inflammatory molecules to enhance the survival of surrounding neurons (Elkabes *et al.*, 1996; Liao *et al.*, 2005; Morgan *et al.*, 2004).

Despite the lack of clear evidence supporting classical hallmarks of inflammation in glaucoma, glial cells from the retina and the optic nerve in the glaucomatous optic neuropathy show a chronic activation (Tezel & the Fourth ARVO/Pfizer Ophthalmics Research Institute Conference,Working Group, 2009), a situation that is commonly accepted as a sign of neuroinflammation in the CNS.

Under normal conditions, the retina, as a part of the CNS, does not prompt an immunological rejection reaction due to an immune privilege that allows tissue to survive. To preserve this immune privilege, under pathological conditions, glial cells need to be capable of responding rapidly to any damage and consequently become activated (Tezel *et al.*, 2007). Microglial cells play fundamental roles in local immune responses and immunosurveillance. On the other hand, astrocytes are involved in maintaining the integrity of the blood-brain barrier (BBB), thus preserving the CNS immune privilege. The BBB, composed of endothelial cells, pericytes, and macroglial cells, represents both a physical and a functional separation of circulating blood components from the CNS. This barrier restricts the diffusion of some damaging molecules that could alter the nerve-tissue integrity and allow the active transport of other metabolic products and substances. In the retina this barrier is called blood-retinal barrier (BRB), which under pathological conditions could be altered, leading to a loss of the immune privilege.

Both the microglia and the astrocytes are able to protect neurons from potentially damaging effects of an inflammatory immune response (Tezel & the Fourth ARVO/Pfizer Ophthalmics Research Institute Conference, Working Group, 2009). An initial immunological response to the CNS injury is possibly associated with cleaning and tissue repair, but an inappropriate immune response could be involved in several autoimmune diseases, perhaps finally being a harmful response against the CNS.

The continuous nature of glial activation in the glaucomatous retina and optic-nerve head therefore appears to be crucial in determining the outcome of an immune response as being neurodestructive rather than neurosupportive to RGCs (Tezel & the Fourth ARVO/Pfizer Ophthalmics Research Institute Conference, Working Group, 2009). It has been suggested that early, moderate, and transient well-controlled activation of local glia correlate with protective immunity in the injured CNS by providing tissue cleaning and tissue repair. However, the widespread and persistent nature of glial activation in glaucomatous human eyes may lead to tissue damage through proinflammatory cytokines, facilitating the progression of RGC neurodegeneration in the glaucomatous eyes (Tezel & the Fourth ARVO/Pfizer Ophthalmics Research Institute Conference, Working Group, 2009). This would support the contention that, as resident immunoregulatory cells, glia have the potential to start the stimulation of an immune response during glaucomatous neurodegeneration and therefore a secondary autoimmune component may be involved in this neurodegenerative injury (Tezel, 2013).

Resident glia alter their gene-expression profile during activation (Bosco *et al.*, 2011). Glial response in glaucomatous eyes reportedly involves the activation of a glial immunoregulatory function and antigen-presenting ability (Steele *et al.*, 2006). Glial cells are capable of producing numerous immune mediators in human glaucoma and in animal models of the disease (Johnson *et al.*, 2007; Kompass *et al.*, 2008; Luo *et al.*, 2010; Panagis *et al.*, 2011; Steele *et al.*, 2006; Tezel *et al.*, 2010; Yang et al., 2011). In glaucomatous patients, an upregulation of TNF-α (Tezel *et al.*, 2001) and other proinflammatory cytokines has been demonstrated (Kuchtey *et al.*, 2010). In addition, the involvement of different complement components (Kuehn *et al.*, 2006; Stasi *et al.*, 2006), the presence of an abnormal subset of T cells Yang *et al.*, 2001), an increase of the titres of serum auto-antibodies (Dervan *et al.*, 2010; Joachim *et al.*, 2008), and an increased expression of glial MHC class II molecules have been detected in human glaucoma (Yang *et al.*, 2001).

MHC class-II molecules are critical to start the specific immune response and are confined to professional antigen-presenting cells (APCs). In the healthy CNS parenchyma, MHC- II molecules are not constitutively expressed in neural cells but, in an environment rich in inflammatory cytokines, of which interferon-γ (IFN-γ) is the most potent (Holling *et al.*, 2004), MHC II expression can be induced in non-professional APCs.

Human and animal studies have demonstrated that in the retina and optic nerve the expression of MHC II in glial cells is minimal or absent and, when present, is restricted to some microglia (Aloisi, 2001; Gallego *et al.*, 2012; Hayes *et al.*, 1987) and a few astrocytes (Gallego *et al.*, 2012). However, a significant correlation has been established between glaucomatous disease progression and MHC class-II expression by resident cells of the organ involved (Tezel *et al.*, 2007). Under virtually all inflammatory and neurodegenerative diseases, microglia have been shown to upregulate MHC class-II expression and MHC class-II+ astrocytes, and Müller cells have been detected (Crish & Calkins, 2011).

2   Anatomy of the Retina

2.1   Retinal Cell Layers

The primary function of the retina is to convert light into nerve impulses which are transferred to the brain via the optic nerve. The retina comprises the retinal pigment epithelium (RPE) and the neurosensory retina, the latter containing neurons, glial cells, and components of the vascular system. Various types of neurons are present, such as: photoreceptors, bipolar cells, ganglion cells, amacrine cells, and horizontal cells (Hogan *et al.*, 1971) (Fig.1).

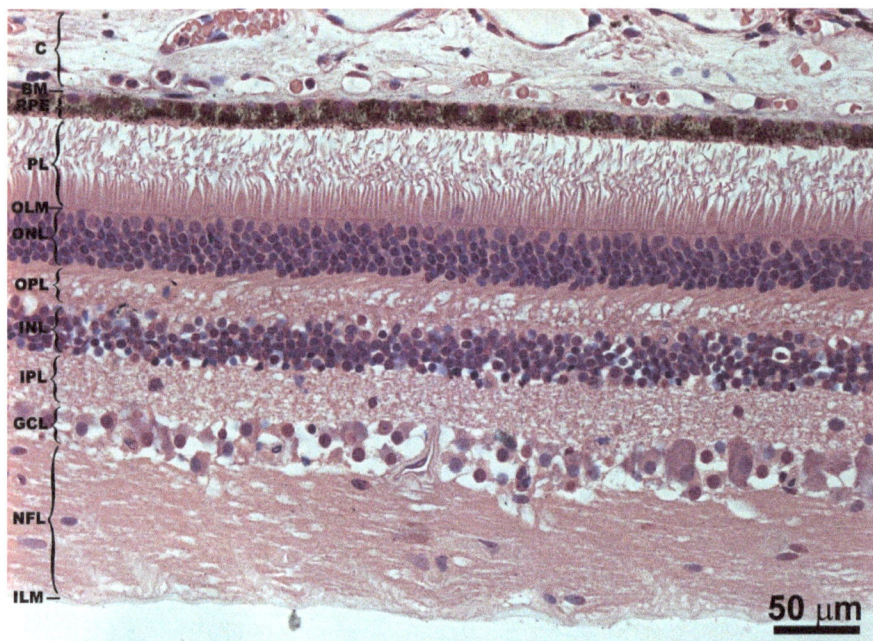

Figure 1: Histological section of the human retina. Hematoxylin/eosin. C: Choroid; BM: Bruch's membrane; RPE: retinal pigment epithelium; PL: photoreceptor layer; OLM: outer limiting membrane; ONL: outer nuclear layer; OPL: outer plexiform layer; INL: inner nuclear layer; IPL: inner plexiform layer; GCL: ganglion-cell layer; NFL: nerve-fibre layer; ILM: inner limiting membrane.

The coding function of the retina depends not only on photoreceptors but also on neurons, glial cells, and RPE, which amplify the signal (Fourgeux *et al.*, 2011). Photoreceptors are cells that capture light and are situated at the most external side of the neurosensory retina, in the vicinity of the RPE. These cells are of two types: rods (for scotopic vision) and cones (for photopic vision) (Hogan *et al.*, 1971). The photoreceptors can convert light photons into an electrical signal because they contain a photopigment in their outer segments. These segments consist of a stack of disk membranes that are synthesised in the proximal portion of the outer segment and shed at its apical size (Fourgeux *et al.*, 2011). Photoreceptors form contacts with horizontal and bipolar cells in the outer plexiform layer (OPL). Coupling between neighbouring rods and cones in OPL allows the first stage of visual processing. The inner nuclear layer (INL) contains cell bodies of Müller glial, bipolar, amacrine, and horizontal cells. The inner plexiform layer (IPL) consists of a synaptic connections between the axons of bipolar cells and dendrites of ganglion and amacrine cells. The retinal ganglion cell layer (GCL) contains the cell bodies of retinal ganglion cells, certain displaced amacrine cells, and astrocytes. Inside the eye, ganglion-cell axons run along the retinal surface towards the optic-nerve head forming the nerve fibre layer (NFL) (Fourgeux *et al.*, 2011; Sharma, 2007) (Fig. 1).

2.2   Retinal Macroglial Cells

The neural retina also contains two types of macroglial cells: Müller cells and astrocytes (Fig. 2). Müller cells are long, radially oriented cells which span the width of the neural retina from the outer limiting membrane (OLM), where their apical ends are located, to the inner limiting membrane (INL), where their basal endfeet terminate. In the nuclear layers, the lamellar processes of the Müller cells can be seen to form basket-like structures which enclose the cell bodies of photoreceptors and neural cells. In plexiform layers, fine processes of these cells are interwoven between the synaptic processes of neural cells. In both the plexiform and nuclear layers, Müller cell processes cover most but not all of the neural surfaces (Newman, 1986).

Astrocytes are located mainly in the NFL and GCL in most mammals (e.g. human [Fig. 2], rabbit, rats and mouse) (Gallego *et al.*; Ramírez *et al.*, 1994; Triviño *et al.*, 1997). Astrocyte morphology differs between species. In humans, two types of astrocytes can be distinguished: elongated (located in the NFL) (Fig. 2A) and star-shaped (located in GCL) astrocytes (Fig. 2B). In mice (Fig. 8) and rats the astrocytes are star-shaped.

Macroglial cells perform various essential roles for the normal physiology of the retina, maintaining a close and permanent relationship with the neurons (Ramírez *et al.*, 1998) (Fig. 3). Thus every aspect of the development, homeostasis, and function of the visual system involves a neuron-glia partnership. Glial cells insulate neurons, provide physical support for them, and supplement them with several metabolites and growth factors. These cells are also important in axon guidance and the control of synaptogenesis (Pfrieger, 2002; 2003). Under normal conditions, astrocytes and Müller cells maintain the homeostasis of extracellular ions, glucose, and other metabolites, water, pH and neurotransmitters such as glutamate and GABA (Johnson & Morrison, 2009). These cells also produce a great quantity of cytokines and growth factors (basic fibroblast growth factor (bFGF), transformation growth factor beta (TGF-β), and neuronal-survival growth factor such as the nerve growth factor (NGF) (Pena *et al.*, 1999; 2001)), which may contribute both to neurotoxic as well as to neuroprotective effects. In addition, they produce laminin, fibronectin, and tropoelastin, the percursor of elastin (Pena *et al.*, 2001). It has also been demonstrated that macroglial cells are more resistant to oxidative damage than are neurons, this characteristic protecting them against such damage. This potential is due to the fact that these cells contain high concentrations of antioxidants such as reduced glutathione and vitamin (Wilson, 1997). Conse quently, a depression of these cellular activities could lead to neuronal dysfunction (Triviño *et al.*, 2005).

Macroglial cells induce the properties of barrier in the retinal capillaries (the BRB) (Abbott *et al.*, 2006; Tout *et al.*, 1993), as they release substances that stabilize the close tight junctions between endothelial vascular cells (Tout *et al.*, 1993), securing immune privilege to protect neurons from potentially damaging effects of an inflammatory immune response. Finally, glial cells play fundamental roles in local immune responses and immunosurveillance (Aloisi, 2001; Dong & Benveniste, 2001).

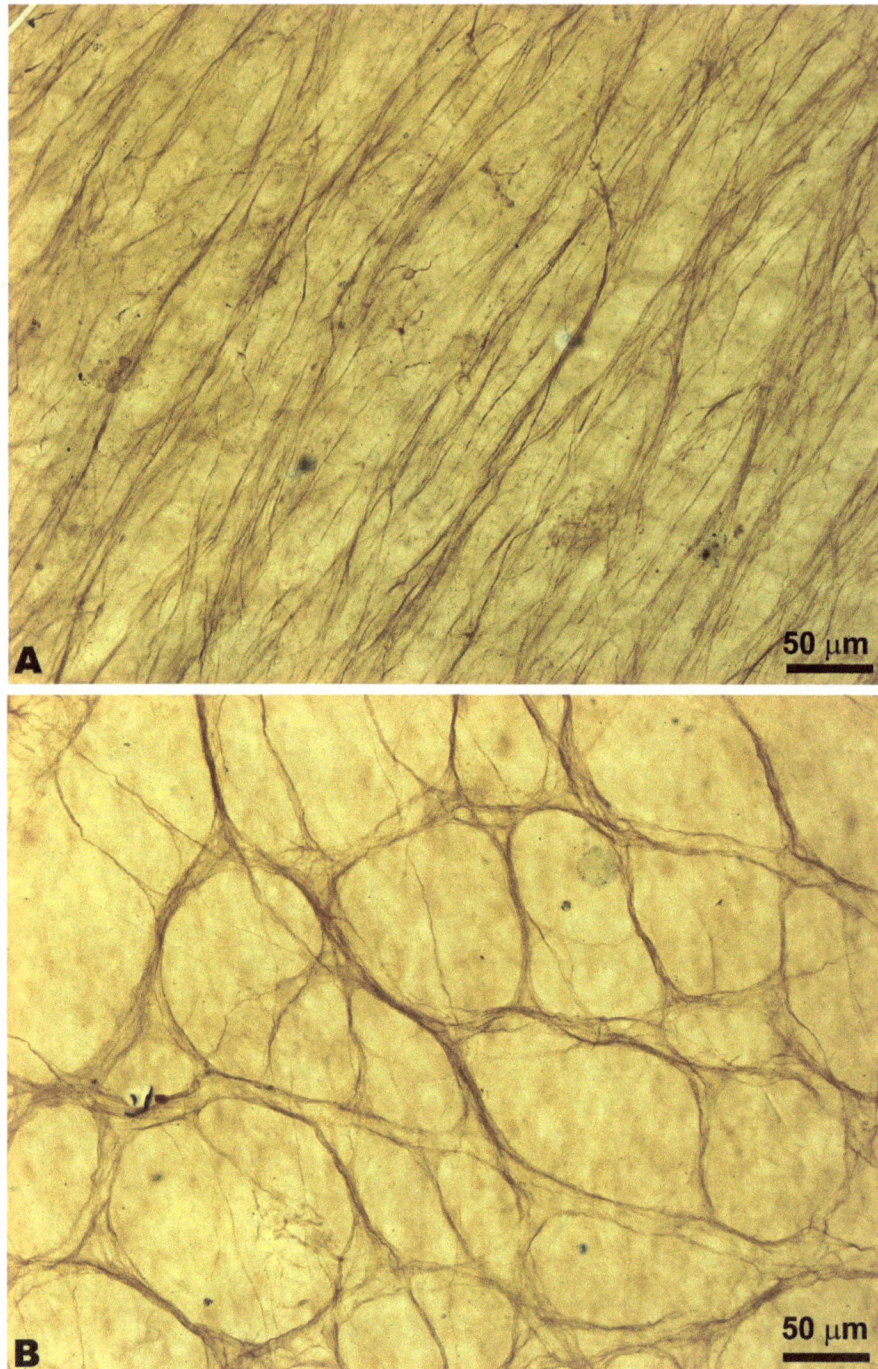

Figure 2: Astrocytes on the nerve-fibre-RCG layer of the human retina. Immunohistochemistry, anti-GFAP. Retinal whole-mount. A. In the NFL, the astrocytes form astroglial bundles parallel to the ganglion cell axons. B. In the GCL astrocytes form a homogeneous honeycomb plexus constituted by stellate cells.

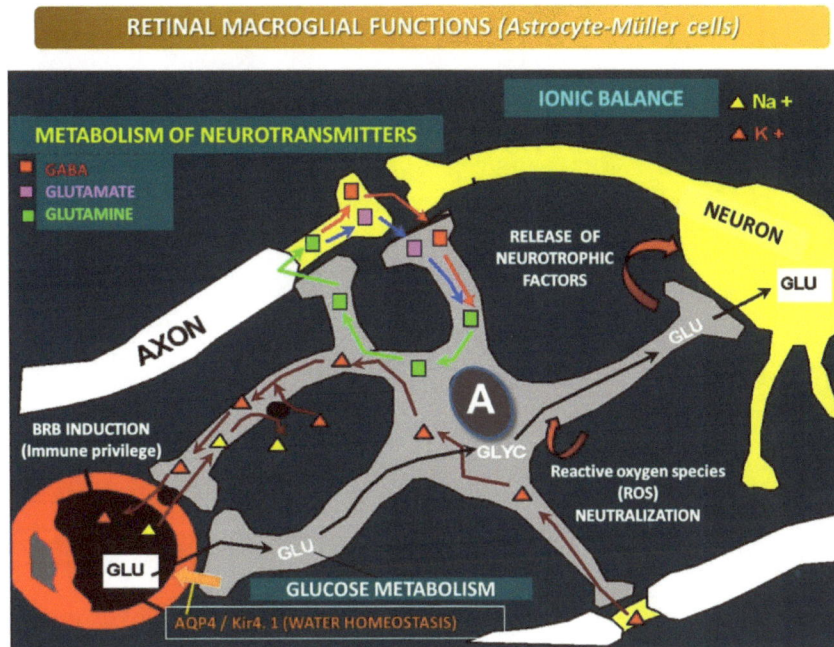

Figure 3: Scheme illustrating the links between the macroglia, the blood-retinal barrier and retinal neurons.

Macroglial cells also take part in pathological processes in the CNS. Glial cells in the CNS have been implicated in the pathological course of neuronal damage after mechanical, ischaemic, and various other insults. Glial-cell activation is a hallmark of CNS injury, characterized by an increase in size and number of glial cells and upregulation of GFAP, with additional cellular changes that may cause or relieve neuronal impairment. These reactive cells also have higher metabolic activity (Ames, 2000). After injury, reactive glial cells participate in the formation of a glial scar, in which there is an accumulation of enlarged astrocyte bodies and a thick network of processes with increased expression of GFAP and vimentin. Macroglial cells become reactive in response to a wide variety of stimuli, including inflammation as well as oxidative and mechanical stress (Zhong *et al.*, 2007).

2.3   Retinal Vascularization

Retinal vasculature is mostly a bi-layered system, i.e. a superficial network (Fig. 4) and a deep capillary plexus; however, there are multiple layers of capillaries in the peripapillary region, known as the radial peripapillary capillaries (Ryan *et al.*, 2013). The inner retinal layers have their own blood supply coming from the blood vessels entering the retina at the optic-nerve head (Fig. 4), while the outer retina is supplied only by the choroidal vasculature (Fig. 5). The retinal vascularization is supplied by the central retina artery and has an end-arterial hierarchy: arteries branch to arterioles, which supply a capillary network that is drained by venules, and then veins remove the blood from the retina (Ryan *et al.*, 2013) (Fig. 4). Capillaries have a lumen diameter of 3.5 to 6 μm and perivascular pericytes. The retina has the highest endothelial cell-to-pericyte ratio in the body, 1:1 (Cogan & Kuwabara, 1967).

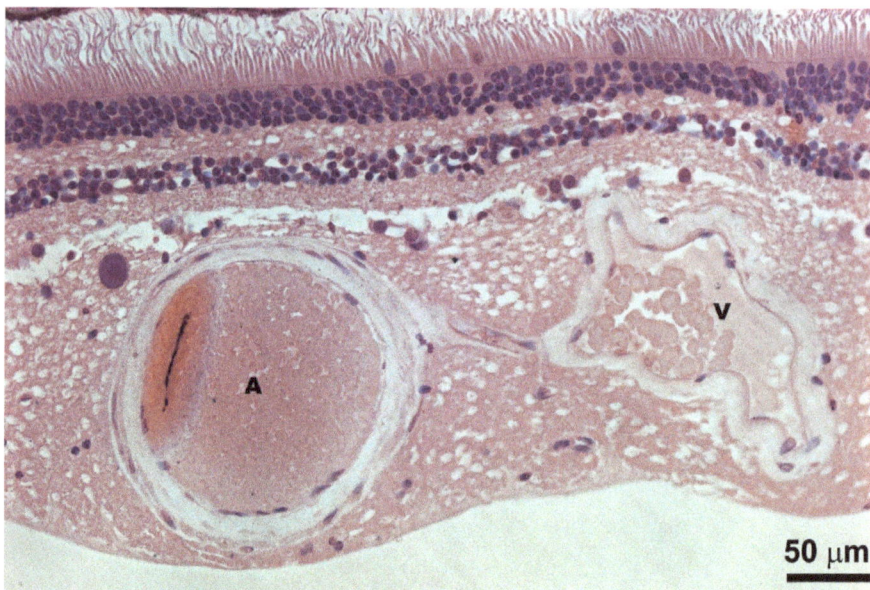

Figure 4: Histological section of the human retina. Retinal vessels. Hematoxylin/eosin. Microphotography of an arteriole (A) and a venule (V) of the superficial vascular network in the nerve fiber layer.

The choroidal vasculature provides oxygen and nutrients to the photoreceptors via the choriocapillaris. The choriocapillaris is made up of capillaries situated between the medium-sized vessel layer (Sattler's layer) and Bruch's membrane (Fig. 5). This array of these capillaries, flattened and elliptical in transverse section, creates a large surface for metabolic exchange with the retina. With the same purpose, the vessels of the choriocapillaris are composed of tubes of endothelial cells (EC) and pericytes that do not completely surround it, appearing only towards the scleral side. Meanwhile, the ratio of pericytes:endothelial cells in the choriocapillaris is 1:6 (Bron *et al.*, 1997). Given the contractile nature of these cells, which enables the blood supply to be regulated in other tissues, their lower number in the choriocapillaris could suggest that the regulation of the choroidal blood flow is regulated by the autonomic nervous system (Bill, 1975) and the contribution of pericyte contraction is practically nil (Bron *et al.*, 1997).

The EC presents fenestrations in the side oriented towards Bruch's membrane and RPE (Melamed *et al.*, 1980; Spitznas, 1974; Spitznas & Reale, 1975). These fenestrations are of great physiological importance, as they permit the passage of nutrients towards the retina. The choroid capillaries are permeable to small molecules such as glucose (20-fold more than in cardiac muscle and 80-fold more than in skeletal muscle) (Bill *et al.*, 1980) and amino acids (Törnquist, 1979), as well as large molecules such as γ-immunoglobulin and vitamin A (Bill, 1975; 1980; 1983).

2.4   Blood-retinal barriers

The retina is physiologically and immunologically segregated from the rest of the body by tight junctions between vascular endothelial cells (inner BRB) and RPE cells (outer BRB). This situation is responsible for intraocular tissue to be an immune-privileged site, thus protecting the eye from the innocent-bystander effect of inflammation (Sharma, 2007).

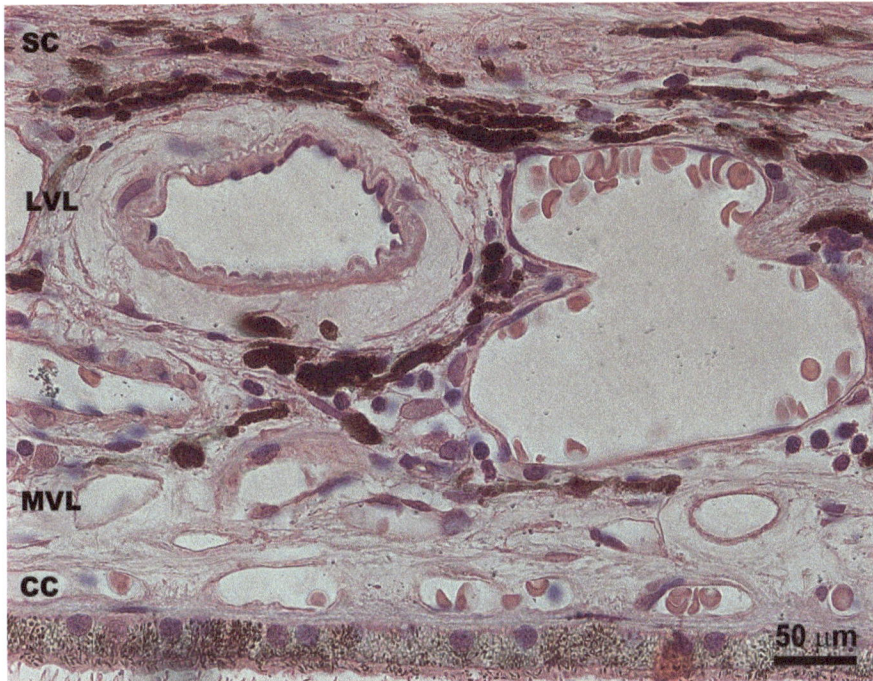

Figure 5: Histological section of the human choroid. Hematoxylin/eosin. SC: suprachoroid; LVL: large-size vessel layer; MVL: medium-size vessel layer; CC: choriocapillary.

In addition, only small molecules can cross these barriers, making it difficult for many drugs to reach ocular tissue. Astrocytes and Müller cells induce the BRB (Janzer & Raff, 1987). Retinal capillaries are closely ensheathed by glial processes. Usually, Müller cells enhance the barrier function of vascular endothelia by the secretion of factors such as PEDF, thrombospondin-1, and glial-cell line-derived neurotrophic factor (GDNF) (Eichler *et al.*, 2004; Nishikiori *et al.*, 2007). However, in response to hypoxia, inflammation, or glucose deprivation, Müller cells produce factors such as vascular endothelial-growth factor (VEGF) and tumour-necrosis factor, which increase vascular permeability (Aiello *et al.*, 1995; Eichler *et al.*, 2004; Noda *et al.*, 2005). Müller cells are also a source of matrix metaloproteinases (Behzadian *et al.*, 2001; Noda *et al.*, 2005) which degrade the tight-junction protein, occluden (Giebel *et al.*, 2005).

3   Immune Privilege of the Eye

Immune privilege is the condition in which selected immune responses are suppressed or excluded in certain organs. Immune privilege is well developed in three regions of the body: the eye, the brain and the pregnant uterus (Niederkorn, 2006). Immune privilege was first described by Peter Medawar in his study of allogenic skin grafts placed hereterotypically in the anterior chamber of the eye and into the brains of rabbits (Medawar, 1948). Immune privilege is a property of certain tissues in which immune responses to foreign antigens, particularly alloantigens are suppressed, end even completely inhibited. It is widely believed that immune privilege is an adaptation for reducing immune-mediated injury to cells that have limited or no capacity for regeneration (Niederkorn & Stein-Streilein, 2010). Immune privilege normally serves as a homeostatic mechanism that preserves normal function in tissues, particularly those that are highly specialized or have limited capacity for renewal, such as the eye and brain (Forrester, 2013). In the eye, immune privilege was described over 130 years ago, but its significance was not appreciated until the early 1950s. Investigations beginning in the 1970s ushered in a new era, revealing that ocular immune privilege is due to anatomical, physiological, and immunoregulatory processes that prevent the induction and expression of immune-mediated inflammation (Niederkorn & Stein-Streilein, 2010).

In the eye, immune privilege promotes the survival of intraocular tumour grafts by inhibiting both adaptive and innate immune effectors (Streilein, 2003), whereas such grafts at conventional body sites leads to acute, irreversible immune rejection (Ohta *et al.*, 1999). To achieve immune privilege, the eye and the immune system use several different but related strategies that prevent or alter innate and adaptive immune responses in eyes: immunological ignorance, peripheral tolerance of eye-derived antigens, and the development of an intraocular immunosuppressive microenvironment (Streilein, 2003). By limiting intraocular inflammation, immune privilege preserves the integrity of the visual axis and thereby prevents blindness (Ohta *et al.*, 1999). Visual axis integrity is essential to focus light images precisely on the retina. Another important advantage of ocular immune privilege is that certain cells components of the eyes (corneal endothelium and neurosensory retina) are incapable of replication and cannot regenerate after injury and loss after destructive inflammation (Streilein, 2003). The anterior chamber, the vitreous cavity, and the subretinal space are immune-privileged ocular compartments (Jiang *et al.*, 1993; Niederkorn *et al.*, 1981; Wenkel, *et al.*, 1999). In addition, certain ocular tissues function as immune-privileged sites. This is true of the cornea (Hori *et al.*, 2000), RPE (Wenkel & Streilein, 2000), and the neuronal retina (Streilein *et al.*, 2002).

It is becoming increasingly clear that immune privilege is not aimed at entirely suppressing immune responses in the target organ, but rather at maintaining a specialized, tightly regulated immunological niche to preserve the integrity of especially vulnerable organs, such as the brain and the eye (Niederkorn, 2006; Streilein, 2003). In contrast to the previous view that immune privilege is maintained by immune-cell exclusion, it is now increasingly accepted that the privileged status is preserved by local active mechanisms that suppress responses to antigens within the privileged tissues (Niederkorn & Stein-Streilein, 2010). In the eye, one such mechanism is anterior-chamber-associated immunodeviation (ACAID) (Streilein, 1987). The systemic unresponsiveness elicited by introducing antigens in the anterior chamber of the eye was first reported by Kaplan *et al.* in 1975. ACAID was defined as an antigen-specific, stereotypic, deviant systemic immune response in which the effectors of Th1-type immunogenic inflammation (T cells that mediate delayed hypersensitivity and B cells that secrete complement-fixing antibodies) (Coffman *et al.*, 1988) are selectively deficient (Niederkorn, 1990; Niederkorn, 2002; Streilein, 1987; Wilbanks & Streilein, 1990). We know now that ACAID results in the activation of an altered antibody response with T-cell suppression of the Th1 and Th2 responses (Katagiri *et al.*, 2002). Other mechanisms that contributed to mantaining the immune-privileged state of the eye include the reduced expression of MHC molecules on ocular cells, and the existence of an intraocular anti-inflammatory environment (Benhar *et al.*, 2012).

Immune privilege is mediated by both active and passive mechanisms (Streilein, 2003). The eye is privileged in part because of the blood-ocular barriers that include the iris, ciliary body, and retinal-pigment epithelium as well as the retinal vasculature (Qiao *et al.*, 2009). Because blood-ocular barriers are not completely impermeable, innate and adaptive immune cells and molecules can still gain access to the internal compartments of the eye. In response to this threat to vision, the eye has soluble and cell-surface immunomodulatory and anti-inflammatory factors in ocular fluids and on parenchymal cell surfaces (Qiao *et al.*, 2009). Thus, the aqueous humour contains vasoactive intestinal peptide (VIP), somatastatine, α-melanocyte-stimulating hormone (α-MSH), calcitonin gen-related peptide (CGRP), macrophage migration inflammatory factor (MIF), the mediator of apoptosis Fas ligand (CD95L), and TGF-β2 (Streilein, 2003). Ocular parenchymal cells expressing molecules that can modulate immune effector mechanisms include the cornea, retinal-pigment epithelium, and iris. Among the cell-surface molecules that promote ocular IP are CD95L, inhibitors of the complement (CD46, CD55, CD59, and complement receptor-related protein, Crry) the immune co-stimulator B7-2 (Cd86) or the cytotoxic T lymphocyte antigen 4 (CTLA4) (Streilein, 2003).

Although the eye is an immunoprivileged site and has mechanisms to interfere the development of immune inflammation, under certain pathological conditions, ocular immune privilege is terminated and severe inflammation occurs (Niederkorn, 2006; Streilein, 2003). This process contributes to the pathogenesis of many ocular diseases (Qiao *et al.*, 2009).

4 Glaucomatous Optic Neuropathy

This pathology may begin by an increase in intraocular pressure (IOP) or by a vascular dysregulation, which would provoke a series of incipient changes, such as: the obstruction of the axoplasmic flow of the RGCs, microvascular and glial alterations, and disturbances of the connective tissue (at the level of the lamina cribosa) and the immune system. In turn, these incipient changes would bring about a number of secondary problems, including: 1) excitotoxic damage, provoked by the glutamate released by the injured neurons; 2) neurotrophin deprivation; 3) oxidative damage, for the excess of free radicals; and 4) neurotoxicity, for the excess of nitrous oxide (NO) (Agarwal *et al.*, 2009). The overall result will be the dysfunction and subsequent death of the RGCs with the subsequent loss of their axons towards the lateral geniculate body, which ultimately leads to the irreversible loss of vision.

4.1 Risk Factors and Physiopathological Mechanisms

4.1.1 Increase in the IOP

There is a close relationship between the increase in the IOP and the death of RGCs by apoptosis (Quigley *et al.*, 1989; Quigley, 1999). However, between 30 and 40% of the patients with glaucomatous visual field defects have a normal IOP and are diagnosed as normotensional glaucomas (Agarwal *et al.*, 2009; Caprioli & Spaeth, 1985). Therefore, the rise in the IOP is an important factor but not the only one responsible for damaging the optic nerve.

The axons of the RGC exit the eye posteriorly through the lamina cribosa (LC), the site where the main damage to the axons of the RGCs occurs in glaucoma (Fig. 6). The LC is a structure of porous connective tissue composed of lamellas cribiformes through which the bundles of axons leave the eyeball (Fig. 2) (Salazar, 1994). It has two components, the cellular one and extracellular matrix (ECM). The ECM is composed of specific macromolecules assembled to provide strength, flexibility, and elasticity to the tissue. Among its components, different types of collagen (I, III, IV, V, and VI), elastin, proteoglycans, hyaluronic acid, integrins, and laminin can be distinguished (Elkington *et al.*, 1990; Hernandez *et al.*, 1991). The cell component is constituted by astrocytes, which coat the cribiforme pores and that provide the metabolic support, contribute to the maintenance of the extracellular environment, and confront mechanical and ischaemic damage (Triviño *et al.*, 1996). Also, there are other types of cells such as fibroblasts and microglial cells (Salazar, 1994).

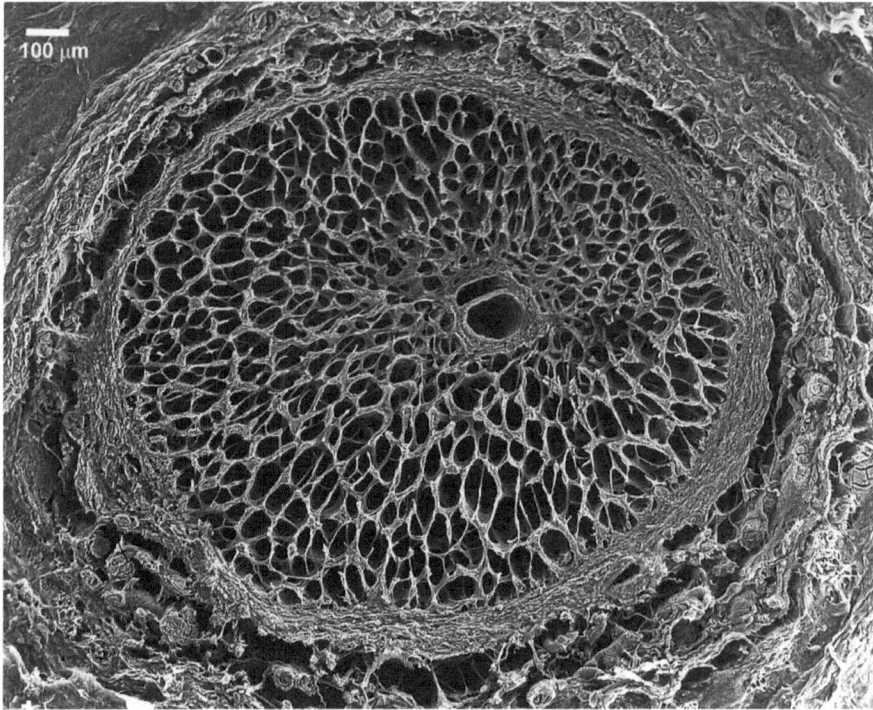

Figure 6: Human lamina cribosa. Scanning electron microscopy of trypsine digested nervous tissue.

The arteries supplying the eye have a relatively high blood pressure. At the origin of the retina and cilliary arteries, blood pressure is about 65-70 mmHg (Neetens, 1979). There is a direct relationship between vessel caliber and pressure of intraocular vessels. The drop in the pressure from the small arteries and arterioles to the capillaries is greater in the choroid than in the retina (Weigelin, 1972) . It is well known that a whatershed zone, as an area of poor vascularity, is most vulnerable to ischemia (Hayreh, 1990). The vascularization of the LC depends on the Zinn-Haller circle (branches of the posterior ciliary arteries). The posterior ciliary arteries are end-arteries, so they have a watershed zone between them; an issue that could increase the vulnerability of the LC to decreases in blood flow. The LC is an area of biomechanical interest since a discontinuity occurs there in the corneal-scleral cover, this being a weak point in the mechanical load systems and therefore a site where tension or stress concentrates (Sigal *et al.*, 2010).

Higher IOP can act mechanically in the eye tissues, causing deformations and stress, which augment or abate depending on the geometry and the material properties of each eye. When the levels of stress and tension exceed the physiological tolerance of the tissue cells, these induce a remodelling of the connective tissue (increased production or elimination of collagen and elastin), in an attempt to reestablish mechanical homeostasis (Downs *et al.*, 2011; Grytz *et al.*, 2011). This increase in connective tissue could seriously alter the blood flow by compression, and therefore the nutrition in this laminar region. It should be taken into account that all this could occur with IOP within the normal range in eyes that are particularly susceptible to the stress related to IOP (Grytz *et al.*, 2012; Sigal *et al.*, 2012).

IOP-related alterations in connective tissue may cause the most anterior cribiforme lamellae to give way or be destroyed, thereby transferring the load (weight) to adjacent lamellae in a cascade of damage that, together with the loss of axons, helps provoking glaucomatous excavation (Burgoyne, 2011; Downs *et al.*, 2011; Sigal, 2009; Sigal *et al.*, 2010; 2012).

As stated above, the mechanical stress generated by the IOP causes the reactivation of the astrocytes, the main cells of the optic-nerve head, prompting a remodelling of the ECM (Hernandez, 2000; Morgan, 2000; Varela & Hernandez, 1997). The integrins would act as mechanosensors intercommunicating the astrocytes with the ECM (Morrison, 2006). During this remodelling, type IV and VI collagens increase (the former type being a constituent of the basal astrocyte membrane) which modifies the original structure of the cribiforme pores (Hernandez *et al.*, 2008). Furthermore, the proteoglycans and glycosaminoglycans are altered and the elastic fibres degenerate (Morrison, 2006). All this leads to the biochemical change of the tissue described above.

The ECM is also responsible for providing adhesion signals to control the cell functions and cell survival. Reactive astrocytes increase the activity of matrix metalloproteinases (MMPs) (Agapova *et al.*, 2001; Yan *et al.*, 2000), enzymes involved in the remodelling of the ECM, in such a way that they can degrade the cell-adhesion molecules to permit cell mobility. On the other hand, the changes in the specific components of the ECM (greater MMP-9, laminina loss, etc.) can interrupt cell-cell and cell-ECM interactions, which in turn could, in the case of the RGCs, provoke cell death by apoptosis (Agarwal *et al.*, 2009).

Because of the deformation, mechanical stress, and the subsequent increased collagen in the LC, the axons may also undergo deformation and mechanical stress on passing through the pores of the LC. This can trigger mitochondrial dysfunction, depressing energy production and blocking axonal transport of molecules (Crish & Calkins, 2011), including neurotrophic factors (such as BDNF), which originate in the brain and are transported towards the soma of the RGCs (Crish *et al.*, 2013; Quigley, 1999). These factors, important for the regulation of the metabolism and for cell survival, if diminished, could lead to the progressive death of the RGCs by apoptosis (Nickells, 1996). This would be considered one of the first events to induce apoptosis of the RGCs.

4.1.2   Alteration of Ocular Blood Flow

In healthy eyes, the retina and the optic-nerve head require a constant blood flow to maintain their high metabolic needs. On the contrary, patients with glaucoma generally suffer reduced ocular blood flow (Flammer *et al.*, 2002; Satilmis *et al.*, 2003). However, the restricted flow reportedly leads to optic atrophy (as occurs in other pathologies) but not to glaucomatous damage. Therefore, the connection between glaucoma and blood flow would not therefore be the diminished flow but rather its instability, which inflicts repetitive damage of ischaemia-reperfusion (Flammer & Mozaffarieh, 2007). There is a relation between the progressive glaucomatous damage and the fluctuations in the IOP, the drops in blood pressure, and the alterations of self-regulation (e.g. in the primary vascular dysregulation syndrome) (Martínez, 2013; Martinez & Sanchez, 2005; Siesky *et al.*, 2012).

The severe decrease in blood flow to a tissue or organ causes an infarction (which may be due to an inflammation of the vessels or to atherosclerosis). If the flow reduction is not so severe and is reversible, damage occurs by ischaemia-reperfusion (Flammer & Mozaffarieh, 2007). The absence of oxygen and nutrients in a tissue create conditions in which the re-establishment of circulation provokes inflammation and oxidative damage instead of restoring normal functioning. An example of this situation is the release of inflammatory factors, such as interleukins or free radicals, by white blood cells which arrive again to the tissue. In addition, the entry of oxygen, when the blood flow is restored, can cause the formation of reactive oxygen species that can damage proteins and/or lipids and therefore the plasma membrane. This cell damage induces the release of more free radicals (Karageuzyan, 2005). In the optic-nerve head the ischaemia-reperfusion lead to a repeated mild reperfusion injury (Flammer & Mozaffarieh, 2007).

In glaucoma patients, high concentrations of MMP-9 and ET-1 have been recorded in plasma (Cellini *et al.*, 2012; Emre *et al.*, 2005; Flammer *et al.*, 2001). Both molecules can spread from the choroid to the optic-nerve head and provoke vasoconstriction (ET-1) (Rader *et al.*, 1994) as well as the weakening of the secondary BRB with proteolytic degradation (MMP-9) (Grieshaber & Flammer, 2007). This latter repercussion, in extreme situations, leads to splinter hemorrhages (Grieshaber *et al.*, 2006), which appear in some glaucoma patients. The increase in ET-1 provokes another series of alterations related to glaucoma (Good & Kahook, 2010; Prasanna *et al.*, 2011), such as: the remodelling of the extracellular matrix (ET-1 increases the expression of MMPs and their inhibitors), the alteration in the anterograde axonal transport, or astrogliosis (ET-1 is a powerful glial mitogen). Also, the episodes of ischaemia reperfusion activate macroglial cells, both in the retina (astrocytes and Müller glia) as well as the optic-nerve head (Prasanna *et al.*, 2002), resulting in the tissue changes discussed below.

4.1.3   Participation of Glial Cells in Glaucomatous Damage

The macroglial cells of the retina (astrocytes and Müller glia) and the optic nerve (astrocytes, one of the most numerous cell types in the optic-nerve head) fulfil key functions for the maintenance and survival of both tissues and therefore of the RGCs (Ramirez *et al.*, 1996).

In the case of damage, as with glaucoma (mechanical stress, ischaemia-reperfusion), the astrocytes and the Müller glia become reactive, characterized generally by hypertrophia, hyperplasia, and increased expression of gliofibrillary acid protein (GFAP) (Hernandez & Pena, 1997; Hernandez, 2000; Inman & Horner, 2007). In an effort to limit the lesion and promote the reparation of the tissue in the glaucomatous eyes, the moderate and transitory activation of the glial cells can have a protective function through to the supply of certain metabolites, growth factors such as BDNF, ciliary neurotrophic factor (CNTF) or the pigment epithelium-derived factor from the retina (PEDF), the expression of antiapoptotic proteins (e.g. BCL-2) and other anti-inflammatory substances, as well as the elimination of neurotoxic substances of the environment (e.g. glutamate) (Johnson & Morrison, 2009; Munemasa & Kitaoka, 2012; Ridet & Privat, 2000),

The chronic activation of the macroglia, a situation observed in glaucoma (Hernandez & Pena, 1997; Neufeld, 1999a; Ramírez *et al.*, 2010; Tezel *et al.*, 2003; Wang *et al.*, 2002), spurs a number of changes in the tissues (retina and optic nerve) that can result in dysfunction and death of the RGCs (Tezel & the Fourth ARVO/Pfizer Ophthalmics Research Institute Conference,Working Group, 2009). These changes include (Fig. 5):

- Remodelling of the extracellular matrix, boosting the production of collagens IV and VI, and increasing the expression of MMPs (MMP-2, MMP-9) and their inhibitors at the level of the optic nerve head (Agapova *et al.*, 2001; Yan *et al.*, 2000). Furthermore, in parallel, this increase in MMPs can provoke alterations in the function of the barrier of the endothelial vascular cells by proteolytic degradation of the occludin proteins present in the tight junctions.

- In addition, in a parallel way, this surge in MMPs can alter the barrier function of the endothelial vascular cells by proteolytic degradation of occludin proteins present in these tight junctions (Grieshaber *et al.*, 2006; Grieshaber & Flammer, 2007).

- Secretion of inflammatory cytokines as tumoural necrosis factor-α (TNF-α), and IL-1 beta, which mediate the death of RGCs through several pathways: the activation of nuclear factor (NF)-κB, nitric oxide synthesis and inflammatory assembly (Johnson *et al.*, 2011; Sappington & Calkins, 2008; Tezel *et al.*, 2012; Yan *et al.*, 2000; Yang *et al.*, 2011; Yuan & Neufeld, 2000).

- Overproduction of NO. Under normal conditions, astrocytes communicate using NO as the neurotransmitter (Neufeld, 1999b). In stress situations, cytokines increase the expression of NOS-2 in astrocytes, stimulating a burst in NO production. This brings about the formation of toxic peroxynitrates for the axons, favouring the death of RGCs by apoptosis (Boehm *et al.*, 2011; Liu & Neufeld, 2000; Neufeld *et al.*, 1997b; Polazzi & Contestabile, 2002; Tezel & Wax, 2000b; Yan *et al.*, 2000).

- Loss of the capacity to regulate glutamate homeostasis for the reduced biosynthesis of glutamate transporters (GLAST), so that glutamate accumulates in the intercellular space, provoking neuronal death (Aronica *et al.*, 2003; Naskar *et al.*, 2000; Rieck, 2013; Vorwerk *et al.*, 1999).

- Capacity to act as antigen-presenting cells on expressing the class II major histocompatibility complex (MHCII) (molecule necessary for the presentation of the antigen to the T cells), thereby contributing to the immune response that could cause the destruction of the RGCs (Gallego *et al.*, 2012; Johnson & Morrison, 2009).

- Increase in size and number of processes, which favor the accumulation of glutamate, H+, and K+ in the intercellular space and that afterwards is introduced into the astrocyte cytoplasm, giving rise to cell oedema. This oedema prompts the disinsertion of the intermediate filaments and cell death (Ramírez *et al.*, 2001).

4.1.4   Secondary Alterations that Cause Ganglion-cell Death in Glaucoma

In glaucoma, most of the RGCs die by apoptosis, though necrosis can contribute in the final phases. The neurons respond directly to three main causes, such as: the loss of trophic support, the increase in excitatory amino acids (such as glutamate) and oxidative stress (Osborne, 2008; Wax & Tezel, 2002). The death of RGCs occurs in two phases. In the first and more rapid phase, the cells die from apoptosis. In the second phase, which is slower, the neuronal loss is due to the toxic effects of the primary neurons degenerated in addition to the continual exposure to high IOP (Munemasa & Kitaoka, 2012).

Apoptosis of the RGCs results from the activation of the tumour-suppressor protein p53, which activates the caspase pathway. Caspases are central regulatory proteases of apoptosis (Wax *et al.*, 2008). These enzymes are present as inactive zymogens and once activated commence an organized cascade, which leads to the proteolysis of key cytosolic and nuclear components which trigger the destruction of the cell. Caspases can be activated by an extrinsic or intrinsic pathway. The extrinsic pathway involves the interaction of specific ligands, such as TNF-α, with pro-apoptotic receptors of the cell surface. However, the intrinsic pathway is regulated by pro-apoptotic molecules released by the mitochondria (Chowdhury *et al.*, 2008; Earnshaw *et al.* 1999; Pop & Salvesen, 2009).

It has been postulated that in RGCs, as in other neurons, "compartmentalized self-destruction" occur; suggesting that depending on the nature and location of the initial damage, the death of the soma can be preceded by a series of degenerative processes that affect the axons, the dendrites, and the neuronal synapses (Munemasa & Kitaoka, 2012). One of these self-destructive processes is the Wallerian degeneration, which occurs in severe cases of axonal damage (axonal crushing, axonal shearing), which extends synchronously through the axon in days (Coleman & Freeman, 2010; Tse, 2012). The second self-destructive process, called "dying back", is prompted by general neuronal stress without an acute neuronal trauma. It begins with a disconnection of the synapses followed by an asynchronous progression of the destructive process towards the soma. In the case of the dying back, the neuron has an opportunity to return if the neuronal stress diminishes but, in Wallerian degeneration, the soma death by apoptosis is inevitable (Vidal-Sanz et al., 2002; Whitmore et al., 2005).

4.1.5   Neurotoxicity Mediated by Glutamate in RGCs

Glutamate is the most important excitatory neurotransmitter of the retina in vertebrates and its interactions with its specific membrane receptors are essential in retinal visual transduction. For physiological conditions to be maintained, excesses of glutamate must be eliminated from the extracellular environment. Glial cells, in particular astrocytes and Müller cells, gather this neurotransmitter through the GLAST transporter (Agarwal et al., 2009; Moreno et al., 2005a). In glaucoma the mediated extracellular glutamate concentration augments, either due to its release by RGCs that die, or else due to a failure in the regathering mechanism, because of the lower expression of the GLAST transporter in the reactive astrocytes (Dreyer et al., 1994; Lipton, 2001; Rieck, 2013). Consequently, the ionotrophic glutamate receptors (mainly the NMDA type) become overstimulated, unleashing a massive entry of calcium into the neurons. This calcium overload contributes to the neurotoxicity and the death of ganglion cells by apoptosis (Dreyer, 1998; Sucher et al., 1997).

4.1.6   Deprivation of Neurotrophins as the Death Mechanisms of the RGCs

RGCs project their axons towards specific cerebral regions where neurotrophins, which are vital for neuronal survival, are actively secreted. Neurotrophins are transported continuously, in a retrograde manner, from the superior colliculus to the soma of these cells. RGCs respond to a great variety of neurotrophins, but the main ones are: brain-derived neurotrophic factor (BDNF), ciliary neurotrophic factor (CNTF), glia-derived neurotrophic factor (GDNF)(Johnson, et al., 2011; Thanos & Emerich, 2005).

The interruption of axoplasm flow, with the subsequent deviation in the transport of neurotrophins (as occurs in glaucoma), can compromise the survival of RGCs, starting an apoptotic process (Nickells, 1996). However, in the retina, the glial cells (astrocytes and Müller glia) can synthesise diverse neurotrophins, notably BDNF. As mentioned above, the activation of glial cells in glaucoma could favour the secretion of neurotrophins, which may contribute to enhance the survival of the RGCs. Therefore, while the ocular hypertension may block a proper axoplasmic flow and therefore the arrival of neurotrophins, in a retrograde manner (Minckler et al., 1976; Quigley et al., 2000), the provision of neurotrophic factors by glial cells could in a certain way offset this initial deficit (Di Polo et al., 1998; Peinado-Ramon et al., 1996; Thanos & Emerich, 2005).

4.1.7   Neurotoxicity Mediated by the Free Radicals in the RGCs

In oxygen metabolism, oxygen reactive species are inevitably produced in association with the mitochondrial respiratory chain: superoxide anion, peroxide, and hydroxylic radicals. These are detoxified in the retina by very effective endogenous antioxidants, including several enzymes (Alarma-Estrany & Pintor, 2007; Erb & Heinke, 2011; Ghanem et al., 2010; Lundmark et al., 2006; Majsterek et al., 2011; Pinazo-Duran et al., 2013), such as superoxide dismutase (SOD), catalase or glutathione peroxidase (GPX), and other substances such as glutathione, ascorbic acid, β-carotene, melatonin and vitamin E.

During periods of hypoxia, metabolic stress, and other types of cell stress, the reactive oxygen species can accumulate to a critical point in which the cell functions are altered (Johnson & Morrison, 2009). These free radicals inflict severe damage, not only in the mitochondria but also in cell proteins, lipids, and nucleic acids, promoting cell death (Munemasa & Kitaoka, 2012). The excessive formation of free radicals is an etiopathological factor of many ocular diseases such as glaucoma (Agarwal *et al.*, 2009), in which vascular dysregulation or ischaemia can favour oxidative stress (Flammer, Haefliger, Orgul, & Resink, 1999). This can prompt a proliferation of proteins that cannot be repaired, an accelerated expression of MMP-9, and the overexpression of ET-1(Dalle-Donne *et al.*, 2005).

In principle, free radicals could stimulate the endogenous neuroprotective mechanisms, but in more advanced phases, this effect is lost. Therefore, in glaucoma, the antioxidant capacity declines, and levels of glutathione, superoxide dismutase, catalase, and melatonin fall (Gherghel *et al.*, 2005; Gherghel, Mroczkowska, & Qin, 2013; Moreno *et al.*, 2004; Yildirim *et al.*, 2005).

4.1.8   Role of Nitrous Oxide (NO)

At adequate physiological concentrations, NO is crucial in the organism. NO is produced by a wide variety of cell types. In the neurons, it can function as a neurotransmitter and its release by endothelial cells stimulates the smooth-muscle vascular cells and causes vasodilation.

NO is synthesised by the action of the enzyme nitric oxide synthase (NOS). There are three forms of NOS: two called constitutive, the endothelial (NOS-1) and the neuronal (NOS-3) isoforms; and an inducible one (NOS-2), which is not expressed or only very weakly under physiological conditions, but when it is expressed it can provoke excess NO in the tissues (Bredt & Snyder, 1994; Knott & Bossy-Wetzel, 2009; Lowenstein, Dinerman, & Snyder, 1994; Yun, *et al.*, 1997; Zhang & Snyder, 1995). In normal eyes, NOS-1 is sparsely present in astrocytes throughout the optic nerve head. In glaucomatous optic nerve heads, almost every astrocyte is positive for NOS-1. NOS-1 immunoreactivity is abundantly present throughout the prelaminar region and the lamina cribrosa and is localized inside the diminished nerve fiber bundles (Neufeld, *et al.*, 1997a). In glaucoma, an increase has been reported in the expression of NOS-2 by reactive astrocytes (Liu & Neufeld, 2000; Neufeld *et al.*, 1997b), being present in a few cells in the disorganized lamina cribrosa of the glaucomatous eye and is not present at all in normal tissue. NOS-3 is present in normal eyes in the vascular endothelia of small blood vessels of the prelaminar region. In glaucomatous tissue, NOS-3 is present in astrocytes and in the vascular endothelia of large and small vessels (Neufeld *et al.*, 1997a). NO in high concentrations can be neurotoxic. Furthermore, it can reach the axons of the ganglion cells, where there are high concentrations of superoxide anion (free radical generated by damage from ischaemia-reperfusion), and can form peroxynitrates. The superoxide anion and the peroxynitrites are trapped in the axons and are spread by the axon towards the retina and the lateral geniculate body, inducing apoptosis in the neurons (Flammer & Mozaffarieh, 2007; Neufeld, 1999b).

4.2   Inflammation as a Physiopathological Mechanism

The pathogenic mechanisms of glaucoma include the inflammatory mechanisms triggered by the immune response. In human and experimental glaucoma, a chronic activation of the microglia in the retina and in the optic nerve has been reported, as well as an alteration of the T cells, increased autoantibody production, immunoglobulin deposits in the retina, and activation of the complement (Rieck, 2013; Tezel *et al.*, 2007).

Although the immune response in glaucomatous patients may initially be beneficial to repair tissue, the failure of immunoregulatory mechanisms related to chronic stress of this pathology could have neurodegenerative consequences. Microglia would be involved in this immune response (Bosco *et al.*, 2011; Tezel, 2013). In the CNS, the main function of the microglia is the continuous surveillance over the nerve parenchyma. In this way, it takes care of cleaning tissue and limiting the neurodegenerative consequences of stress (Boya *et al.*, 1979).

The activation of the microglia is a sign that an inflammatory process is under way in the CNS (Block *et al.*, 2007). The activated microglia act as a phagocyte, eliminating the apoptotic neurons (the RGCs in the case of glaucoma), cell remains, and pathogens. These latter are recognized by the microglia through the toll-like receptors (TLR), the activation of which causes the secretion of proinflammatory cytokines (e.g. TNF-α), NO and prostaglandins that induce the neurodegenerative process (Gonzalez-Scarano & Baltuch, 1999).

In the human glaucomatous optic-nerve heads, microglia can reportedly express several MMPs and their inhibitors, suggesting that they could participate in the remodelling of the extracellular matrix, which is key in the physiopathology of glaucoma (Yuan & Neufeld, 2001; Yuan & Neufeld, 2000). Furthermore, these cells, as discussed above, can secrete TNF-α, reactive oxygen species and NO, which have been found to be involved as mediators of neuronal damage in glaucoma (Yuan & Neufeld, 2001). Moreover, increased expression of TLRs 2, 3, and 4, heat-shock proteins (HSP) HSP27, HSP60, and HSP72, as well as adapter proteins and kinases characteristic of the TLR signalling cascade has been found in human glaucoma (Tezel *et al.*, 1998; Tezel *et al.*, 2000; Tezel & Wax, 2000b; Yang *et al.*, 2011). In this way, the TRLs and the increase in the HSPs could contribute to the activation of the innate immune system in this pathology (Tezel *et al.*, 2010).

It has been postulated that the onset of glaucoma could also be mediated by an autoimmune mechanism. In human glaucoma, as mentioned above, the amount of HSPs is high (Tezel *et al.*, 1998; 2000; Tezel & Wax, 2000b). These proteins are components of cell-defence mechanisms and are overexpressed under pathological conditions. Some have a neuroprotective effect (HSP27 and HSP70) and can be induced by ischaemia in retinal glia. However, others can induce apoptosis (HSP60) (Tezel *et al.*, 2004).

In glaucoma patients, high concentrations of antibodies against neuron γ-enolase, rhodopsin and α-crystalin, and HSPs, among others, have been found (Maruyama *et al.*, 2000; Romano *et al.*, 1995; Tezel *et al.*, 2000). The presence of antibodies against HSPS could be explained because these proteins are phylogenetically highly conserved proteins and therefore present molecular similarities between the host and the pathogens, causing at times crossed reactions (Rieck, 2013). Other theories seek to explain the presence of antigens and specific autoantibodies of the CNS in peripheral blood. The oxidised proteins, by reactive oxygen species, or fragmented by metalloproteinases, could serve as autoantigens (e.g. HSP27, HSP70, or HSP90) (Cauwe *et al.*, 2009).

Autoantibodies can bind to antigens on the surface of the cells or capture circulating antigens, forming immunocomplexes that can accumulate in the lymph nodes or in different organs. The immunocomplexes have the potential of activating the cascade of the complement by the classical pathway (Ren & Danias, 2010; Ricklin *et al.*, 2010). Autoantibodies can be destructive but also protective, inasmuch as they can help eliminate cell damage and promote cell repair (Bell *et al.*, 2013). In this line, they can mask the self-recognition against the pathogenic autoantibodies, neutralize inflammatory cytokines such as TNFα, through antibodies against cytokines, and have an immuno-modulating function (Wax & Tezel, 2009). The decrease in reactivity of these protective autoantibodies could provoke a loss of immune defence, increasing the risk of developing experimental (Grus & Sun, 2008; Wax *et al.*, 2008) and human (Grus & Sun, 2008; Wax *et al.*, 2008) glaucoma.

The participation of the cell immune response against neuronal components has been confirmed by the presence of T cells and macrophages in the brain of patients with neurodegenerative diseases (Rieck, 2013). The inflammatory process in the CNS can occur when the T cells and the autoantibodies gain access to the CNS through the blood, by the alteration of the BBB (Grieshaber & Flammer, 2007). These T lymphocytes are again reactivated by antigen-presenting cells (e.g. microglia), provoking the release of inflammatory cytokines and therefore the maintenance of the immune response (Rieck, 2013).

Antibodies bind to the neuronal antigens, altering their function, causing cell stress, and finally apoptosis of the neuron. The microglia go to the site of the inflammation, eliminating the cell remains by endocytosis and presenting their antigens on the surface, activating the adaptive immune response. In fact, in unilateral laser- induced glaucoma, the overexpression of MHC-II by the microglia has been demonstrated (Gallego *et al.*, 2012). The adaptive immunity activates the T CD4+cells, specific of the antigen, and the differentiation of the B cells in plasma cells that produce antibodies, in the peripheral tissues. The antibodies cross the BBB mainly under pathological conditions (e.g. elevated IOP) (Nguyen *et al.*, 2002; Rieck, 2013). These immunoglobulins can bind to the cell surface or else enter the cell by a receptor or by endocytosis (e.g. anti-HSP27). Once in the cytoplasm of the neurons, the immunoglobulins cause apoptosis (Tezel & Wax, 2000b). The recurrent release of cytokines and presentation of antigen starts the vicious circle in the inflammatory mechanism.

In conclusion, in glaucoma the chronic stress that results in the retina and the optic nerve, through the overexpression of heat-shock proteins and ROS generation, are determinant in the immune response. The alterations in the interactions between the glia cells and the neurons under stress conditions, together with an increase in the antigenicity of the damaged tissue, as well as the increase in the presenting activity of the antigen in the resident glial cells have a determining role in the behaviour of the immune system in glaucoma.

5   Animal Models of Glaucoma

A variety of natural-occurring glaucoma models have been described in different animal species. Albino New Zealand rabbits exhibit spontaneous alterations in trabecular mesh development that could be the cause of elevated IOP (Kolker, *et al.*, 1963). Other dog models of closed-angle glaucoma in beagles, cocker spaniels, and basset hounds have been reported. Cockers develop glaucoma at an early age, whereas beagles and bassets begin to develop the disease between 6 and 12 months of age. Beagles expressing autosomal recessive phenotype present a pre-glaucoma stage characterized by increased IOP and an open angle (Gelatt, *et al.*, 1977).

Models of induced glaucoma were developed for non-human primates by inducing elevated IOP via intraocular injections of the proteolytic enzyme alpha chymotrypsin (Kalvin *et al.*, 1966). Alpha chymotrypsin, however, produced highly variable IOP responses depending on the doses (Fernández-Durango *et al.*, 1991). Developed laser induced scar formation of the trabecular meshwork (TM) with an Argon laser (Gaasterland & Kupfer, 1974). Recently, the use of laser to induce experimental glaucoma in non-human primates was implemented with a high-power diode laser (Wang *et al.*, 1998). The injection of latex microspheres into the anterior chamber of the rhesus monkey eye introduced a new, inexpensive technique (Weber & Zelenak, 2001).

The pig model is more accessible than non-human primates. The retina is more similar to the human retina than that of other larger mammals. This constitutes a model for eye diseases and has been extensively studied. The IOP in the pig and minipig was increased by episcleral vein cauterization (Shareef *et al.*, 1995) or by the injection of latex fluorospheres into the anterior chamber (Ruiz-Ederra *et al.*, 2005). Experimental rodent models have been used to study glaucomatous neuropathy because they are inexpensive and easier to handle than other animal models (dog and rabbit). The most relevant rodent models of experimental glaucomatous optic neuropathy are those that obstruct aqueous humour outflow. In rats, this can be accomplished by retrograde injections of hypertonic saline into the aqueous humour outflow pathways via episcleral veins (Morrison *et al.*, 1997) or using external laser to the anterior chamber angle (Levkovitch-Verbin *et al.*, 2002; Ueda *et al.*, 1998; WoldeMussie *et al.*, 2001). In addition, intracameral injections of foreign substances, including hyaluronic acid (Moreno *et al.*, 2005b) and latex microspheres were used as methods of elevating IOP and obstructing aqueous outflow (Sappington *et al.*, 2010). In mice, hypertonic saline injection, external laser and injection of microspheres induce higher IOP (Aihara *et al.*, 2003; Sappington *et al.*, 2010; Walsh *et al.*, 2009). Another model, using cautery of one or more large external episcleral veins immediately intensifies pressure, which gradually returns to normal after one or more months (Grozdanic *et al.*, 2003; Mittag *et al.*, 2000; Neufeld *et al.*, 1999; Sawada *et al.*, 1999; Shareef *et al.*, 1995).

The DBA/2J mouse line, is the most well-characterized of the spontaneous rodent glaucoma models (John, 2005; John *et al.*, 1998; Libby *et al.*, 2005). In this model, mutations of 2 genes results in iris stroma atrophy and pigment dispersion in the anterior segment and the trabecular meshwork, which results in reduced aqueous humour outflow. In most animals, IOP increases at about 7-8 months of age, although its extent varies among animals of the same age, and between the two eyes of a single animal (Schlamp *et al.*, 2006). More recently, other transgenic mouse models have been developed, including one with a targeted mutation in the gene for the alpha-1 subunit of collagen type 1, which demonstrates a gradual rise in IOP and progressive optic-nerve axon loss (Mabuchi *et al.*, 2004). The transgenic mouse expressing a mutant form of human myocilin protein has also been described (Senatorov *et al.*, 2006; Zhou *et al.*, 2008). Finally, mutations affecting a serine protease (PRSS56) cause a mouse phenotype resembling closed-angle glaucoma (Nair *et al.*, 2011).

It has been suggested that Foxc1+/− and Foxc2+/− mice may lead to the identification of genes that interact with Foxc1 and Foxc2 to produce a phenotype with elevated IOP and glaucoma (Smith *et al.*, 2000). Expression of ODAG (ocular development-associated gene) under the control of the mouse Crx promoter significantly raised the IOP (approximately 50% above control) (Sasaki *et al.*, 2009).

6   Glial and Retinal Ganglion Cells in Experimental Unilateral Laser-induced Ocular Hypertension

Altered crosstalk between RGCs and microglia, astrocytes or, oligodendrocytes has been proposed as an early factor in the pathophysiology of glaucoma (Bosco *et al.*, 2011). The lack of agreement concerning the role played by the glia in ganglion cells has raised the need for research on both the location and the discrimination of responses which take place simultaneously in the RGCs and glia (Johnson & Morrison, 2009).

It has been suggested that reactive glial cells could help protect retinal ganglion cells, as they can be a source of neurotrophic factors (Di Polo *et al.*, 1998). On the contrary, reactive glial cells can exacerbate neuronal damage and may become one of the aetiologies of experimental glaucoma through the release of cytokines, reactive oxygen species, and functional disorders of the glutamate uptake in Müller cells (Kawasaki *et al.*, 2000). This could negatively influence ganglion cells, which could lose their normal functional support (Johnson *et al.*, 2007). In this regard, the colocalization of caspase 3 and GFAP in astrocytes and Müller glia in experimental glaucomatous retinas has indicated that these cells may be involved in the apoptosis process, in which the increase of nitric oxide (NO) and tumour-necrosis factor (TNF-α) produced by glial cells would lead to the death of retinal ganglion cells exposed to stressful conditions (Tezel & Wax, 2000a; Wang & Tay, 2005).

In a recent study in a mouse model of ocular hypertension (OHT), both the eye with laser-induced OHT and the contralateral eye (Gallego *et al.*, 2012) were analysed for the purpose of identifying concurrent responses of macroglial and retinal ganglion cells and whether there was an inflammatory reaction to OHT and then comparing them with retinas from naïve eyes. These findings correspond to changes observed after 15 days of lasering the treated eye. Although the experimental conditions of this study do not completely mimic or serve as a model for human glaucomatous optic neuropathy, they can be used to investigate OHT-induced changes undergone by retinal macroglia, microglia, and ganglion cells. In this model of laser-induced OHT, a substantial rise in the IOP was evident 24 h after lasering, this continuing for 4 days and then gradually returning to the basal value after the fifth day, so that by one week after lasering, the IOP values in the treated animals were comparable for both eyes (Salinas-Navarro *et al.*, 2009).

Numerous in vitro and in vivo studies have shown GFAP to be essential for several astrocyte functions such as proliferation, differentiation, extension of processes, vesicle trafficking, astrocyte-neuron interaction (Middeldorp & Hol, 2011), astrogliosis (Perez-Alvarez *et al.*, 2008), and protection against cerebral ischaemia (Middeldorp & Hol, 2011).The intermediate filament protein GFAP of astrocytes is considered to be an early marker for retinal injury and is commonly used as an index of gliosis-hypertrophy (Hernandez, 2000; Ramírez *et al.*, 2001; Varela & Hernandez, 1997). Two relevant morphological alterations in gliotic Müller cells are hypertrophy and the expression of the filament protein GFAP (Reichenbach & Bringmann, 2010).

In the above-mentioned model of laser-induced OHT (Gallego *et al.*, 2012), it has been reported that OHT induces a differential GFAP-expression pattern in the macroglial cells of the retina, reduces GFAP-IR in astrocytes, and increases GFAP-IR in Müller cells (Fig. 7). Such opposite reactions in astrocytes and Müller cells in terms of GFAP-IR has been reported in OHT eyes of two models of laser induced glaucoma in rats (Kanamori *et al.*, 2005; Ramírez *et al.*, 2010) and in models of experimental diabetes in rats (Barber *et al.*, 2000).

In addition, the laser-induced OHT-model in mouse has revealed astrocyte changes, consisting of fewer secondary processes, decreased GFAP-labelled retinal area (Fig. 8C1,C2) (Gallego *et al.*, 2012), changes also demonstrated in laser-induced experimental glaucoma in rats that could impair the neuro-supportive role of astrocytes (Lorber *et al.*, 2012) and could participate in the death of RGCs (Salinas-Navarro *et al.*, 2009). In experimental glaucoma models this reactive, non-proliferative gliotic response (Gallego *et al.*, 2012; Bolz *et al.*, 2008; Inman & Horner, 2007; Ramírez *et al.*, 2010) is the consequence of slow degeneration, while rapid degeneration leads to a proliferative gliosis (Bolz *et al.*, 2008; Inman & Horner, 2007; Soto *et al.*, 2008).

NF-200 is a component of the neuronal cytoskeleton. Under normal conditions, anti-NF-200 labels RGC axons but rarely RGC somas (Bizzi *et al.*, 1991). It is known that an elevated IOP has been associated with the disruption of the axonal transport (Mabuchi *et al.*, 2004) in different animal models (Anderson *et al.*, 1974; Minckler *et al.*, 1976; Pease *et al.*, 2000; Quigley & Anderson, 1977; Quigley, *et al.*, 1981). A factor deeply involved in axonal transport is phosphorylation of the heavy neurofilament subunit (NF-H) (Lee & Cleveland, 1996; Nixon & Sihag, 1991; Pant & Veeranna, 1995). In a monkey model of laser- induced chronic ocular hypertension (Kashiwagi *et al.*, 2003), most NF-Hs in RGC axons in the glaucomatous eyes were significantly dephosphorylated by high IOP, which may be a sign of damaged axonal transport. In a mouse model of laser-induced ocular hypertension (OHT) (Gallego *et al.*, 2012), it has been reported that the number of NF-200+RGCs significantly augmented in OHT-eyes in comparison to naïve and contralateral eyes. These RGCs that had accumulated NF-200 in their cell bodies, proximal axon, and primary dendrites (Fig. 9) most probably represented functionally impaired RGCs as a consequence of the disruption of the axonal transport (Gallego *et al.*, 2012; Salinas-Navarro *et al.*, 2009).

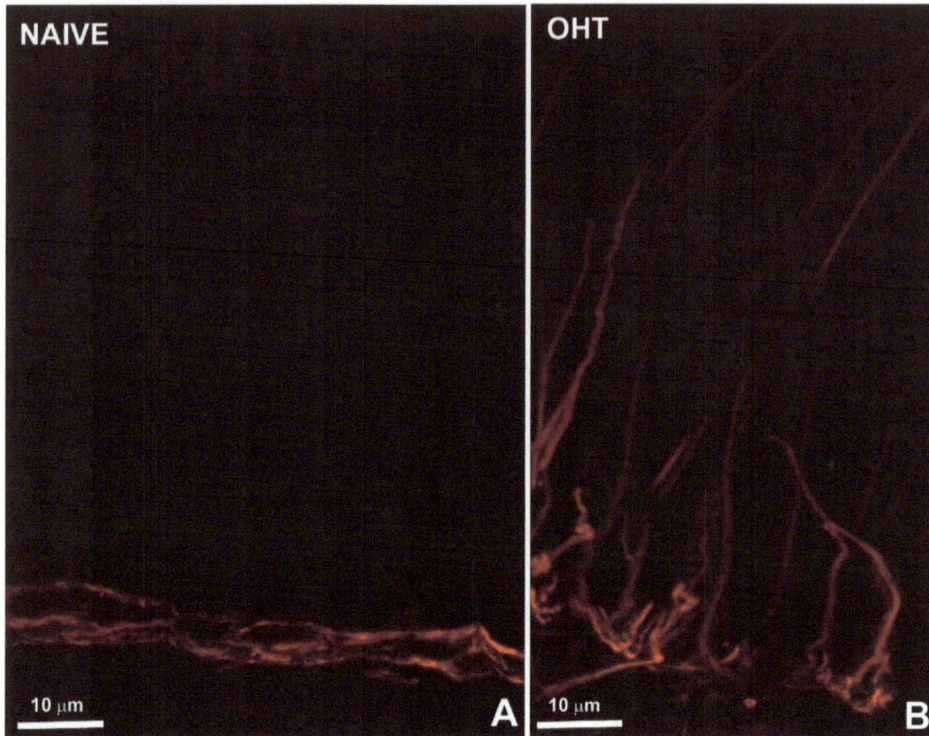

Figure 7: Macroglial cells of the mice retina. Immunostaining for GFAP (red). The pressure exerted by the cover glass on the retinal whole-mount, produced a retinal-like section effect in some retinal borders. A. GFAP+ astrocytes in the nerve-fibre-RCG layer in a normal mice retina (naive). B. After 15 days of laser-induced OHT, GFAP expression in Müller cells is upregulated. Müller cells exhibit a radial morphology that creates a columnar matrix that maintains the laminar structure of the retina [GFAP: glial fibrillary acidic protein; OHT: ocular hypertension]. Fluorescence microscopy and image acquisition using the ApoTome.

Notably, in this mouse model of laser-induced ocular hypertension (OHT), the NF-200+RGC somas of the OHT eyes tended to be more abundant in areas of the retina having less GFAP-labelled retinal area (Gallego *et al.*, 2012). As demonstrated in rodent an impairment of axonal support exerted by astrocytes could possibly increase the vulnerability of the axon to IOP-nduced stress (Morrison *et al.*, 2011; Dibas *et al.*, 2008) offered a possible explanation, according to which rat reinas with OHT showed a dowregulation of AQP4 protein and an accumulation of ubiquitin in astrocytes which might not be appropriately transferred to adjacent RGCs. The attenuation of ubiquitination in axons may result in the accumulation of several proapoptotic proteins (i.e. caspases, Bax and Bad) (Dahlmann, 2007) and thus contributes to axonal degeneration in glaucoma. It is known that a severe axon insult can result in a rapid Wallerian degeneration of the distal axon (Conforti *et al.*, 2007). On the contrary, milder insults may result in degeneration via the slower process of axonal dying back and greater functional connectivity between the soma, proximal axon, and the distal axon segments (Buckingham *et al.*, 2008; Crish *et al.*, 2010; Fu & Sretavan, 2010; Howell *et al.*, 2007; Schlamp *et al.*, 2006; Whitmore *et al.*, 2005). This situation involving the NF-200+RGCs in OHT-eyes (Fig. 9) could represent RGCs that, after having suffered an insult, retain their fundamental homeostatic mechanisms (Gallego *et al.*, 2012; Soto *et al.*, 2008; Soto *et al.*, 2011) , which might provide an opportunity for therapeutic rescue in the human disease.

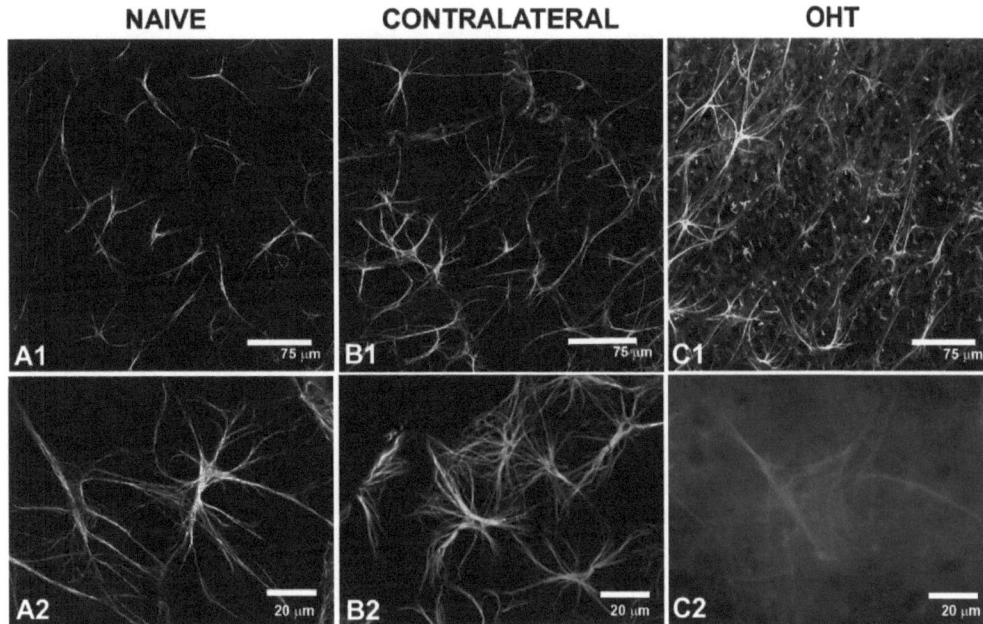

Figure 8: GFAP immunostaining of equivalent areas of the mice retinal whole-mounts. Astrocyte morphology and GFAP-IR of macroglial cells in naïve and in contralateral and OHT-eyes after 15 days of laser-induced OHT. A. In naïve eyes the astrocytes form a homogeneous plexus on the nerve-fiber-RCG layer of GFAP+ cells regularly distributed throughout the retina (A1). The astrocytes have a rounded body from which numerous primary and secondary processes extended (A2). B. In contralateral eyes astrocytes form a honeycomb network (B1) and are more robust (B2) than in naïve eyes. C. Astrocyte morphology in OHT-eyes is not uniform (C1), with astrocytes in which primary and secondary processes could be observed and astrocytes in which only primary processes could be observed (C2). [GFAP: glial fibrillary acidic protein; OHT: ocular hypertension; RGC: retinal ganglion cells]. Confocal microscopy (A1, B1, C1). Fluorescence microscopy and image acquisition using the Apo-Tome (A2, B2, C2).

A striking feature in mice retina contralateral to experimental glaucoma was that macroglia exhibited morphological signs of reactivity that differed from naïve (Fig.8A) and OHT-eyes (Fig. 8B): astrocytes were more robust, formed a honeycomb-like network, and had an increase in GFAP-labelled retinal area (Gallego *et al.*, 2012) (Fig. 8B). By contrast, the contralateral retinas of two laser-induced models of glaucoma in rats exhibited a decrease in both the retinal area occupied by astrocytes (Ramírez *et al.*, 2010) and the GFAP-IR in astrocytes (Kanamori *et al.*, 2005; Ramírez *et al.*, 2010). The different behaviour of the retinal macroglia of the contralateral eyes between mice and rats could be a species-related phenomenon or could depend on the experimental model, such as differences in time to build pressure or time to return to normal values, among other possibilities (Morrison *et al.*, 2011).

It has been reported that the glial-activation response in experimental and human glaucomatous eyes involves the activation of a glial immunoregulatory function and antigen-presenting ability (Steele *et al.*, 2006; Tezel & the Fourth ARVO/Pfizer Ophthalmics Research Institute Conference,Working Group, 2009). The expression of MHC-II in glial cells, required for antigen presentation to T cells, is upregulated in the glaucomatous human retina and optic-nerve head (Tezel *et al.*, 2003; Tezel & the Fourth ARVO/Pfizer Ophthalmics Research Institute Conference,Working Group, 2009; Yang *et al.*, 2001).

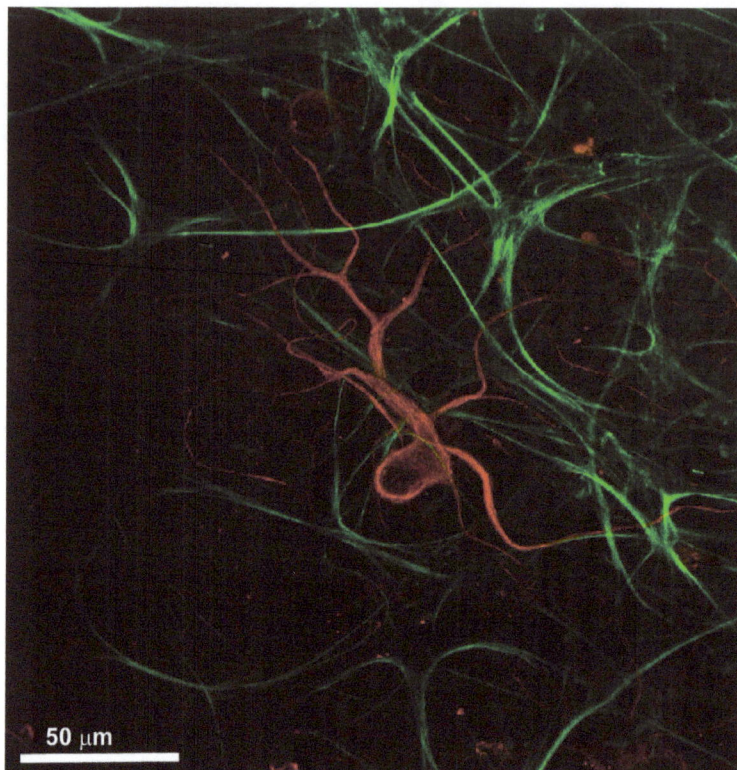

Figure 9: Retinal whole-mount. Double immunostaining for NF-200 and GFAP after 15 days of laser-induced OHT. RGCs (red). Astrocyte (green). Abnormal staining of cell bodies and primary dendrites of RGCs in OHT-eyes. [GFAP: glial fibrillary acidic protein; NF-200: neurofilament of 200kD; OHT: ocular hypertension; RGCs: retinal ganglion cells]. Confocal microscopy.

In addition, microglial activation has been demonstrated in human eyes with glaucoma (Neufeld, 1999a), in experimental models of OHT (Gallego *et al.*, 2012; Johnson & Morrison, 2009; Naskar *et al.*, 2002; Tezel *et al.*, 2003; Wang *et al.*, 2000) (Fig. 10) and in a genetic mouse model of glaucoma (Inman & Horner, 2007). Also, MHC-II immunoreaction in Müller cells supports the idea of immune activation in the eyes with laser-induced OHT (Gallego *et al.*, 2012) (Fig. 11).

A lack of relation between immune responses in DBA/2J mice retina and greater IOP has been reported (Fan *et al.*, 2010) and recently corroborated by Bosco *et al.* (2011), who saw no strict correlation between higher IOP and early microglia activation. These researchers concluded that a rise in IOP may not be a contributing factor in these initial changes (Bosco *et al.*, 2011). It bears mentioning that most microglial cells of the retinas contralateral to laser-induced experimental glaucoma (normal IOP values) showed morphological changes and MHC-II upregulation in comparison with naïve eyes (Gallego *et al.*, 2012). This MHC-II upregulation was detected in the three retinal glial types (astrocyte, Müller cells, microglia) (Fig. 10, 11) (Gallego *et al.*, 2012), which were not temporally related to surgical eyeball manipulations, leading to the postulation that an immunologically mediated process was taking place in retinas contralateral to experimental glaucoma. This glial response may contribute to the maintainance of tissue homeostasis, perhaps in an effort to protect optic axons from a compromised BBB (Bosco *et al.*, 2011; Neufeld, 1999a). A more sustained insult or prolonged neuronal stress may lead to glial changes that could potentially contribute to neuronal decline.

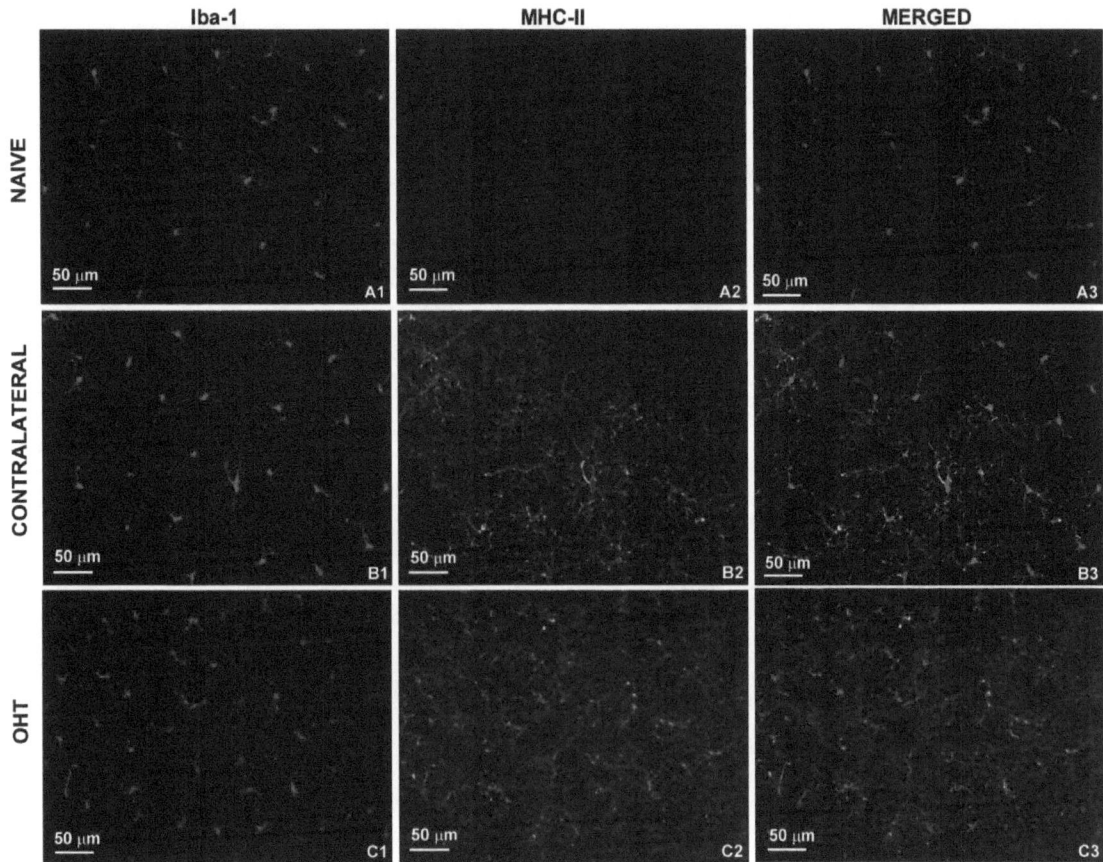

Figure 10: MHC-II expression of Iba-1+ cells in retinal whole-mounts after 15 days of laser-induced OHT. Double immunofluorescence staining for Iba-1 (red) and MHC-II (green). A. in naïve retinas, a constitutive weak expression of MHC-II is observed in some Iba-1+ cells throughout the retina. B. in contralateral eyes, Iba-1+ microglial cells of the retina have morphological signs of activation and show a stronger expression of MHC-II immunoreactivity throughout the retina in comparison with naïve. C. Iba+1 cell in OHT-eyes have a similar up-regulation of MHC-II as did contralateral. In comparison with contralateral retinas, the cell bodies are larger and the processes thicker and more retracted. Fluorescence microscopy and image acquisition using the ApoTome. [Iba-1: ionized calcium-binding adapter molecule 1; MHC-II: major histocompatibility complex class II molecule; OHT: ocular hypertension].

In a model of laser-induced OHT RGC loss was documented using a retrograde tracer applied to both superior colliculi one week prior to animal processing. In that study, the contralateral retinas showed the typical distribution of RGCs throughout the retina (Salinas-Navarro *et al.*, 2009). Based on this data, macroglial activation as well as MHC-II expression on astrocytes and Müller cells of contralateral retinas to experimental glaucoma could have exerted a neuroprotective effect (Fig. 11) (Gallego *et al.*, 2012). It has been suggested that the expression of modest levels of MHC-II may inhibit the activation of invading T cell, whereas overexpression of these molecules may promote the activation of autoimmune T cells, thereby augmenting the inflammatory cascade, leading to tissue damage (Shao *et al.*, 2007; Tezel & the

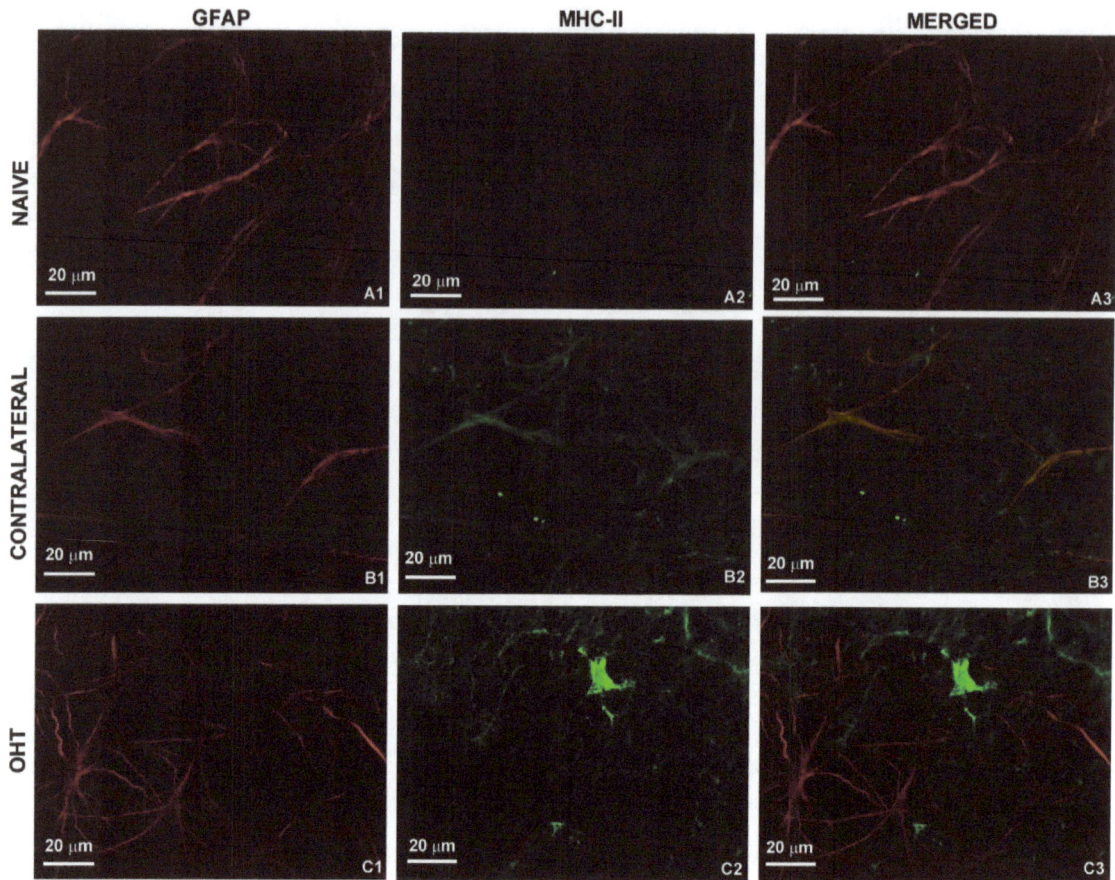

Figure 11: MHC-II expression of GFAP+ cells in retinal whole-mounts after 15 days of laser-induced OHT. Double immunostaining for GFAP (red) and MHC-II (in green). A. A weak constitutive MHC-II expression is found rarely in the naïve retina. B. In contralateral eyes, MHC-II immunoreactivity of astrocytes and Müller cells is increased with respect to naïve eyes. C. In OHT-eyes, MHC-II immunoreactivity of Müller cells is notably upregulated in comparison with contralateral eyes. Fluorescence microscopy and image acquisition using the ApoTome. [GFAP: glial fibrillary acidic protein; MHC-II: major histocompatibility complex class II molecule; OHT: ocular hypertension].

Fourth ARVO/Pfizer Ophthalmics Research Institute Conference, Working Group, 2009) The gliotic behaviour in eyes contralateral to experimental glaucoma could be related to the immune response. The absence of NF-200+RGCs (sign of RGC degeneration) leads to the postulation that the MHC-II upregulation in contralateral eyes could bolster neuroprotection (Gallego *et al.*, 2012).

7   Conclusions

Glaucoma, the second leading cause of blindness in the world, is a multifactorial neurodegenerative disease characterized by an irreversible decrease of retinal-ganglion cells of the retina (RGCs) and their axons. Many of the proposed mechanisms in the development and progression of this pathology are linked to increased intraocular pressure (IOP). Although IOP was considered a major factor responsible for the glaucomatous neuropathy, today the role has been relieved for multiple factors: aging, vascular dysregulation, and the involvement of the immune system. Glial cells from the retina and the optic nerve in the glaucomatous optic neuropathy show a chronic activation. The increased antigen-presenting activity in macro- and microglial cells may be key in the role of the immune system in glaucoma. Persistent changes in GFAP and MHC-II expression took place in macro- and microglial cells, both in the contralateral and OHT eyes of adult Swiss mice. These changes could be related to inmune-system activation in the glaucomatous neuropathy. Knowledge of the role of the immune system en the glaucoma physiopathology could lead to the development of more effective neuroprotective treatments for modulating the immune response in order to achieve, on the one hand, tissue repair and neuronal survival and, on the other, decreased immune-mediated neurodegenerative damage.

References

Abbott, N. J., Rönnbäck, L., & Hansson, E. (2006). Astrocyte–endothelial interactions at the blood–brain barrier. *Nature Reviews Neuroscience, 7, 41-53.*

Agapova, O. A., Ricard, C. S., Salvador-Silva, M., & Hernandez, M. R. (2001). Expression of matrix metalloproteinases and tissue inhibitors of metalloproteinases in human optic nerve head astrocytes. *Glia, 33, 205-216.*

Agarwal, R., Gupta, S., Agarwal, P., Saxena, R., & Agrawal, S. (2009). Current concepts in the pathophysiology of glaucoma. *Indian Journal of Ophthalmology, 57, 257-266.*

Aiello, L. P., Northrup, J. M., Keyt, B. A., Takagi, H., & Iwamoto, M. A. (1995). Hypoxic regulation of vascular endothelial growth factor in retinal cells. *Archives of Ophthalmology, 113, 1538.*

Aihara, M., Lindsey, J. D., & Weinreb, R. N. (2003). Experimental mouse ocular hypertension: Establishment of the model. *Investigative Ophthalmology & Visual Science, 44, 4314-4320.*

Alarma-Estrany, P., & Pintor, J. (2007). Melatonin receptors in the eye: Location, second messengers and role in ocular physiology. *Pharmacology & Therapeutics, 113, 507-522.*

Aloisi, F. (2001). Immune function of microglia. *Glia, 36, 165-179.*

Ames III, A. (2000). CNS energy metabolism as related to function. *Brain Research Reviews, 34, 42-68.*

Anderson, D. R., & Hendrickson, A. (1974). Effect of intraocular pressure on rapid axoplasmic transport in monkey optic nerve. *Investigative Ophthalmology & Visual Science, 13, 771-783.*

Aronica, E., Gorter, J. A., Ijlst-Keizers, H., Rozemuller, A. J., Yankaya, B., Leenstra, S., & Troost, D. (2003). Expression and functional role of mGluR3 and mGluR5 in human astrocytes and glioma cells: Opposite regulation of glutamate transporter proteins. *European Journal of Neuroscience, 17, 2106-2118.*

Barber, A. J., Antonetti, D. A., & Gardner, T. W. (2000). Altered expression of retinal occludin and glial fibrillary acidic protein in experimental diabetes. the penn state retina research group. *Investigative Ophthalmology & Visual Science, 41, 3561-3568.*

Behzadian, M. A., Wang, X., Windsor, L. J., Ghaly, N., & Caldwell, R. B. (2001). TGF-β increases retinal endothelial cell permeability by increasing MMP-9: Possible role of glial cells in endothelial barrier function. *Investigative Ophthalmology & Visual Science, 42, 853-859.*

Bell, K., Gramlich, O. W., Von Thun Und Hohenstein-Blaul, N., Beck, S., Funke, S., Wilding, C., Pfeiffer, N., & Grus, F. H. (2013). Does autoimmunity play a part in the pathogenesis of glaucoma? *Progress in Retinal and Eye Research, 36, 199-216.*

Benhar, I., London, A., & Schwartz, M. (2012). The privileged immunity of immune privileged organs: The case of the eye. *Frontiers in Immunology, 3, 296.*

Bill, A. (1975). Blood circulation and fluid dynamics in the eye. Physiological Reviews, 55, 383-417.

Bill, A., Sperber, G., & Ujiie, K. (1983). Physiology of the choroidal vascular bed. International Ophthalmology, 6, 101-107.

Bill, A., Tornquist, P., & Alm, A. (1980). Permeability of the intraocular blood vessels. Transactions of the Ophthalmological Societies of the United Kingdom, 100, 332-336.

Bizzi, A., Schaetzle, B., Patton, A., Gambetti, P., & Autilio-Gambetti, L. (1991). Axonal transport of two major components of the ubiquitin system: Free ubiquitin and ubiquitin carboxyl-terminal hydrolase PGP 9.5. Brain Research, 548, 292-299.

Block, M. L., Zecca, L., & Hong, J. S. (2007). Microglia-mediated neurotoxicity: Uncovering the molecular mechanisms. Nature Review Neuroscience, 8, 57-69.

Boehm, M. R., Oellers, P., & Thanos, S. (2011). Inflammation and immunology of the vitreoretinal compartment. Inflammation & Allergy Drug Targets, 10, 283-309.

Bolz, S., Schuettauf, F., Fries, J. E., Thaler, S., Reichenbach, A., & Pannicke, T. (2008). K(+) currents fail to change in reactive retinal glial cells in a mouse model of glaucoma. Graefe's Archive for Clinical and Experimental Ophthalmology, 246, 1249-1254.

Bosco, A., Steele, M. R., & Vetter, M. L. (2011). Early microglia activation in a mouse model of chronic glaucoma. Journal of Comparative Neurology, 519(4), 599-620.

Boya, J., Calvo, J., & Prado, A. (1979). The origin of microglial cells. Journal of Anatomy, 129, 177-186.

Bredt, D. S., & Snyder, S. H. (1994). Nitric oxide: A physiologic messenger molecule. Annual Review of Biochemistry, 63, 175-195.

Bringmann, A., Pannicke, T., Grosche, J., Francke, M., Wiedemann, P., Skatchkov, S. N., Osborne, N.N., Reichenbach, A. (2006). Muller cells in the healthy and diseased retina. Progress in Retinal and Eye Research, 25, 397-424.

Bron, A. J., Tripathi, R. C., & Tripathi, B. J. (1997). The choroid and uveal vessels. In A. J. Bron, R. C. Tripathi & B. J. Tripathi (Eds.), Wolff's anatomy of the eye and orbit (eighth edition). (pp. 371-410). London.: Chapman & Hall Medical.

Buckingham, B. P., Inman, D. M., Lambert, W., Oglesby, E., Calkins, D. J., Steele, M. R., Vetter, M.L., Marsh-Armstrong, N., & Horner, P. J. (2008). Progressive ganglion cell degeneration precedes neuronal loss in a mouse model of glaucoma. Journal of Neuroscience, 28, 2735-2744.

Burgoyne, C. F. (2011). A biomechanical paradigm for axonal insult within the optic nerve head in aging and glaucoma. Experimental Eye Research, 93, 120-132.

Caprioli, J., & Spaeth, G. L. (1985). Comparison of the optic nerve head in high- and low-tension glaucoma. Archives of Ophthalmology, 103, 1145-1149.

Cauwe, B., Martens, E., Proost, P., & Opdenakker, G. (2009). Multidimensional degradomics identifies systemic autoantigens and intracellular matrix proteins as novel gelatinase B/MMP-9 substrates. Integrative Biology, 1, 404-426.

Cellini, M., Strobbe, E., Gizzi, C., Balducci, N., Toschi, P. G., & Campos, E. C. (2012). Endothelin-1 plasma levels and vascular endothelial dysfunction in primary open angle glaucoma. Life Sciences, 91, 699-702.

Chowdhury, I., Tharakan, B., & Bhat, G. K. (2008). Caspases - an update. Comparative Biochemistry and Physiology. Part B, Biochemistry & Molecular Biology, 151, 10-27.

Coffman, R. L., Seymour, B. W., Lebman, D. A., Hiraki, D. D., Christiansen, J. A., Shrader, B., Cherwinski, H.M., Savelkoul, H.F., Finkelman, F.D., & Bond, M. W. (1988). The role of helper T cell products in mouse B cell differentiation and isotype regulation. Immunological Reviews, 102, 5-28.

Cogan, D. G., & Kuwabara, T. (1967). The mural cell in perspective. Archives of Ophthalmology, 78, 133-139.

Coleman, M. P., & Freeman, M. R. (2010). Wallerian degeneration, wld(s), and nmnat. Annual Review of Neuroscience, 33, 245-267

Conforti, L., Adalbert, R., & Coleman, M. P. (2007). Neuronal death: Where does the end begin? Trends in Neurosciences,

30, 159-166.

Crish, S. D., & Calkins, D. J. (2011). *Neurodegeneration in glaucoma: Progression and calcium-dependent intracellular mechanisms. Neuroscience, 176, 1-11.*

Crish, S. D., Dapper, J. D., MacNamee, S. E., Balaram, P., Sidorova, T. N., Lambert, W. S., & Calkins, D. J. (2013). *Failure of axonal transport induces a spatially coincident increase in astrocyte BDNF prior to synapse loss in a central target. Neuroscience, 229, 55-70.*

Crish, S. D., Sappington, R. M., Inman, D. M., Horner, P. J., & Calkins, D. J. (2010). *Distal axonopathy with structural persistence in glaucomatous neurodegeneration. Proceedings of the National Academy of Sciences, 107, 5196-5201.*

Dalle-Donne, I., Scaloni, A., Giustarini, D., Cavarra, E., Tell, G., Lungarella, G., Colombo, R., Rossi, R., & Milzani, A. (2005). *Proteins as biomarkers of oxidative/nitrosative stress in diseases: The contribution of redox proteomics. Mass Spectrometry Reviews, 24, 55-99.*

Dervan, E. W., Chen, H., Ho, S. L., Brummel, N., Schmid, J., Toomey, D., Haralambova, M., Gould, E., Wallace, D.M., Prehn, J.H., O'Brien, C.J., & Murphy, D. (2010). *Protein macroarray profiling of serum autoantibodies in pseudoexfoliation glaucoma. Investigative Ophthalmology & Visual Science, 51, 2968-2975.*

Di Polo, A., Aigner, L. J., Dunn, R. J., Bray, G. M., & Aguayo, A. J. (1998). *Prolonged delivery of brain-derived neurotrophic factor by adenovirus-infected muller cells temporarily rescues injured retinal ganglion cells. Proceedings of the National Academy of Sciences of the United States of America, 95, 3978-3983.*

Dibas, A., Yang, M. H., He, S., Bobich, J., & Yorio, T. (2008). *Changes in ocular aquaporin-4 (AQP4) expression following retinal injury. Molecular Vision, 14, 1770-1783.*

Dong, Y., & Benveniste, E. N. (2001). *Immune function of astrocytes. Glia, 36, 180-190.*

Downs, J. C., Roberts, M. D., & Sigal, I. A. (2011). *Glaucomatous cupping of the lamina cribrosa: A review of the evidence for active progressive remodeling as a mechanism. Experimental Eye Research, 93, 133-140.*

Dreyer, E. B. (1998). *A proposed role for excitotoxicity in glaucoma. Journal of Glaucoma, 7, 62-67.*

Dreyer, E. B., Pan, Z. H., Storm, S., & Lipton, S. A. (1994). *Greater sensitivity of larger retinal ganglion cells to NMDA-mediated cell death. Neuroreport, 5, 629-631.*

Earnshaw, W. C., Martins, L. M., & Kaufmann, S. H. (1999). *Mammalian caspases: Structure, activation, substrates, and functions during apoptosis. Annual Review of Biochemistry, 68, 383-424.*

Eichler, W., Yafai, Y., Wiedemann, P., & Reichenbach, A. (2004). *Angiogenesis-related factors derived from retinal glial (Müller) cells in hypoxia. Neuroreport, 15, 1633-1637.*

Elkabes, S., DiCicco-Bloom, E. M., & Black, I. B. (1996). *Brain microglia/macrophages express neurotrophins that selectively regulate microglial proliferation and function. Journal of Neuroscience, 16, 2508-2521.*

Elkington, A. R., Inman, C. B., Steart, P. V., & Weller, R. O. (1990). *The structure of the lamina cribrosa of the human eye: An immunocytochemical and electron microscopical study. Eye, 4, 42-57.*

Emre, M., Orgul, S., Haufschild, T., Shaw, S. G., & Flammer, J. (2005). *Increased plasma endothelin-1 levels in patients with progressive open angle glaucoma. British Journal of Ophthalmology, 89, 60-63.*

Erb, C., & Heinke, M. (2011). *Oxidative stress in primary open-angle glaucoma. Frontiers in Bioscience, 3, 1524-1533.*

Fan, W., Li, X., Wang, W., Mo, J. S., Kaplan, H., & Cooper, N. G. (2010). *Early involvement of immune/inflammatory response genes in retinal degeneration in DBA/2J mice. Ophthalmology and Eye Diseases, 1, 23-41.*

Fernández-Durango, R., Ramírez, J. M., Triviño, A., Sánchez, D., Paraiso, P., García De Lacoba, M., Ramírez, A.I., Salazar, J.J., Fernández-Cruz, A., & Gutkowska, J. (1991). *Experimental glaucoma significantly decreases atrial natriuretic factor (ANF) receptors in the ciliary processes of the rabbit eye. Experimental Eye Research, 53, 591-596.*

Flammer, J., Haefliger, I. O., Orgul, S., & Resink, T. (1999). *Vascular dysregulation: A principal risk factor for glaucomatous damage? Journal of Glaucoma, 8, 212-219.*

Flammer, J., Orgul, S., Costa, V. P., Orzalesi, N., Krieglstein, G. K., Serra, L. M., Renard, J.P., & Stefansson, E. (2002). *The impact of ocular blood flow in glaucoma. Progress in Retinal and Eye Research, 21, 359-393.*

Flammer, J., Pache, M., & Resink, T. (2001). Vasospasm, its role in the pathogenesis of diseases with particular reference to the eye. Progress in Retinal and Eye Research, 20, 319-349.

Flammer, J., & Mozaffarieh, M. (2007). What is the present pathogenetic concept of glaucomatous optic neuropathy? Survey of Ophthalmology, 52, S162-S173.

Forrester, J. V. (2013). Bowman lecture on the role of inflammation in degenerative disease of the eye. Eye, 27, 340-352.

Fourgeux, C., Bron, A., Acar, N., Creuzot-Garcher, C., & Bretillon, L. (2011). 24S-hydroxycholesterol and cholesterol-24S-hydroxylase (CYP46A1) in the retina: From cholesterol homeostasis to pathophysiology of glaucoma. Chemistry and Physics of Lipids, 164, 496-499.

Fu, C. T., & Sretavan, D. (2010). Laser-induced ocular hypertension in albino CD-1 mice. Investigative Ophthalmology Visual Science, 51, 980-990.

Gaasterland, D., & Kupfer, C. (1974). Reports: Experimental glaucoma in the rhesus monkey. Investigative Ophthalmology & Visual Science, 13, 455-457.

Gallego, B. I., Salazar, J. J., de Hoz, R., Rojas, B., Ramírez, A. I., Salinas-Navarro, M., Ortín-Martínez, A., Valiente-Soriano, F., Avilés-Trigueros, M., Villegas-Perez, M.P., Vidal-Sanz, M., Triviño, A., & Ramírez, J.M.. (2012). IOP induces upregulation of GFAP and MHC-II and microglia reactivity in mice retina contralateral to experimental glaucoma. Journal of Neuroinflammation, 9, 92.

Gelatt, K. N., Peiffer, R., Gwin, R. M., Gum, G. G., & Williams, L. W. (1977). Clinical manifestations of inherited glaucoma in the beagle. Investigative Ophthalmology & Visual Science, 16, 1135-1142.

Ghanem, A. A., Arafa, L. F., & El-Baz, A. (2010). Oxidative stress markers in patients with primary open-angle glaucoma. Current Eye Research, 35, 295-301.

Gherghel, D., Griffiths, H. R., Hilton, E. J., Cunliffe, I. A., & Hosking, S. L. (2005). Systemic reduction in glutathione levels occurs in patients with primary open-angle glaucoma. Investigative Ophthalmology & Visual Science, 46, 877-883.

Gherghel, D., Mroczkowska, S., & Qin, L. (2013). Reduction in blood glutathione levels occurs similarly in patients with primary-open angle or normal tension glaucoma. Investigative Ophthalmology & Visual Science, 54, 3333-3339.

Giebel, S. J., Menicucci, G., McGuire, P. G., & Das, A. (2005). Matrix metalloproteinases in early diabetic retinopathy and their role in alteration of the blood–retinal barrier. Laboratory Investigation, 85, 597-607.

Gonzalez-Scarano, F., & Baltuch, G. (1999). Microglia as mediators of inflammatory and degenerative diseases. Annual Review of Neuroscience, 22, 219-240.

Good, T. J., & Kahook, M. Y. (2010). The role of endothelin in the pathophysiology of glaucoma. Expert Opinion on Therapeutic Targets, 14, 647-654.

Grieshaber, M. C., Terhorst, T., & Flammer, J. (2006). The pathogenesis of optic disc splinter haemorrhages: A new hypothesis. Acta Ophthalmologica Scandinavica, 84, 62-68.

Grieshaber, M. C., & Flammer, J. (2007). Does the blood-brain barrier play a role in glaucoma? Survey of Ophthalmology, 52, S115-S121.

Grozdanic, S. D., Betts, D. M., Sakaguchi, D. S., Kwon, Y. H., Kardon, R. H., & Sonea, I. M. (2003). Temporary elevation of the intraocular pressure by cauterization of vortex and episcleral veins in rats causes functional deficits in the retina and optic nerve. Experimental Eye Research, 77, 27-33.

Grus, F., & Sun, D. (2008). Immunological mechanisms in glaucoma. Seminars in Immunopathology, 30, 121-126.

Grytz, R., Meschke, G., & Jonas, J. B. (2011). The collagen fibril architecture in the lamina cribrosa and peripapillary sclera predicted by a computational remodeling approach. Biomechanics and Modeling in Mechanobiology, 10, 371-382.

Grytz, R., Girkin, C. A., Libertiaux, V., & Downs, J. C. (2012). Perspectives on biomechanical growth and remodeling mechanisms in glaucoma. Mechanics Research Communications, 42, 92-106.

Hayes, G. M., Woodroofe, M. N., & Cuzner, M. L. (1987). Microglia are the major cell type expressing MHC class II in *human white matter. Journal of the Neurological Sciences, 80, 25-37.*

Hayreh, S. S. (1990). In vivo choroidal circulation and its watershed zones. Eye, 4, 273-289.

Hernandez, M. R., Wang, N., Hanley, N. M., & Neufeld, A. H. (1991). Localization of collagen types I and IV mRNAs in human optic nerve head by in situ hybridization. Investigative Ophthalmology & Visual Science, 32(8), 2169-2177.

Hernandez, M. R. (2000). The optic nerve head in glaucoma: Role of astrocytes in tissue remodeling. Progress in Retinal and Eye Research, 19(3), 297-321. doi:DOI: 10.1016/S1350-9462(99)00017-8

Hernandez, M. R., & Pena, J. D. (1997). The optic nerve head in glaucomatous optic neuropathy. Archives of Ophthalmology, 115, 389-395.

Hernandez, M. R., Miao, H., & Lukas, T. (2008). Astrocytes in glaucomatous optic neuropathy. Progress in Brain Research, Volume 173, 353-373.

Hogan, M. J., Alvarado, J. A., & Weddell, J. E. (1971). Histology of the human eye: An atlas and textbook.. Toronto.: W.B. Saunders Company Ed.

Holling, T. M., Schooten, E., & van Den Elsen, P. J. (2004). Function and regulation of MHC class II molecules in T-lymphocytes: Of mice and men. Human Immunology, 65, 282-290.

Hori, J., Joyce, N. C., & Streilein, J. W. (2000). Immune privilege and immunogenicity reside among different layers of the mouse cornea. Investigative Ophthalmology & Visual Science, 41, 3032-3042.

Howell, G. R., Libby, R. T., Jakobs, T. C., Smith, R. S., Phalan, F. C., Barter, J.W., Barbay, J.M., Marchant, J.K., Mahesh, N., Whitmore, A.V., Masland, R.H., & John, S. W. (2007). Axons of retinal ganglion cells are insulted in the optic nerve early in DBA/2J glaucoma. Journal of Cell Biology, 179, 1523-1537.

Inman, D. M., & Horner, P. J. (2007). Reactive nonproliferative gliosis predominates in a chronic mouse model of glaucoma. Glia, 55, 942-953.

Janzer, R. C., & Raff, M. C. (1987). Astrocytes induce blood–brain barrier properties in endothelial cells. Nature, 325, 253-257.

Jiang, L. Q., Jorquera, M., & Streilein, J. W. (1993). Subretinal space and vitreous cavity as immunologically privileged sites for retinal allografts. Investigative Ophthalmology & Visual Science, 34, 3347-3354.

Joachim, S. C., Reichelt, J., Berneiser, S., Pfeiffer, N., & Grus, F. H. (2008). Sera of glaucoma patients show autoantibodies against myelin basic protein and complex autoantibody profiles against human optic nerve antigens. Graefe's Archive for Clinical and Experimental Ophthalmology, 246, 573-580.

John, S. W. (2005). Mechanistic insights into glaucoma provided by experimental genetics the cogan lecture. Investigative Ophthalmology & Visual Science, 46, 2650-2661.

John, S., Smith, R. S., Savinova, O. V., Hawes, N. L., Chang, B., Turnbull, D., Davisson, M., Roderick, T.H., & Heckenlively, J. R. (1998). Essential iris atrophy, pigment dispersion, and glaucoma in DBA/2J mice. Investigative Ophthalmology & Visual Science, 39, 951-962.

Johnson, E. C., Jia, L., Cepurna, W. O., Doser, T. A., & Morrison, J. C. (2007). Global changes in optic nerve head gene expression after exposure to elevated intraocular pressure in a rat glaucoma model. Investigative Ophthalmology & Visual Science, 48, 3161-3177.

Johnson, E. C., & Morrison, J. C. (2009). Friend or foe? resolving the impact of glial responses in glaucoma. Journal of Glaucoma, 18, 341-353.

Johnson, E. C., Doser, T. A., Cepurna, W. O., Dyck, J. A., Jia, L., Guo, Y., Lambert, W.S., & Morrison, J. C. (2011). Cell proliferation and interleukin-6–Type cytokine signaling are implicated by gene expression responses in early optic nerve head injury in rat glaucoma. Investigative Ophthalmology & Visual Science, 52, 504-518.

Johnson, E. C., Guo, Y., Cepurna, W. O., & Morrison, J. C. (2009). Neurotrophin roles in retinal ganglion cell survival: Lessons from rat glaucoma models. Experimental Eye Research, 88, 808-815.

Johnson, T. V., Bull, N. D., & Martin, K. R. (2011). Neurotrophic factor delivery as a protective treatment for glaucoma. Experimental Eye Research, 93, 196-203.

Kalvin, N., Hamasaki, D., & Gass, J. (1966). Experimental glaucoma in Monkeys. I. Relationship between intraocular pressure and cupping of the optic disc and cavernous atrophy of the optic nerve. Archives of Ophthalmology, 76, 82-93.

Kanamori, A., Nakamura, M., Nakanishi, Y., Yamada, Y., & Negi, A. (2005). Long-term glial reactivity in rat retinas ipsilateral and contralateral to experimental glaucoma. Experimental Eye Research, 81, 48-56.

Kaplan, H. J., Stevens, T. R., & Streilein, J. W. (1975). Transplantation immunology of the anterior chamber of the eye I. an intra-ocular graft-vs-host reaction (immunogenic anterior uveitis). Journal of Immunology, 115, 800-804.

Karageuzyan, K. G. (2005). Oxidative stress in the molecular mechanism of pathogenesis at different diseased states of organism in clinics and experiment. Current Drug Targets.Inflammation and Allergy, 4, 85-98.

Kashiwagi, K., Ou, B., Nakamura, S., Tanaka, Y., Suzuki, M., & Tsukahara, S. (2003). Increase in dephosphorylation of the heavy neurofilament subunit in the monkey chronic glaucoma model. Investigative Ophthalmology Visual Science, 44, 154-159.

Katagiri, K., Zhang-Hoover, J., Mo, J. S., Stein-Streilein, J., & Streilein, J. W. (2002). Using tolerance induced via the anterior chamber of the eye to inhibit Th2-dependent pulmonary pathology. Journal of Immunology, 169, 84-89.

Kaushik, S., Pandav, S. S., & Ram, J. (2003). Neuroprotection in glaucoma. Journal of Postgraduate Medicine, 49, 90-95.

Kawasaki, A., Otori, Y., & Barnstable, C. J. (2000). Muller cell protection of rat retinal ganglion cells from glutamate and nitric oxide neurotoxicity. Investigative Ophthalmology & Visual Science, 41, 3444-3450.

Kerrigan-Baumrind, L. A., Quigley, H. A., Pease, M. E., Kerrigan, D. F., & Mitchell, R. S. (2000). Number of ganglion cells in glaucoma eyes compared with threshold visual field tests in the same persons. Investigative Ophthalmology & Visual Science, 41, 741-748.

Kimelberg, H. K., & Nedergaard, M. (2010). Functions of astrocytes and their potential as therapeutic targets. Neurotherapeutics, 7, 338-353.

Knott, A. B., & Bossy-Wetzel, E. (2009). Nitric oxide in health and disease of the nervous system. Antioxidants & Redox Signaling, 11, 541-554.

Kolker, A. E., Moses, R. A., Constant, M. A., & Becker, B. (1963). The development of glaucoma in rabbits. Investigative Ophthalmology & Visual Science, 2, 316-321.

Kompass, K., Agapova, O. A., Li, W., Kaufman, P., Rasmussen, C., & Hernandez, M. R. (2008). Bioinformatic and statistical analysis of the optic nerve head in a primate model of ocular hypertension. BMC Neuroscience, 9, 93.

Kuchtey, J., Rezaei, K. A., Jaru-Ampornpan, P., Sternberg, P.,Jr, & Kuchtey, R. W. (2010). Multiplex cytokine analysis reveals elevated concentration of interleukin-8 in glaucomatous aqueous humor. Investigative Ophthalmology & Visual Science, 51, 6441-6447.

Kuehn, M. H., Kim, C. Y., Ostojic, J., Bellin, M., Alward, W. L., Stone, E. M., . . . Kwon, Y. H. (2006). Retinal synthesis and deposition of complement components induced by ocular hypertension. Experimental Eye Research, 83, 620-628.

Kumpulainen, T., Dahl, D., Korhonen, L. K., & Nystrom, S. H. (1983). Immunolabeling of carbonic anhydrase isoenzyme C and glial fibrillary acidic protein in paraffin-embedded tissue sections of human brain and retina. Journal of Histochemistry and Cytochemistry, 31, 879-886.

Lee, M. K., & Cleveland, D. W. (1996). Neuronal intermediate filaments. Annual Review of Neuroscience, 19, 187-217.

Levkovitch-Verbin, H., Quigley, H. A., Martin, K. R., Valenta, D., Baumrind, L. A., & Pease, M. E. (2002). Translimbal laser photocoagulation to the trabecular meshwork as a model of glaucoma in rats. Investigative Ophthalmology & Visual Science, 43, 402-410.

Liao, H., Bu, W. Y., Wang, T. H., Ahmed, S., & Xiao, Z. C. (2005). Tenascin-R plays a role in neuroprotection via its distinct domains that coordinate to modulate the microglia function. Journal of Biological Chemistry, 280, 8316-8323.

Libby, R. T., Anderson, M. G., Pang, I., Robinson, Z. H., Savinova, O. V., Cosma, I. M., Snow, A., Wilson, L.A., Smith, R.S.,Clark, A.F., & John, S.W. (2005). Inherited glaucoma in DBA/2J mice: Pertinent disease features for studying the neurodegeneration. Visual Neuroscience, 22, 637.

Lipton, S. A. (2001). *Retinal ganglion cells, glaucoma and neuroprotection. Progress in Brain Research, 131, 712-718.*

Liu, B., & Neufeld, A. H. (2000). *Expression of nitric oxide synthase-2 (NOS-2) in reactive astrocytes of the human glaucomatous optic nerve head. Glia, 30, 178-186.*

Lorber, B., Guidi, A., Fawcett, J. W., & Martin, K. R. (2012). *Activated retinal glia mediated axon regeneration in experimental glaucoma. Neurobiology of Disease, 45, 243-252.*

Lowenstein, C. J., Dinerman, J. L., & Snyder, S. H. (1994). *Nitric oxide: A physiologic messenger. Annals of Internal Medicine, 120, 227-237.*

Lundmark, P. O., Pandi-Perumal, S. R., Srinivasan, V., & Cardinali, D. P. (2006). *Role of melatonin in the eye and ocular dysfunctions. Visual Neuroscience, 23, 853-862.*

Luo, C., Yang, X., Kain, A. D., Powell, D. W., Kuehn, M. H., & Tezel, G. (2010). *Glaucomatous tissue stress and the regulation of immune response through glial toll-like receptor signaling. Investigative Ophthalmology & Visual Science, 51, 5697-5707.*

Mabuchi, F., Aihara, M., Mackey, M. R., Lindsey, J. D., & Weinreb, R. N. (2004). *Regional optic nerve damage in experimental mouse glaucoma. Investigative Ophthalmology Visual Science, 45, 4352-4358.*

Majsterek, I., Malinowska, K., Stanczyk, M., Kowalski, M., Blaszczyk, J., Kurowska, A. K., Kaminska, A., & Szaflik, J. (2011). *Evaluation of oxidative stress markers in pathogenesis of primary open-angle glaucoma. Experimental and Molecular Pathology, 90, 231-237.*

Martínez, A. (2013). *Papel de las alteraciones hemodinámicas sistémicas y oculares en el glaucoma. Revista Española de Glaucoma e Hipertensión Ocular, 3, 6-16.*

Martinez, A., & Sanchez, M. (2005). *Predictive value of colour doppler imaging in a prospective study of visual field progression in primary open-angle glaucoma. Acta Ophthalmologica Scandinavica, 83,*

Maruyama, I., Ohguro, H., & Ikeda, Y. (2000). *Retinal ganglion cells recognized by serum autoantibody against gamma-enolase found in glaucoma patients. Investigative Ophthalmology & Visual Science, 41, 1657-1665.*

Medawar, P. (1948). *Immunity to homologous grafted skin. III. the fate of skin homographs transplanted to the brain, to subcutaneous tissue, and to the anterior chamber of the eye. British Journal of Experimental Pathology, 29, 58.*

Melamed, S., Ben-Sira, I., & Ben-Shaul, Y. (1980). *Ultrastructure of fenestrations in endothelial choriocapillaries of the rabbit--a freeze-fracturing study. British Journal of Ophthalmology, 64, 537-543.*

Middeldorp, J., & Hol, E. M. (2011). *GFAP in health and disease. Progress in Neurobiology, 93, 421-443.*

Minckler, D. S., Tso, M. O., & Zimmerman, L. E. (1976). *A light microscopic, autoradiographic study of axoplasmic transport in the optic nerve head during ocular hypotony, increased intraocular pressure, and papilledema. American Journal of Ophthalmology, 82, 741-757.*

Mittag, T. W., Danias, J., Pohorenec, G., Yuan, H., Burakgazi, E., Chalmers–Redman, R., Podos, S.M., & Tatton, W. G. (2000). *Retinal damage after 3 to 4 months of elevated intraocular pressure in a rat glaucoma model. Investigative Ophthalmology & Visual Science, 41, 3451-3459.*

Moreno, M. C., Campanelli, J., Sande, P., Sanez, D. A., Keller Sarmiento, M. I., & Rosenstein, R. E. (2004). *Retinal oxidative stress induced by high intraocular pressure. Free Radical Biology & Medicine, 37, 803-812.*

Moreno, M. C., Sande, P., Marcos, H. A., de Zavalia, N., Keller Sarmiento, M. I., & Rosenstein, R. E. (2005a). *Effect of glaucoma on the retinal glutamate/glutamine cycle activity. FASEB Journal, 19, 1161-1162.*

Moreno, M. C., Marcos, H. J. A., Oscar Croxatto, J., Sande, P. H., Campanelli, J., Jaliffa, C. O., Benozzi, J., & Rosenstein, R. E. (2005b). *A new experimental model of glaucoma in rats through intracameral injections of hyaluronic acid. Experimental Eye Research, 81, 71-80.*

Morgan, J. E. (2000). *Optic nerve head structure in glaucoma: Astrocytes as mediators of axonal damage. Eye, 14, 437-444.*

Morgan, S. C., Taylor, D. L., & Pocock, J. M. (2004). *Microglia release activators of neuronal proliferation mediated by activation of mitogen-activated protein kinase, phosphatidylinositol-3-kinase/akt and delta-notch signalling cas-*

cades. Journal of Neurochemistry, 90, 89-101.

Morrison, J. C. (2006). *Integrins in the optic nerve head: Potential roles in glaucomatous optic neuropathy (an american ophthalmological society thesis). Transactions of the American Ophthalmological Society, 104, 453-477.*

Morrison, J. C., Cepurna Ying Guo, W. O., & Johnson, E. C. (2011). *Pathophysiology of human glaucomatous optic nerve damage: Insights from rodent models of glaucoma. Experimental Eye Research, 93, 156-164.*

Morrison, J. C., Moore, C. G., Deppmeier, L. M., Gold, B. G., Meshul, C. K., & Johnson, E. C. (1997). *A rat model of chronic pressure-induced optic nerve damage. Experimental Eye Research, 64, 85-96.*

Munemasa, Y., & Kitaoka, Y. (2012). *Molecular mechanisms of retinal ganglion cell degeneration in glaucoma and future prospects for cell body and axonal protection. Frontiers in Cellular Neuroscience, 6, 60.*

Nag, S. (2011). *Morphology and properties of astrocytes. Methods in Molecular Biology, 686, 69-100.*

Nair, K. S., Hmani-Aifa, M., Ali, Z., Kearney, A. L., Salem, S. B., Macalinao, D. G., Cosma, I.M., Bouassida, W., Hakim, B., Benzina, Z., Soto, I., Söderkvist, P., Howell, G.R., Smith, R.S., Ayadi, H., John, S.V. (2011). *Alteration of the serine protease PRSS56 causes angle-closure glaucoma in mice and posterior microphthalmia in humans and mice. Nature Genetics, 43, 579-584.*

Naskar, R., Vorwerk, C. K., & Dreyer, E. B. (2000). *Concurrent downregulation of a glutamate transporter and receptor in glaucoma. Investigative Ophthalmology & Visual Science, 41, 1940-1944.*

Naskar, R., Wissing, M., & Thanos, S. (2002). *Detection of early neuron degeneration and accompanying microglial in the retina of a rat model of glaucoma. Investigative Ophthalmology Visual Science, 43, 2962-2968.*

Neetens, A. (1979). *The vascular problem in glaucoma. In J. G. Bellows (Ed.), Glaucoma: Contemporary international concepts (pp. 49-99). USA: Masson Publishing USA.*

Neufeld, A. H. (1999a). *Microglia in the optic nerve head and the region of parapapillary chorioretinal atrophy in glaucoma. Archives of Ophthalmology, 117, 1050-1056.*

Neufeld, A. H. (1999b). *Nitric oxide: A potential mediator of retinal ganglion cell damage in glaucoma. Survey of Ophthalmology, 43, S129-35.*

Neufeld, A. H., Hernandez, M. R., & Gonzalez, M. (1997a). *Nitric oxide synthase in the human glaucomatous optic nerve head. Archives of Ophthalmology, 115, 497-503.*

Neufeld, A. H., Hernandez, M. R., & Gonzalez, M. (1997b). *Nitric oxide synthase in the human glaucomatous optic nerve head. Archives of Ophthalmology, 115, 497-503.*

Neufeld, A. H., Sawada, A., & Becker, B. (1999). *Inhibition of nitric-oxide synthase 2 by aminoguanidine provides neuroprotection of retinal ganglion cells in a rat model of chronic glaucoma. Proceedings of the National Academy of Sciences, 96, 9944-9948.*

Newman, E. A. (1986). *The müller cell. In S. Federoff, & A. Vernadakis (Eds.), Development, morphology and regional specialization of astrocytes (pp. 149-171). Orlando: Academic Press, Inc.*

Newman, E. A. (2004). *A dialogue between glia and neurons in the retina: Modulation of neuronal excitability. Neuron Glia Biology, 1, 245-252.*

Nguyen, M. D., Julien, J. P., & Rivest, S. (2002). *Innate immunity: The missing link in neuroprotection and neurodegeneration? Nature Reviews Neuroscience, 3, 216-227.*

Nickells, R. W. (1996). *Retinal ganglion cell death in glaucoma: The how, the why, and the maybe. Journal of Glaucoma, 5, 345-356.*

Niederkorn, J. Y. (1990). *Immune privilege and immune regulation in the eye. Advances in Immunology, 48, 191-226.*

Niederkorn, J. Y. (2002). *Immune privilege in the anterior chamber of the eye. Critical Reviews in Immunology, 22, 13-46*

Niederkorn, J. Y. (2006). *See no evil, hear no evil, do no evil: The lessons of immune privilege. Nature Immunology, 7(4), 354-359.*

Niederkorn, J. Y., & Stein-Streilein, J. (2010). *History and physiology of immune privilege. Ocular Immunology and In-*

flammation, 18, 19-23.

Niederkorn, J., Streilein, J. W., & Shadduck, J. A. (1981). Deviant immune responses to allogeneic tumors injected intra-camerally and subcutaneously in mice. Investigative Ophthalmology & Visual Science, 20, 355-363.

Nishikiori, N., Osanai, M., Chiba, H., Kojima, T., Mitamura, Y., Ohguro, H., & Sawada, N. (2007). Glial Cell–Derived cytokines attenuate the breakdown of vascular integrity in diabetic retinopathy. Diabetes, 56, 1333-1340.

Nixon, R. A., & Sihag, R. K. (1991). Neurofilament phosphorylation: A new look at regulation and function. Trends in Neurosciences, 14, 501-506.

Noda, K., Ishida, S., Shinoda, H., Koto, T., Aoki, T., Tsubota, K., Oguchi, Y., Okada, Y., & Ikeda, E. (2005). Hypoxia induces the expression of membrane-type 1 matrix metalloproteinase in retinal glial cells. Investigative Ophthalmology & Visual Science, 46, 3817-3824.

Nork, T. M., Ver Hoeve, J. N., Poulsen, G. L., Nickells, R. W., Davis, M. D., Weber, A. J., Vaegan., Sarks, S.H., Lemley, H.L., & Millecchia, L.L. (2000). Swelling and loss of photoreceptors in chronic human and experimental glaucomas. Archives of Ophthalmology, 118, 235-245.

Ohta, K., Wiggert, B., Taylor, A. W., & Streilein, J. W. (1999). Effects of experimental ocular inflammation on ocular immune privilege. Investigative Ophthalmology & Visual Science, 40, 2010-2018.

Osborne, N. N. (2008). Pathogenesis of ganglion "cell death" in glaucoma and neuroprotection: Focus on ganglion cell axonal mitochondria. Progress in Brain Research, 173, 339-352.

Panagis, L., Zhao, X., Ge, Y., Ren, L., Mittag, T. W., & Danias, J. (2011). Retinal gene expression changes related to IOP exposure and axonal loss in DBA/2J mice. Investigative Ophthalmology & Visual Science, 52, 7807-7816.

Pant, H. C., & Veeranna. (1995). Neurofilament phosphorylation. Biochemistry and Cell Biology, 73, 575-592.

Pease, M. E., McKinnon, S. J., Quigley, H. A., Kerrigan-Baumrind, L. A., & Zack, D. J. (2000). Obstructed axonal transport of BDNF and its receptor TrkB in experimental glaucoma. Investigative Ophthalmology & Visual Science, 41, 764-774.

Peinado-Ramon, P., Salvador, M., Villegas-Perez, M. P., & Vidal-Sanz, M. (1996). Effects of axotomy and intraocular administration of NT-4, NT-3, and brain-derived neurotrophic factor on the survival of adult rat retinal ganglion cells. A quantitative in vivo study. Investigative Ophthalmology & Visual Science, 37, 489-500.

Pena, J. D., Taylor, A. W., Ricard, C. S., Vidal, I., & Hernandez, M. R. (1999). Transforming growth factor beta isoforms in human optic nerve heads. British Journal of Ophthalmology, 83, 209-218.

Pena, J. D. O., Agapova, O., Gabelt, B. T., Levin, L. A., Lucarelli, M. J., Kaufman, P. L., & Hernandez, M. R. (2001). Increased elastin expression in astrocytes of the lamina cribrosa in response to elevated intraocular pressure. Invest.Ophthalmol.Vis.Sci., 42, 2303-2314.

Perez-Alvarez, M. J., Isiegas, C., Santano, C., Salazar, J. J., Ramírez, A. I., Triviño, A., Ramírez, J.M., Albar, J.P., de la Rosa, E.J., & Prada, C. (2008). Vimentin isoform expression in the human retina characterized with the monoclonal antibody 3CB2. Journal of Neuroscience Research, 86, 1871-1883.

Pfrieger, F. W. (2002). Role of glia in synapse development. Current Opinion in Neurobiology, 12, 486-490.

Pfrieger, F. W. (2003). Role of cholesterol in synapse formation and function. Biochimica et Biophysica Acta, 1610, 271-280.

Pinazo-Duran, M. D., Zanon-Moreno, V., Garcia-Medina, J. J., & Gallego-Pinazo, R. (2013). Evaluation of presumptive biomarkers of oxidative stress, immune response and apoptosis in primary open-angle glaucoma. Current Opinion in Pharmacology, 13, 98-107.

Polazzi, E., & Contestabile, A. (2002). Reciprocal interactions between microglia and neurons: From survival to neuropathology. Reviews in the Neurosciences, 13, 221-242.

Pop, C., & Salvesen, G. S. (2009). Human caspases: Activation, specificity, and regulation. Journal of Biological Chemistry, 284, 21777-21781.

Prasanna, G., Krishnamoorthy, R., Clark, A. F., Wordinger, R. J., & Yorio, T. (2002). Human optic nerve head astrocytes *as a target for endothelin-1. Investigative Ophthalmology & Visual Science, 43, 2704-2713.*

Prasanna, G., Krishnamoorthy, R., & Yorio, T. (2011). *Endothelin, astrocytes and glaucoma. Experimental Eye Research, 93, 170-177.*

Qiao, H., Lucas, K., & Stein-Streilein, J. (2009). *Retinal laser burn disrupts immune privilege in the eye. American Journal of Pathology, 174, 414-422.*

Quigley, H. A. (1999). *Neuronal death in glaucoma. Progress in Retinal and Eye Research, 18, 39-57.*

Quigley, H. A. (2001). *Selective citation of evidence regarding photoreceptor loss in glaucoma. Archives of Ophthalmology, 119, 1390-1391.*

Quigley, H. A., Addicks, E. M., Green, W. R., & Maumenee, A. E. (1981). *Optic nerve damage in human glaucoma. II. the site of injury and susceptibility to damage. Archives of Ophthalmology, 99, 635-649.*

Quigley, H. A., & Anderson, D. R. (1977). *Distribution of axonal transport blockade by acute intraocular pressure elevation in the primate optic nerve head. Investigative Ophthalmology & Visual Science, 16, 640-644.*

Quigley, H. A., Dunkelberger, G. R., & Green, W. R. (1989). *Retinal ganglion cell atrophy correlated with automated perimetry in human eyes with glaucoma. American Journal of Ophthalmology, 107, 453-464.*

Quigley, H. A., McKinnon, S. J., Zack, D. J., Pease, M. E., Kerrigan-Baumrind, L. A., Kerrigan, D. F., & Mitchell, R. S. (2000). *Retrograde axonal transport of BDNF in retinal ganglion cells is blocked by acute IOP elevation in rats. Investigative Ophthalmology & Visual Science, 41, 3460-3466.*

Rader, J., Feuer, W. J., & Anderson, D. R. (1994). *Peripapillary vasoconstriction in the glaucomas and the anterior ischemic optic neuropathies. American Journal of Ophthalmology, 117, 72-80.*

Ramírez, A. I., Salazar, J. J., de Hoz, R., Rojas, B., Gallego, B. I., Salinas-Navarro, M., Alarcón-Martínez, L., Ortín-Martínez, A., Avilés-Trigueros, M., Vidal-Sanz, M., Triviño, A., & Ramírez, J. M. (2010). *Quantification of the effect of different levels of IOP in the astroglia of the rat retina ipsilateral and contralateral to experimental glaucoma. Investigative Ophthalmology & Visual Science, 51, 5690-5696.*

Ramírez, J. M., Ramírez, A. I., Salazar, J. J., de Hoz, R., & Triviño, A. (2001). *Changes of astrocytes in retinal ageing and age-related macular degeneration. Experimental Eye Research, 73, 601-615.*

Ramírez, J. M., & Salazar, J. J. (2008). *Implications of astroglia in glaucomatous damage. [Implicacion de la astroglia en el dano glaucomatoso]. Archivos de la Sociedad Española de Oftalmologia, 83, 339-342.*

Ramírez, J. M., Triviño, A., Ramírez, A. I., & Salazar, J. J. (1998). *Organization and function of astrocytes in human retina. In B. Castellano, B. Gonzalez & M. Nieto-Sampedro (Eds.), Understanding glial cells (pp. 47--62). Boston: Kluwer Academic Publishers.*

Ramírez, J. M., Triviño, A., Ramírez, A. I., Salazar, J. J., & García-Sánchez, J. (1994). *Immunohistochemical study of human retinal astroglia. Vision Research, 34, 1935-1946.*

Ramírez, J. M., Triviño, A., Ramírez, A. I., Salazar, J. J., & García-Sánchez, J. (1996). *Structural specializations of human retinal glial cells. Vision Research, 36, 2029-2036.*

Reichenbach, A., & Bringmann, A. (2010). *Müller cells in the diseased retina. In A. Reichenbach, & A. Bringmann (Eds.), Müller cells in the healthy and diseased retina (pp. 215). New York: Springer.*

Ren, L., & Danias, J. (2010). *A role for complement in glaucoma? Advances in Experimental Medicine and Biology, 703, 95-104.*

Ricklin, D., Hajishengallis, G., Yang, K., & Lambris, J. D. (2010). *Complement: A key system for immune surveillance and homeostasis. Nature Immunology, 11, 785-797.*

Ridet, J., & Privat, A. (2000). *Reactive astrocytes, their roles in CNS injury, and repair mechanisms. Advances in Structural Biology, 6, 147-185.*

Rieck, J. (2013). *The pathogenesis of glaucoma in the interplay with the immune system. Investigative Ophthalmology & Visual Science, 54, 2393-2409.*

Romano, C., Barrett, D. A., Li, Z., Pestronk, A., & Wax, M. B. (1995). *Anti-rhodopsin antibodies in sera from patients with normal-pressure glaucoma. Investigative Ophthalmology & Visual Science, 36, 1968-1975.*

Ruiz-Ederra, J., García, M., Hernández, M., Urcola, H., Hernández-Barbáchano, E., Araiz, J., & Vecino, E. (2005). The pig eye as a novel model of glaucoma. Experimental Eye Research, 81, 561-569.

Ryan, S. J., Hinton, D. R., & Sadda, s. R. (2013). Retina: Vol. 1, retinal imaging and diagnostics.basic science and translation to therapy. London, [etc]: Saunders-Elsevier.

Salazar, J. J. (1994). Glioarquitectura de la cabeza del nervio óptico humano estudio inmunohistoquímico con anti-PGFA. Madrid : Universidad Complutense de Madrid, Servicio de Publicaciones.

Salinas-Navarro, M., Alarcón-Martinez, L., Valiente-Soriano, F. J., Ortín-Martinez, A., Jimenez-Lopez, M., Aviles-Trigueros, M., Villegas-Pérez, M.P., de la Villa, P., & Vidal-Sanz, M. (2009). Functional and morphological effects of laser-induced ocular hypertension in retinas of adult albino swiss mice. Molecular Vision, 15, 2578-2598.

Sappington, R. M., & Calkins, D. J. (2008). Contribution of TRPV1 to microglia-derived IL-6 and NFkappaB translocation with elevated hydrostatic pressure. Investigative Ophthalmology & Visual Science, 49, 3004-3017.

Sappington, R. M., Carlson, B. J., Crish, S. D., & Calkins, D. J. (2010). The microbead occlusion model: A paradigm for induced ocular hypertension in rats and mice. Investigative Ophthalmology Visual Science, 51, 207-216.

Sasaki, T., Watanabe, W., Muranishi, Y., Kanamoto, T., Aihara, M., Miyazaki, K., Tamura, H., Saeki, T., Oda, H., Souchelnytskyi, N., Souchelnytskyi, S., Aoyama, H., Honda, Z., Furukawa, T., Mishima, H.K., Kiuchi, Y., & Honda, H., N. (2009). Elevated intraocular pressure, optic nerve atrophy, and impaired retinal development in ODAG transgenic mice. Investigative Ophthalmology & Visual Science, 50, 242-248.

Satilmis, M., Orgul, S., Doubler, B., & Flammer, J. (2003). Rate of progression of glaucoma correlates with retrobulbar circulation and intraocular pressure. American Journal of Ophthalmology, 135, 664-669.

Sawada, A., & Neufeld, A. H. (1999). Confirmation of the rat model of chronic, moderately elevated intraocular pressure. Experimental Eye Research, 69, 525-531.

Schlamp, C. L., Li, Y., Dietz, J. A., Janssen, K. T., & Nickells, R. W. (2006). Progressive ganglion cell loss and optic nerve degeneration in DBA/2J mice is variable and asymmetric. BMC Neuroscience, 7, 66.

Senatorov, V., Malyukova, I., Fariss, R., Wawrousek, E. F., Swaminathan, S., Sharan, S. K., & Tomarev, S. (2006). Expression of mutated mouse myocilin induces open-angle glaucoma in transgenic mice. Journal of Neuroscience, 26, 11903-11914.

Shao, H., Kaplan, H. J., & Sun, D. (2007). Major histocompatibility complex molecules on parenchymal cells of the target organ protect against autoimmune disease. Chemical Immunology and Allergy, 92, 94-104.

Shareef, S. R., Garcia-Valenzuela, E., Salierno, A., Walsh, J., & Sharma, S. C. (1995). Chronic ocular hypertension following episcleral venous occlusion in rats. Experimental Eye Research, 61, 379-382.

Sharma, R. K. (2007). Molecular neurobiology of retinal degeneration. In A. Lajtha, & D. Johnson (Eds.), Handbook of neurochemistry and molecular neurobiology (pp. 47-92) Springer US.

Siesky, B. A., Harris, A., Amireskandari, A., & Marek, B. (2012). Glaucoma and ocular blood flow: An anatomical perspective. Expert Review of Ophthalmology 7, 325-340.

Sigal, I. A. (2009). Interactions between geometry and mechanical properties on the optic nerve head. Investigative Ophthalmology Visual Science, 50, 2785-2795.

Sigal, I. A., Bilonick, R. A., Kagemann, L., Wollstein, G., Ishikawa, H., Schuman, J. S., & Grimm, J. L. (2012). The optic nerve head as a robust biomechanical system. Investigative Ophthalmology & Visual Science, 53, 2658-2667.

Sigal, I.A., Flanagan, J.G., Tertinegg, I., & Ethier, C. R. (2010). 3D morphometry of the human optic nerve head. Experimental Eye Research, 90, 70-80.

Smith, R. S., Zabaleta, A., Kume, T., Savinova, O. V., Kidson, S. H., Martin, J. E., .Nishimura, D.Y., Alward, W.L., Hogan, B.L., &. John, S. W. (2000). Haploinsufficiency of the transcription factors FOXC1 and FOXC2 results in aberrant ocular development. Human Molecular Genetics, 9, 1021-1032.

Sofroniew, M., & Vinters, H. (2010). Astrocytes: Biology and pathology. Acta Neuropathologica, 119(1), 7-35.*

Soto, I., Oglesby, E., Buckingham, B. P., Son, J. L., Roberson, E. D., Steele, M. R., Inman, D.M., Vetter, M.L., Horner, P.J., & Marsh-Armstrong, N. (2008). Retinal ganglion cells downregulate gene expression and lose their axons within the optic nerve head in a mouse glaucoma model. The Journal of Neuroscience, 28(2), 548-561.

Soto, I., Pease, M. E., Son, J. L., Shi, X., Quigley, H. A., & Marsh-Armstrong, N. (2011). Retinal ganglion cell loss in a rat ocular hypertension model is sectorial and involves early optic nerve axon loss. Investigative Ophthalmology & Visual Science, 52, 434-441.

Spitznas, M. (1974). The fine structure of the chorioretinal border tissues of the adult human eye. Advances in Ophthalmology, 28, 78-174.

Spitznas, M., & Reale, E. (1975). Fracture faces of fenestrations and junctions of endothelial cells in human choroidal vessels. Investigative Ophthalmology, 14, 98-107.

Stasi, K., Nagel, D., Yang, X., Wang, R. F., Ren, L., Podos, S. M., Mittag, T., & Danias, J. (2006). Complement component 1Q (C1Q) upregulation in retina of murine, primate, and human glaucomatous eyes. Investigative Ophthalmology & Visual Science, 47, 1024-1029.

Steele, M. R., Inman, D. M., Calkins, D. J., Horner, P. J., & Vetter, M. L. (2006). Microarray analysis of retinal gene expression in the DBA/2J model of glaucoma. Investigative Ophthalmology & Visual Science, 47, 977-985.

Streilein, J.W. (1987). Immune regulation and the eye: A dangerous compromise. The FASEB Journal, 1, 199-208.

Streilein, J.W. (2003). Ocular immune privilege: Therapeutic opportunities from an experiment of nature. Nature Reviews Immunology, 3, 879-889.

Streilein, J.W., Ma, N., Wenkel, H., Fong Ng, T., & Zamiri, P. (2002). Immunobiology and privilege of neuronal retina and pigment epithelium transplants. Vision Research, 42, 487-495.

Sucher, N. J., Lipton, S. A., & Dreyer, E. B. (1997). Molecular basis of glutamate toxicity in retinal ganglion cells. Vision Research, 37, 3483-3493.

Tezel, G. (2013). Immune regulation toward immunomodulation for neuroprotection in glaucoma. Current Opinion in Pharmacology, 13, 23-31.

Tezel, G., Chauhan, B. C., LeBlanc, R. P., & Wax, M. B. (2003). Immunohistochemical assessment of the glial mitogen-activated protein kinase activation in glaucoma. Investigative Ophthalmology & Visual Science, 44, 3025-3033.

Tezel, G., Hernandez, M. R., & Wax, M. B. (2000). Immunostaining of heat shock proteins in the retina and optic nerve head of normal and glaucomatous eyes. Archives of Ophthalmology, 118, 511-518.

Tezel, G., Li, L. Y., Patil, R. V., & Wax, M. B. (2001). TNF-alpha and TNF-alpha receptor-1 in the retina of normal and glaucomatous eyes. Investigative Ophthalmology & Visual Science, 42, 1787-1794.

Tezel, G., Seigel, G., & Wax, M. (1998). Autoantibodies to small heat shock proteins in glaucoma. Investigative Ophthalmology Visual Science, 39, 2277-2287.

Tezel, G., & Wax, M. B. (2000a). Increased production of tumor necrosis factor-alpha by glial cells exposed to simulated ischemia or elevated hydrostatic pressure induces apoptosis in cocultured retinal ganglion cells. Journal of Neuroscience, 20, 8693-8700.

Tezel, G., & Wax, M. B. (2000b). The mechanisms of hsp27 antibody-mediated apoptosis in retinal neuronal cells. Journal of Neuroscience, 20(10), 3552-3562.

Tezel, G., & Wax, M. B. (2007). Glaucoma. Chemical Immunology and Allergy, 92, 221-227.

Tezel, G., Yang, X., Luo, C., Cai, J., & Powell, D. W. (2012). An astrocyte-specific proteomic approach to inflammatory responses in experimental rat glaucoma Investigative Ophthalmology & Visual Science, 53, 4220-4233.

Tezel, G., Yang, X., Luo, C., Kain, A. D., Powell, D. W., Kuehn, M. H., & Kaplan, H. J. (2010). Oxidative stress and the regulation of complement activation in human glaucoma. Investigative Ophthalmology & Visual Science, 51, 5071-5082.

Tezel, G., Yang, X., Luo, C., Peng, Y., Sun, S. L., & Sun, D. (2007). Mechanisms of immune system activation in glaucoma: Oxidative stress-stimulated antigen presentation by the retina and optic nerve head glia. Investigative Ophthalmolo-

gy & Visual Science, 48, 705-714.

Tezel, G., Yang, J., & Wax, M. B. (2004). *Heat shock proteins, immunity and glaucoma. Brain Research Bulletin, 62(6), 473-480.*

Tezel, G., & the Fourth ARVO/Pfizer Ophthalmics Research Institute Conference,Working Group. (2009). *The role of glia, mitochondria, and the immune system in glaucoma. Investigative Ophthalmology Visual Science, 50, 1001-1012.*

Thanos, C., & Emerich, D. (2005). *Delivery of neurotrophic factors and therapeutic proteins for retinal diseases. Expert Opinion on Biological Therapy, 5, 1443-1452.*

Törnquist, P. (1979). *Capillary permeability in cat choroid, studied with the single injection technique (II). Acta Physiologica Scandinavica, 106, 425-430.*

Tout, S., Chan-Ling, T., Hollander, H., & Stone, J. (1993). *The role of Müller cells in the formation of the blood-retinal barrier. Neuroscience, 55, 291-301.*

Triviño, A., Ramírez, A. I., Salazar, J. J., Rojas, B., De Hoz, R., & Ramírez, J. M. (2005). *Retinal changes in age-related macular degeneration. In O. R. Ioseliane (Ed.), Focus on eye research (pp. 1-37). New York: Nova science publishers.*

Triviño, A., Ramírez, J. M., Ramírez, A. I., Salazar, J. J., & García-Sánchez, J. (1997). *Comparative study of astrocytes in human and rabbit retinae. Vision Research, 37, 1707-1711.*

Triviño, A., Ramírez, J. M., Salazar, J. J., Ramírez, A. I., & García-Sánchez, J. (1996). *Immunohistochemical study of human optic nerve head astroglia. Vision Research, 36, 2015-2028.*

Tse, M. T. (2012). *Axon degeneration: A new pathway emerges. Nature Reviews.Neuroscience, 13, 516.*

Ueda, J., Sawaguchi, S., Hanyu, T., Yaoeda, K., Fukuchi, T., Abe, H., & Ozawa, H. (1998). *Experimental glaucoma model in the rat induced by laser trabecular photocoagulation after an intracameral injection of india ink. Japanese Journal of Ophthalmology, 42, 337-344.*

Varela, H. J., & Hernandez, M. R. (1997). *Astrocyte responses in human optic nerve head with primary open-angle glaucoma. Journal of Glaucoma, 6, 303-313.*

Vidal-Sanz, M., Aviles-Trigueros, M., Whiteley, S. J., Sauve, Y., & Lund, R. D. (2002). *Reinnervation of the pretectum in adult rats by regenerated retinal ganglion cell axons: Anatomical and functional studies. Progress in Brain Research, 137, 443-452.*

Vorwerk, C. K., Gorla, M. S., & Dreyer, E. B. (1999). *An experimental basis for implicating excitotoxicity in glaucomatous optic neuropathy. Survey of Ophthalmology, 43, S142-50.*

Walsh, M. M., Yi, H., Friedman, J., Cho, K., Tserentsoodol, N., McKinnon, S., Searle, K., Yeh, A., & Ferreira, P. A. (2009). *Gene and protein expression pilot profiling and biomarkers in an experimental mouse model of hypertensive glaucoma. Experimental Biology and Medicine, 234, 918-930.*

Wang, L., Cioffi, G. A., Cull, G., Dong, J., & Fortune, B. (2002). *Immunohistologic evidence for retinal glial cell changes in human glaucoma. Investigative Ophthalmology & Visual Science, 43, 1088-1094.*

Wang, R., Schumer, R. A., Serle, J. B., & Podos, S. M. (1998). *A comparison of argon laser and diode laser photocoagulation of the trabecular meshwork to produce the glaucoma monkey model. Journal of Glaucoma, 7, 45-49.*

Wang, X., Ng, Y. K., & Tay, S. S. (2005). *Factors contributing to neuronal degeneration in retinas of experimental glaucomatous rats. Journal of Neuroscience Research, 82, 674-689.*

Wang, X., Tay, S., & Ng, Y. K. (2000). *An immunohistochemical study of neuronal and glial cell reactions in retinae of rats with experimental glaucoma. Experimental Brain Research, 132, 476.-484*

Wax, M. B., & Tezel, G. (2002). *Neurobiology of glaucomatous optic neuropathy: Diverse cellular events in neurodegeneration and neuroprotection. Molecular Neurobiology, 26, 45-55.*

Wax, M. B., & Tezel, G. (2009). *Immunoregulation of retinal ganglion cell fate in glaucoma. Experimental Eye Research, 88, 825-830.*

Wax, M. B., Tezel, G., Yang, J., Peng, G., Patil, R. V., Agarwal, N., Sappington, R.M, & Calkins, D. J. (2008). *Induced autoimmunity to heat shock proteins elicits glaucomatous loss of retinal ganglion cell neurons via activated T-cell-derived fas-ligand. Journal of Neuroscience, 28, 12085-12096.*

Weber, A. J., & Zelenak, D. (2001). *Experimental glaucoma in the primate induced by latex microspheres. Journal of Neuroscience Methods, 111, 39-48.*

Weigelin, E. (1972). *The blood circulation of the retina and the uvea. Advances in Ophthalmology, 25, 2-27.*

Wenkel, H., Chen, P. W., Ksander, B. R., & Streilein, J. W. (1999). *Immune privilege is extended, then withdrawn, from allogeneic tumor cell grafts placed in the subretinal space. Investigative Ophthalmology & Visual Science, 40, 3202-3208.*

Wenkel, H., & Streilein, J. W. (2000). *Evidence that retinal pigment epithelium functions as an immune-privileged tissue. Investigative Ophthalmology & Visual Science, 41, 3467-3473.*

Whitmore, A. V., Libby, R. T., & John, S. W. (2005). *Glaucoma: Thinking in new ways-a role for autonomous axonal self-destruction and other compartmentalised processes? Progress in Retinal and Eye Research, 24, 639-662.*

Wilbanks, G., & Streilein, J. (1990). *Distinctive humoral immune responses following anterior chamber and intravenous administration of soluble antigen. evidence for active suppression of IgG2-secreting B lymphocytes. Immunology, 71, 566-572*

Wilson, J. X. (1997). *Antioxidant defense of the brain: A role for astrocytes. Canadian Journal of Physiology and Pharmacology, 75, 1149-1163.*

WoldeMussie, E., Ruiz, G., Wijono, M., & Wheeler, L. A. (2001). *Neuroprotection of retinal ganglion cells by brimonidine in rats with laser-induced chronic ocular hypertension. Investigative Ophthalmology & Visual Science, 42, 2849-2855.*

Yan, X., Tezel, G., Wax, M. B., & Edward, D. P. (2000). *Matrix metalloproteinases and tumor necrosis factor alpha in glaucomatous optic nerve head. Archives of Ophthalmology, 118, 666-673.*

Yang, J., Yang, P., Tezel, G., Patil, R. V., Hernandez, M. R., & Wax, M. B. (2001). *Induction of HLA-DR expression in human lamina cribrosa astrocytes by cytokines and simulated ischemia. Investigative Ophthalmology Visual Science, 42, 365-371.*

Yang, X., Luo, C., Cai, J., Powell, D. W., Yu, D., Kuehn, M. H., & Tezel, G. (2011). *Neurodegenerative and inflammatory pathway components linked to TNF-α/TNFR1 signaling in the glaucomatous human retina. Investigative Ophthalmology Visual Science, 52, 8442-8454.*

Yildirim, O., Ates, N. A., Ercan, B., Muslu, N., Unlu, A., Tamer, L., Atik, U., & Kanik, A. (2005). *Role of oxidative stress enzymes in open-angle glaucoma. Eye, 19, 580-583.*

Yuan, L., & Neufeld, A. H. (2000). *Tumor necrosis factor-alpha: A potentially neurodestructive cytokine produced by glia in the human glaucomatous optic nerve head. Glia, 32, 42-50.*

Yuan, L., & Neufeld, A. H. (2001). *Activated microglia in the human glaucomatous optic nerve head. Journal of Neuroscience Research, 64, 523-532.*

Yun, H. Y., Dawson, V. L., & Dawson, T. M. (1997). *Nitric oxide in health and disease of the nervous system. Molecular Psychiatry, 2, 300-310.*

Zhang, J., & Snyder, S. H. (1995). *Nitric oxide in the nervous system. Annual Review of Pharmacology and Toxicology, 35, 213-233.*

Zhong, Y. S., Leung, C. K., & Pang, C. P. (2007). *Glial cells and glaucomatous neuropathy. Chinese Medical Journal, 120, 326-335.*

Zhou, Y., Grinchuk, O., & Tomarev, S. I. (2008). *Transgenic mice expressing the Tyr437His mutant of human myocilin protein develop glaucoma. Investigative Ophthalmology & Visual Science, 49, 1932-1939.*

Hypocholesterolemia and Plasma Amino Acids in Sepsis

Carlo Chiarla, Ivo Giovannini
CNR-IASI Center for the Pathophysiology of Shock
Catholic University of the Sacred Heart School of Medicine, Rome, Italy

John H. Siegel
Newark, New Jersey, USA

Maria Vellone, Francesco Ardito, Marino Murazio, Gennaro Clemente
Department of Surgical Sciences
Catholic University of the Sacred Heart School of Medicine, Rome, Italy

Zdenek Zadak
Department of Research and Development
University Hospital, Hradec Kralove, Czech Republic

Felice Giuliante
Department of Surgical Sciences
Catholic University of the Sacred Heart School of Medicine, Rome, Italy

1   Introduction

Sepsis is characterized by an adaptation of plasma lipoprotein patterns which commonly results in hypo-cholesterolemia (Fraunberger *et al.*, 1999; Giovannini *et al.*, 1999; Chiarla *et al.*, 2010) and the degree of hypocholesterolemia is generally related to severity of septic illness. The real pathophysiologic role of hypocholesterolemia is not yet adequately explained. It seems to be an adaptive response among the host defense manifestations of sepsis, however it may also reflect inadequate disposal of substrate for stress hormone, lipoprotein synthesis and for other important synthetic processes (Fraunberger *et al.*, 1999; Giovannini *et al.*, 2005; Marik, 2006; Vyroubal *et al.*, 2008). The relationship between changes in choles-terol and septic metabolic abnormalities has not been satisfactorily evaluated. More extensive assessment would certainly improve our understanding of the patterns of septic acute phase response, and of evolu-tion toward metabolic decompensation, as already demonstrated by study of the correlations with other plasma fat and protein components, and with several amino acids (Chiarla *et al.*, 2004, 2006, 2010; Gio-vannini *et al.*, 2005). The panel of amino acid (AA) abnormalities may reflect adequacy of biochemical, metabolic, organ function processes, evolution of disease and even gene expression (Siegel *et al.*, 1979; Roth & Druml, 2011), and a thorough appraisal of the relationships with cholesterol abnormalities would certainly enhance our understanding of sepsis. These have never been evaluated in detail, at least to our knowledge, and we have performed this evaluation over an extended frame of reference of AA abnormal-ities.

2   Materials and Methods

2.1   Patients

Data from 504 plasma AA measurements with the corresponding metabolic and clinical variables, rec-orded in our patient AA database, were analyzed in detail. These were taken from 19 trauma patients (3 women, 16 men) who developed sepsis (Table 1). All patients had acute injury, caused by road accidents in 16 cases and gunshot wounds in 3 cases, with combinations of abdominal, chest, head and limb le-sions. The cause of sepsis was intra-abdominal, pulmonary or extensive soft tissue infection. The diagno-sis of sepsis was based on the occurrence of a temperature > 38.3°C, white blood cell count >12×10^9/L or < 3×10^9/L and clear evidence of infection verified by positive cultures from blood, surgical drainage of infected areas or sputum in the case of pulmonary sepsis. Median sepsis severity score (Skau, 1985) upon diagnosis of sepsis was 24 (range 11 – 75). Most patients survived, some of them after evolving through near-fatal illness, one patient died of septic metabolic and cardiorespiratory decompensation from multi-ple organ dysfunction, and one died suddenly without multiple organ dysfunction. The patients were re-ceiving total parenteral nutrition (34 ± 14 kcal/kg/24 h, about three fourths glucose and one fourth fat, and 1.4 ± 0.6 g/kg/24 h amino acids).

2.2   Measurements

Serial AA determinations were performed every 8 to 12 hours during sepsis until the clinical criteria for the diagnosis of sepsis persisted, for a total number of 504 determinations (median per patient 23, inter-quartile range 15). The Fischer AA ratio (Freund *et al.*, 1979) was calculated according to the ratio (leu-cine + isoleucine + valine)/ (phenylalanine + tyrosine). The amino-acidograms were available together

Pt	Sex	Age yr	BSA m²*	Injury sites	Source of sepsis	Outcome	Cholesterol, mg/dL median (range)
1	M	27	2.09	Abdomen+chest	Abdomen+lung	Survival	84 (28-220)
2	F	22	1.52	Chest	Lung	Survival	116.5 (65-182)
3	M	34	2.02	Abdomen+chest	Lung	Survival	131 (66-198)
4	M	33	2.18	Abdomen	Abdomen	Survival	105 (99-120)
5	M	17	1.89	Abdomen+chest+head	Lung	Survival	58 (43-94)
6	M	40	2.35	Abdomen+chest+pelvis	Abdomen	Death	100.5 (93-110)
7	M	21	1.82	Abdomen+chest+upper limb	Soft tissue	Survival	88 (69-107)
8	M	21	1.98	Abdomen	Abdomen	Survival	98 (95-98)
9	M	30	1.72	Abdomen	Abdomen	Survival	109.5 (108-111)
10	F	71	2.05	Chest+pelvis	Soft tissue	Death	82 (67-119)
11	M	22	1.98	Abdomen+pelvis	Abdomen	Survival	82 (47-108)
12	M	38	1.89	Abdomen+chest+head+pelvis	Lung	Survival	85.5 (79-103)
13	M	53	2.06	Abdomen+head	Abdomen	Survival	98 (78-126)
14	M	24	1.85	Abdomen+head	Abdomen	Survival	68 (48-74)
15	F	27	1.77	Chest+head	Lung	Survival	76 (54-117)
16	M	18	1.69	Chest+upper limb	Soft tissue	Survival	122 (71-145)
17	M	27	2.11	Abdomen+lower limb	Soft tissue	Survival	112 (79-147)
18	M	16	1.65	Head+upper limb	Soft tissue	Survival	110 (60-131)
19	M	19	1.79	Abdomen	Abdomen	Survival	77 (65-93)

*BSA = body surface area

Table 1: Patients.

with the corresponding plasma cholesterol and alkaline phosphatase measurements. The urinary 3-methylhistidine excretion, the respiratory index (the ratio of alveolar-arterial O_2 tension gradient to arterial O_2 tension) and the Sepsis-related Organ Failure Assessment score (SOFA score) (Vincent, 2006) were also available in a smaller number of cases. The study protocol complied with the 1964 Helsinki declaration.

2.3   Statistical Analysis

Medians and ranges were used as indices of centrality and dispersion of the distributions. The obtained measurements provided a continuous distribution of observations over a wide range of conditions, extending from moderate to extremely severe septic illness, which was well suited to assessing the correlates of cholesterol over an ample area of pathophysiologic abnormalities. The relationships existing between cholesterol, the AA levels and the other variables were explored on two- or three-dimensional graphical displays. Further assessments and validations of the results were performed by least-square regression and covariance analysis, and analyzed for the Pearson correlation coefficient (r), with skewness and kurtosis control, and analysis of residuals (Statgraphics Plus, Manugistics, Rockville, MD). Significance of covariance was assessed by Scheffé criteria (based on confidence intervals and differences in slope and intercept) (Seber, 1977) and with the selection of the simplest possible regression yielding the best control of variability of cholesterol.

3   Results

3.1   Basic Results

Median plasma cholesterol was 88 mg/dL, range 28 – 220 (corresponding to 2.28 mmol/L, range 0.72 – 5.70), and median alkaline phosphatase was 126.5 U/L, range 11 – 784 (n.v. 25 – 100). Plasma AA values are reported in Table 2.

Alanine	272.5	(108-1013)
Arginine	89	(29-280)
Asparagine	42	(15-610)
Aspartic acid	6	(0-72)
Citrulline	11	(4-109)
Cystine	46.5	(18-110)
Glutamine	453	(183-2438)
Glutamic acid	54.5	(6-404)
Glycine	239	(74-1184)
Histidine	75	(3-427)
Hydroxyproline	11.5	(0-76)
Isoleucine	73.5	(22-207)
Leucine	129	(64-296)
Lysine	163	(67-534)
Methionine	39	(4-411)
Ornithine	69	(22-352)
Phosphoethanolamine	8	(0-63)
Phenylalanine	114.5	(18-304)
Proline	187	(13-1445)
Phosphoserine	12	(5-41)
Serine	98	(25-301)
Threonine	107.5	(11-612)
Tryptophan	57	(25-94)
Tyrosine	56	(27-203)
Valine	253	(83-671)

Multiple regression:

Cholesterol = 98.22 + 0.11 (alkaline phosphatase) − 0.43 (phenylalanine) + 0.14 (glutamate) + 0.27 (ornithine)

Multiple $r = 0.74$, $r^2 = 0.55$, $p < 0.001$

Table 2: Medians (ranges) for plasma amino acids in µmol/L, with final regression.

3.2   Correlations with Amino Acids

The correlations between cholesterol and individual plasma AAs were assessed. The best correlate of cholesterol was phenylalanine, which was inversely related to it ($r = -0.46$, $p < 0.001$). Among the other aromatic and the branched chain AAs, tyrosine was also inversely related to cholesterol, although with a lower r value ($r = -0.28$, $p < 0.001$), and the phenylalanine/tyrosine ratio was inversely related to cholesterol ($r = -0.27$, $p < 0.001$), while isoleucine was directly related to cholesterol ($r = 0.36$, $p < 0.001$). No evident or significant correlation was found with the remainder. The inverse correlation with the phenyl-alanine/tyrosine ratio reflected the circumstance that the two AAs were directly correlated one to the other ($r = 0.44$, $p < 0.001$) and both increased with decreasing cholesterol, however the increase in phenylalanine outweighed that of tyrosine. There was an inverse correlation with the Fischer AA ratio, which reached a higher r value ($r = -0.55$, $p < 0.001$) most likely because the ratio cumulatively accounted for the impact of each individual AA. Among the other AAs, the main result was a direct correlation with glutamate ($r = 0.41$, $p < 0.001$), while there were weaker correlations with ornithine (direct relationship), and with phosphoserine, hydroxyproline, proline and alanine (inverse relationships) (absolute $r < 0.24$, $p < 0.001$ for all). In addition, there was an inverse correlation between cholesterol and 3-methylhistidine urinary excretion ($r = -0.34$, $p < 0.001$) in 442 measurements which were selected on the basis of plasma creatinine < 1.7 mg/dL, corresponding to 150 µmol/L, to avoid confounding by the effect of kidney dysfunction, if present. The median 3-methylhistidine urinary excretion for these measurements was 537.2 µmol/24 h, range 100.8 – 2005.0. These correlations were also reconfirmed by evaluating individual patient trends on graphical displays.

3.3   Correlation with Alkaline Phosphatase

Because a basic procedure, when assessing the variability of cholesterol in multiple measurements, is to also account for the simultaneous effect of cholestasis, if present (Giovannini *et al.*, 1999; Chiarla *et al.*, 2010), the analysis was repeated including alkaline phosphatase as an independent variable together with the plasma AAs in multiple regressions. In fact, cholestasis is known to independently increase cholesterol, therefore masking or confounding the effect of the factors which cause hypocholesterolemia (Giovannini *et al.*, 1999, Chiarla *et al.*, 2010). The analysis showed that cholesterol was directly related to alkaline phosphatase ($r = 0.47$, $p < 0.001$), and reconfirmed the significance of the previous panel of AA correlations.

3.4   "Simplest best fit"

Selection of the "simplest best fit", explaining the largest possible variability of cholesterol by using the minimum possible number of variables, yielded a multiple regression which included alkaline phosphatase, phenylalanine, glutamate and ornithine, and these accounted for 55% of the variability of cholesterol (multiple $r = 0.74$, $r^2 = 0.55$, $p < 0.001$, Table 2). This regression was not improved by including as independent variables other plasma AAs, or the parenteral AA infusion rate. Indeed the analysis showed that, although cholesterol in itself was directly related to AA infusion rate ($p < 0.001$), in the multiple regression this effect was already accounted for by the impact of AA infusion rate on both glutamate and ornithine (direct correlations, $p < 0.001$ for both).

Apart from the described statistical analyses and validations, many of the listed correlations were already evident when assessing individual patient trends (Figure 1), or all measurements pooled together on graphical displays.

3.5   Correlations with Respiratory Dysfunction and SOFA Score

Finally, although this study was performed to assess the relationship between hypocholesterolemia and plasma AA changes, a peculiar complementary finding was the tendency of signs of respiratory dysfunction to be associated with decreasing cholesterol and increasing phenylalanine. Indeed, in 251 measurements in which the respiratory index was simultaneously available (median 1.36, range 0.19 – 4.78), this

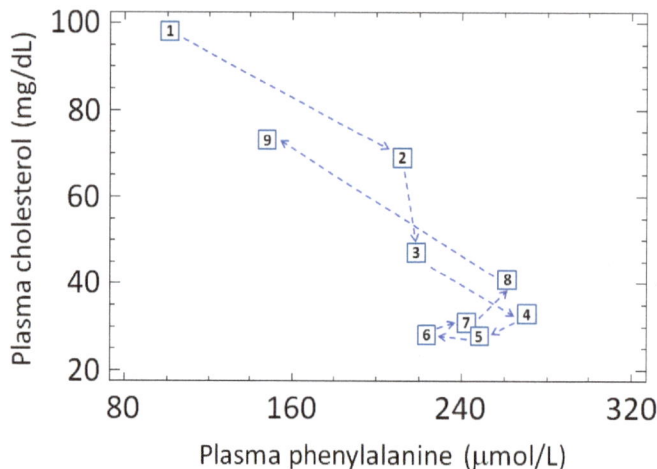

Figure 1: Evolution of plasma cholesterol and phenylalanine in a surviving trauma patient included in the study, who developed transient septic shock, with evident inverse correlation between cholesterol and phenylalanine. The fall in cholesterol, paralleled by increasing phenylalanine, preceded the development of septic shock, with mean blood pressure down to 74 mmHg, followed by improvement of the pattern. The downhill path was paralleled by respiratory dysfunction with respiratory index increasing up to a value of 4.78. Distance between data points 24 h. To convert cholesterol from mg/dL to mmol/L, multiply by 0.0259.

was found to be inversely related to cholesterol ($r = -0.41$, $p < 0.001$) and directly related to phenylalanine ($r = 0.39$, $p < 0.001$). More detailed analysis showed that these correlations were supported by the tendency for a multi-systemic involvement, also implicating a variable degree of respiratory dysfunction, which paralleled the worsening of hypocholesterolemia and of septic metabolic patterns.

This aspect was further verified in correlations with the SOFA score. The score (median 8, range 2 – 16) was inversely and significantly correlated to cholesterol for any given alkaline phosphatase level (multiple $r = 0.72$, $p < 0.001$). Regression analysis on SOFA score and AA levels showed direct correlations between SOFA and phosphoserine, hydroxyproline ($r = 0.60$ for both), phenylalanine, tyrosine ($r = 0.56$ for both), methionine ($r = 0.56$) and cystathionine ($r = 0.50$), and inverse correlations with the Fischer AA ratio ($r = -0.45$), glutamate ($r = -0.40$) and aspartate ($r = -0.32$) ($p < 0.001$ for all). For many other AAs, including alanine and proline, there was a roughly direct correlation, however the distribution of measurements was unsuitable for regression analysis because the transition to the highest SOFA scores was often associated with abrupt hyperaminoacidemia without gradual continuity with previous measurements.

4   Discussion

4.1   Relevance and Determinants of Hypocholesterolemia

Although most of the interest in cholesterol abnormalities regards the implications of *hyper*cholesterolemia, an intriguing issue for several categories of patients is *hypo*cholesterolemia. This is particularly true for surgical septic and critically ill patients, in whom severity of hypocholesterolemia may parallel severity of illness: indeed factors such as acute phase response to trauma, host defense against infectious agents, liver dysfunction and hemodilution from hemorrhage, if present, cumulatively concur to decrease cholesterol (Giovannini *et al.*, 1999; Vyroubal *et al.*, 2008; Chiarla *et al.*, 2010; Hrabovský *et al.*, 2012). In common practice the only adverse factor increasing cholesterol, or moderating the decrease caused by the other factors, is cholestasis. This generally results in a quantifiable direct relationship between cholesterol and alkaline phosphatase, which needs to be taken into account when assessing other determinants of cholesterol level (Chiarla *et al.*, 2010) to avoid confounding. Our present study substantiates and implements the available information on metabolic patterns associated with hypocholesterolemia, with particular regard to the associated panel of amino acid (AA) correlations. As already mentioned, this panel may reflect adequacy of biochemical, metabolic, organ function processes, evolution of disease and even gene expression (Siegel *et al.*, 1979; Roth & Druml, 2011).

4.2   Dominant Amino Acid Correlations

The results have shown that, in spite of the heterogeneous conditions of the patients and of the many uncontrolled factors affecting cholesterol, alkaline phosphatase and three dominant AA variables accounted for as much as 55% of the variability of cholesterol (Table 2, Regression, multiple r = 74, r^2 = 0.55, p < 0.001). The selected best simultaneous AA correlates of cholesterol were phenylalanine (inverse relationship), glutamate and ornithine (direct relationships).

The association between decreasing cholesterol and increasing phenylalanine is consistent with the role of cholesterol as a marker of severity of septic illness, because high phenylalanine mostly reflects the increased load of this AA from endogenous protein catabolism and/or its inadequate metabolic handling, both of which are well known metabolic consequences of deteriorating sepsis (Siegel *et al.*, 1979). This was substantiated by the inverse correlation found with the phenylalanine/tyrosine ratio, which is a substrate/byproduct ratio whose increase reflects impaired phenylalanine metabolism (Wannemacher *et al.*, 1976), and by the inverse correlation found between cholesterol and urinary 3-methylhistidine excretion, which reflected increased endogenous proteolysis at low cholesterol levels. The most likely pathophysiologic explanation is that the cytokine pattern which is held responsible for the amplification of septic acute phase response and severe hypocholesterolemia (Fraunberger *et al.*, 1998; Fraunberger *et al.*, 1999; Gordon *et al.*, 2001; Giovannini *et al.*, 2005; Vyroubal *et al.*, 2008), simultaneously inhibits use of AAs in muscular protein synthesis and enhances proteolytic drive, as reflected by rising urinary 3-methylhistidine excretion and plasma phenylalanine. The rise of the latter is further enhanced by liver dysfunction and impaired phenylalanine hydroxylase activity (Wannemacher *et al.*, 1976), and is often associated with more intense inflammation, encephalopathy, reduction of vascular tone and shock (Eggers *et al.*, 2003; Ploder *et al.*, 2009; Bozza *et al.*, 2013). This situation differs from what may be found in phenylketonuria, where an inverse relationship between cholesterol and phenylalanine may at least in part be explained by an inhibitory effect of phenylalanine on cholesterol synthesis (Colomé *et al.*, 2001; Hargreaves, 2007).

4.3   Additional Amino Acid Correlations

With regard to the other AA correlations found in our septic patients, while some relationship between decreasing cholesterol and increasing proline or alanine may be a predictable pattern depending on severity of illness, the relationship which emerged in this study with increasing phosphoserine is a completely new finding. This is consistent with a previous generic report of higher phosphoserine in lethal compared to non-lethal sepsis (Roth *et al.*, 1982), and with recent evidence suggesting that intensity of acute phase response and septic multiorgan dysfunctions alter the balance between plasma phosphoserine and serine, therefore resulting in higher phosphoserine and phosphoserine/serine ratios in cases with a worse degree of illness (unpublished observations). This topic deserves further specific investigation, to assess the mechanisms which increase phosphoserine, and the performance of this AA as a new biomarker of severity of illness.

4.4   Hypocholesterolemia and Organ Dysfunction

The tendency of hypocholesterolemia to precede, or to be associated with the development of organ dysfunction, was confirmed in our study by the highly significant relationships found between decreasing cholesterol, or increasing phenylalanine, and increasing respiratory index, although an incomplete number of measurements was available for this purpose (n = 261). Of note, some degree of pulmonary dysfunction from ventilation/perfusion mismatch may be a component of the septic multisystemic involvement even in the absence of true parenchymal lesions (Siegel *et al.*, 1979). In these measurements, the tendency of decreasing cholesterol to be associated with organ dysfunctions was substantiated by its simultaneous correlation with increasing SOFA score. Moreover, the relationships observed between AAs and SOFA score basically reconfirmed that the AA abnormalities which were associated with decreasing cholesterol were also associated with increasing SOFA score. Within these abnormalities, the hyperaminoacidemia which characterized the highest SOFA scores was consistent with impaired use of AAs in synthetic processes in the more advanced stages of septic metabolic dysregulation (Cerra *et al.*, 1980).

4.5   Role of Hypocholesterolemia and Clinical Implications

The real pathophysiologic role of hypocholesterolemia is not yet adequately explained. As previously mentioned, it seems to mostly represent an adaptive lipoprotein response among the host defense manifestations of sepsis (Fraunberger *et al.*, 1999; Giovannini *et al.*, 2005; Vyroubal *et al.*, 2008), however it may also reflect inadequate disposal of substrate for important synthetic processes, including lipoprotein, new cell membrane and stress hormone synthesis (Giovannini *et al.*, 2005; Marik, 2006; Vyroubal *et al.*, 2008). Within these considerations, a direct relationship between amino acid supply and cholesterol remains intriguing and unexplained (Giovannini *et al.*, 2005), as remains the direct relationship found between cholesterol and glutamate or ornithine (which should to some extent reflect the wealth of AA pool and disposal) that emerged as the main driving correlations in this study. These results reconfirm and expand some findings which were previously noted in smaller and less heterogeneous groups of measurements included in our same database (Chiarla *et al.*, 2004, 2006). Of course the significance of the described correlations was verified in the remainder of the measurements, therefore strengthening the evidence relating increases in cholesterol (or, more precisely, moderation of the decrease due to sepsis) to availability of amino acid substrate.

In clinical practice the role of hypocholesterolemia as a marker of sepsis should be emphasized more strongly. As a general concept, transient hypocholesterolemia may depend on clearly evident causes such as surgical or nonsurgical trauma, hemodilution from hemorrhage, or easily diagnosable sepsis. However, given the difficulties which may often occur in diagnosing sepsis (Assunção *et al.*, 2010), especially the occult form presenting with light or deceitful manifestations, unexplained hypocholesterolemia may motivate deeper patient assessment looking for concealed infectious sources.

Use of the absolute value of cholesterol as a single marker of severity of septic illness may be limited by some inter-patient variability (Giovannini *et al.*, 1999, 2005; Kruger, 2009; Nuzzo & Giovannini, 2010; Hrabovský *et al.*, 2012) and baseline pre-illness cholesterol should also be considered. In individual patients an important source of variability is cholestasis which increases cholesterol, and therefore moderates the decrease caused by other factors, while the impact of exogenous AAs needs to be more precisely assessed. Nevertheless, these considerations do not prevent serial determinations of plasma cholesterol, in individual patients, from being an inexpensive adjunctive tool to monitor the tendency toward recovery or worsening of sepsis. This better emends and confirms principles and concepts which do not simply regard sepsis in the trauma patients in our study (Figure 2a), but also extend to other conditions of sepsis (Figure 2b).

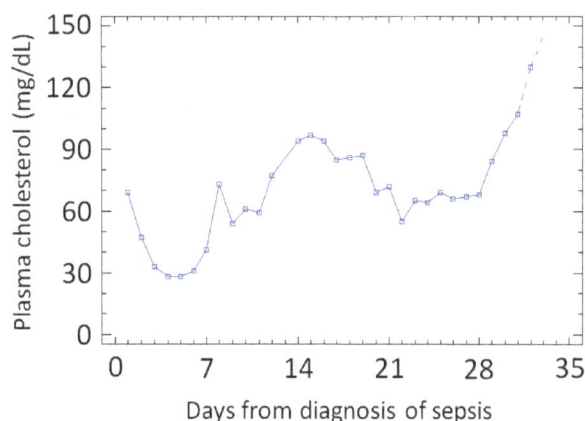

Figure 2a: Evolution of hypocholesterolemia in a trauma patient with sepsis included in the study, showing initial transient improvement, relapse of sepsis and final progression toward recovery. To convert cholesterol from mg/dL to mmol/L, multiply by 0.0259.

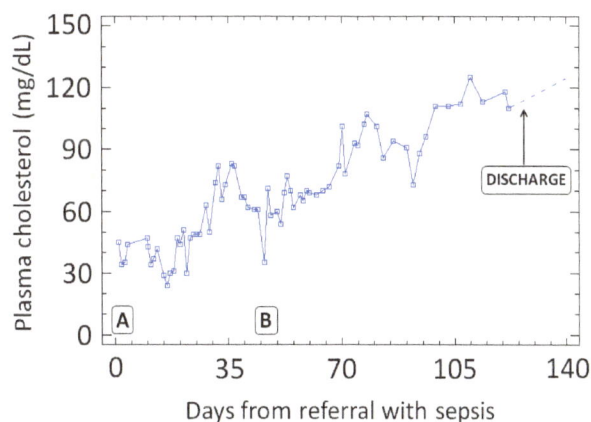

Figure 2b: Evolution of hypocholesterolemia in a different surgical patient, with nearly fatal and persistent abdominal sepsis. Sepsis was due to a complex surgical problem, a cryptic juxta-papillary duodenal fistula within obstructive duodenal scarring, causing recurrent peritonitis and paraduodenal abscesses. **A**. Referral with recurrent peritonitis: surgical, endoscopic and percutaneous treatments followed by unsteady improvement. **B**. Relapse of severe sepsis: surgical drainage of periduodenal abscesses, duodenal exclusion and complete drainage of the whole area, followed by steadier improvement and progressive recovery from sepsis (with transient mild relapses resolved by antibiotic/percutaneous treatments). To convert cholesterol from mg/dL to mmol/L, multiply by 0.0259.

Another important point is that degree of hypocholesterolemia in itself (even as low as 11 mg/dL) may still be associated with good prognosis if hypocholesteromia is rapidly reversed by eradication of the septic focus; on the contrary, persistently severe hypocholesterolemia is more often associated with death (Giovannini *et al.*, 2003, 2007).

4.6   Conclusions

Our study adds some new pieces to the mosaic of knowledge on septic metabolic and cardiorespiratory abnormalities, by quantifying the AA correlations associated with hypocholesterolemia over a large number of measurements in trauma patients who developed sepsis. The correlations found between decreasing cholesterol, changes in AA levels and SOFA score emphasize the role of hypocholesterolemia as a marker of severity of septic metabolic illness, although cholestasis, if present, may moderate degree of hypocholesterolemia. Further study is needed to confirm the correlation with increasing glutamate and ornithine and its clinical significance.

References

Assunção, M., Akamine, N., Cardoso, G.S., Mello, P.V., Teles, J.M., Nunes, A.L., Rea-Neto, A., & Machado, F.R.; SEPSES Study Group (2010). Survey on physicians' knowledge of sepsis: do they recognize it promptly? *Journal of Critical Care*, 25(4), 545-552. Epub 2010 Jun 19.

Bozza, F.A., D'Avila, J.C., Ritter, C., Sonneville, R., Sharshar, T., & Dal-Pizzol F. (2013) Bioenergetics, mitochondrial dysfunction, and oxidative stress in the pathophysiology of septic encephalopathy. *Shock*, 39(Suppl. 1), 10-16.

Cerra, F.B., Siegel, J.H., Coleman, B., Border, J.R., & McMenamy, R.R. Septic autocannibalism. A failure of exogenous nutritional support. *Annals of Surgery* 192(4): 570-579, 1980.

Chiarla C., Giovannini, I., & Siegel, J.H. (2004). The relationship between plasma cholesterol, amino acids and acute phase proteins in sepsis. *Amino Acids*, 27(1), 97-100. Epub 2004 Mar 16.

Chiarla, C., Giovannini, I., & Siegel, J.H. (2006). Plasma arginine correlations in trauma and sepsis. *Amino Acids*, 30(1), 81-86. Epub 2005 May 31.

Chiarla, C., Giovannini, I., Giuliante, F., Zadak, Z., Vellone, M., Ardito, F., Clemente, G., Murazio, M., & Nuzzo, G. (2010). Severe hypocholesterolemia in surgical patients, sepsis, and critical illness. *Journal of Critical Care*, 25(2), 361.e7-361.e12. Epub 2009 Oct 13.

Colomé, C., Artuch, R., Lambruschini, N., Cambra, F.J., Campistol, J., & Vilaseca, M. (2001). Is there a relationship between plasma phenylalanine and cholesterol in phenylketonuric patients under dietary treatment? *Clinical Biochemistry*, 34(5), 373-376.

Eggers, V., Schilling, A., Kox, W.J., & Spies, C. (2003). Septische Enzephalopathie. Differentialdiagnose und therapeutische Einflussmöglichkeiten. *Anaesthesist*, 52(4), 294-303.

Fraunberger, P., Pilz, G., Cremer, P., Werdan, K., & Walli, A.K. (1998). Association of serum tumor necrosis factor levels with decrease of cholesterol during septic shock. *Shock*, 10(5), 359-363.

Fraunberger, P., Schaefer, S., Werdan, K., Walli, A.K., & Seidel, D. (1999). Reduction of circulating cholesterol and apolipoprotein levels during sepsis. *Clinical Chemistry and Laboratory Medicine*, 37(3), 357-362.

Freund, H., Atamian, S., Holroyde, J., & Fischer, J.E. (1979). Plasma amino acids as predictors of the severity and outcome of sepsis. *Annals of Surgery*, 190(5), 571-576.

Giovannini, I., Boldrini, G., Chiarla, C., Giuliante, F., Vellone, M., & Nuzzo, G. (1999). Pathophysiologic correlates of hypocholesterolemia in critically ill surgical patients. *Intensive Care Medicine*, 25(7), 748-751.

Giovannini, I., Chiarla, C., Greco, F., Boldrini, G., & Nuzzo, G. (2003). Characterization of biochemical and clinical correlates of hypocholesterolemia after hepatectomy. Clinical Chemistry, 49(2), 317-319.

Giovannini, I., Chiarla, C., Giuliante, F., Vellone, M., Zadak, Z., & Nuzzo, G. (2005). Hypocholesterolemia in surgical trauma, sepsis, other acute conditions and critical illness. In Trends in Cholesterol Research (Kramer, M.A., editor). New York: Nova Science Publishers Inc (pp. 137-161).

Giovannini, I., Chiarla, C., Giuliante, F., Vellone, M., Ardito, F., Pallavicini, F., & Nuzzo, G. (2007). Biochemical and clinical correlates of hypouricemia in surgical and critically ill patients. Clinical Chemistry and Laboratory Medicine, 45(9), 1207-1210.

Gordon, B.R., Parker, T.S., Levine, D.M., Saal, S.D., Wang, J.C., Sloan, B.J., Barie, P.S., & Rubin, A.L. (2001). Relationship of hypolipidemia to cytokine concentrations and outcomes in critically ill surgical patients. Critical Care Medicine, 29(8), 1563-1568.

Hargreaves, I.P. (2007). Coenzyme Q10 in phenylketonuria and mevalonic aciduria. Mitochondrion, 7(Supplement), S175-S180. Epub 2007 Mar 16.

Hrabovský, V., Zadák, Z., Mendlová, A., Bláha, V., Hyšpler, R., Tichá, A., & Svagera, Z. (2012). Cholesterol metabolism in acute upper gastrointestinal bleeding, preliminary observations. Wiener Klinische Wochenschrift, 124(23-24), 815-821. Epub 2012 Nov 20.

Kruger, P.S. (2009). Forget glucose: what about lipids in critical illness? Critical Care and Resuscitation, 11(4), 305-309.

Marik, P.E. (2006). Dyslipidemia in the critically ill. Critical Care Clinics, 22(1), 151-159, viii.

Nuzzo, G. & Giovannini, I. (2010). Plasma cholesterol level after hepatopancreatobiliary surgery provides information on the postoperative clinical course. Updates in Surgery, 62(3-4), 131-133. Epub 2010 Sep 7.

Ploder, M., Neurauter, G., Spittler, A., Schroecksnadel, K., Roth, E., & Fuchs D. (2008). Serum phenylalanine in patients post trauma and with sepsis correlate to neopterin concentrations. Amino Acids, 35(2), 303-307. Epub 2007 Dec 28.

Roth, E., Funovics, J., Mühlbacher, F., Schemper, M., Mauritz, W., Sporn, P., & Fritsch, A. (1982). Metabolic disorders in severe abdominal sepsis: glutamine deficiency in skeletal muscle. Clinical Nutrition, 1(1), 25-41.

Roth, E. & Druml, W. (2011). Plasma amino acid imbalance: dangerous in chronic diseases? Current Opinion in Clinical Nutrition and Metabolic Care, 14(1), 67-74.

Seber, G.A.F. (1977). Linear regression analysis. New York: Wiley (pp. 369-382).

Siegel, J.H., Cerra, F.B., Coleman, B., Giovannini, I., Shetye, M., Border, J.R. & McMenamy, R.H. (1979). Physiological and metabolic correlations in human sepsis. Invited commentary. Surgery, 86(2), 163-193.

Skau, T. (1985). Severity of illness in intra-abdominal infection. A comparison of two indexes. Archives of Surgery, 120(2), 152-158.

Vincent, J. L. (2006). Organ dysfunction in patients with severe sepsis. Surgical Infections (Larchmt), 7(Supplement 2), S69-S72.

Vyroubal, P., Chiarla, C., Giovannini, I., Hyspler, R., Ticha, A., Hrnciarikova, D., & Zadak, Z. (2008). Hypocholesterolemia in clinically serious conditions—review. Biomedical Papers of the Medical Faculty of the University Palacký Olomouc Czech Republic, 152(2), 181-189.

Wannemacher. R.W., Jr, Klainer, A.S., Dinterman, R.E., & Beisel, W.R. (1976). The significance and mechanism of an increased serum phenylalanine-tyrosine ratio during infection. American Journal of Clinical Nutrition, 29(9), 997-1006.

Novel Cyclic Nucleotide Signals in the Control of Pathologic Vascular Smooth Muscle Growth

David A. Tulis

Department of Physiology, Brody School of Medicine
East Carolina University, Greenville, North Carolina USA

1   Introduction

Cardiovascular disease (CVD) has historically ranked as the primary cause of morbidity and mortality in the United States (American Heart Association, 2012) and worldwide, currently accounting for nearly 30% of all global deaths (World Health Organization, 2011). Despite wide-ranging preventive measures aimed at reducing incidence and severity of CVD, the numbers of individuals suffering and dying from these serious disorders continue to rise. In the next decade it is estimated that the developed world will experience a 15% rise in CVD-related deaths while in less developed countries this increase will approach 70%. Moreover, by the year 2030 it is anticipated that almost 25 million people globally will die from some form of CVD (World Health Organization, 2011). Unfortunately, notwithstanding ample efforts in basic and clinical investigation, failure in the translation of research findings to clinical efficacy shows that the causes of CVD remain incompletely characterized and, in turn, fully effective therapies to curb CVD are lacking.

Of the many forms of CVD, coronary and cerebral artery disease and diseases of the peripheral vasculature constitute the major proportion (Spyridopoulos & Andres, 1998; American Heart Association, 2012). Many different types of blood vessel growth exist including that associated with normal development such as angiogenesis and vasculogenesis or arborization and development of vascular networks. However, foundational to blood vessel disease and/or dysfunction is abnormal growth of vascular smooth muscle (VSM), the normally quiescent and contractile muscular layer in blood vessels. In this pathophysiologic process, normally contractile, non-synthetic VSM cells undergo phenotypic alterations and become proliferative and synthetic and lose their contractile functions (Spyridopoulos & Andres, 1998; Berk, 2001; Marx *et al.*, 2011). These "activated" VSM cells then contribute to loss of normal vessel function and play critical roles in the pathogenesis of primary disorders such as evolution of atherosclerotic plaques and in secondary complications including neointimal development after angioplasty or stenotic luminal injury following stent deployment or bypass grafting (Spyridopoulos & Andres, 1998; Marx *et al.*, 2011). Clearly, the ability to control and attenuate pathologic VSM growth represents a critical approach for reducing vascular disorders and for combatting significant aspects of CVD (World Health Organization, 2011).

A plethora of genetic, molecular and cellular elements have been identified and targeted in basic and clinical investigation with hopes of reducing pathologic VSM growth in the context of CVD. Among these is cyclic nucleotide signaling, comprised of the cyclic adenosine monophosphate (AMP) and cyclic guanosine monophosphate (GMP) pathways. There are manifold elements in these second messenger systems that exert numerous and multifaceted regulatory functions in cardiac and vascular tissues (Beavo & Brunton, 2002; Tsai & Kass, 2009; Beavo *et al.*, 2010; Nossaman *et al.*, 2012). Stimulation of adenylate cyclase (AC) can occur by multiple means including G protein-coupled receptor ligation and activation (via stimulatory G_s), β-stimulation via adrenergic agonists, or through use of pharmacologic ligands such as forskolin or 8-bromo-cyclic AMP. Following AC stimulation, adenosine triphosphate (ATP) becomes dephosphorylated to yield cyclic AMP and pyrophosphate (PPi) (Serezani *et al.*, 2008). The schematic in Figure 1 on the next page briefly summarizes cyclic AMP synthesis following AC stimulation.

In mechanisms similar to cyclic AMP synthesis, following activation of guanylate cyclase (GC) through natriuretic peptides (which activate a particulate isoform, pGC) or via the diatomic gases nitric oxide (NO) or carbon monoxide (CO) (which activate soluble GC, sGC), guanosine triphosphate (GTP) is dephosphorylated to yield cyclic GMP and pyrophosphate (Waldman & Murad, 1987). Interestingly, NO-mediated stimulation of sGC and cyclic GMP synthesis has historically been regarded as the primary source for cyclic GMP in VSM, yet new findings reveal a biological role for heme oxygenase (HO)-derived CO in sGC activation. Moreover, as discussed herein, discovery of novel NO-independent sGC activators and stimulators that operate under heme-dependent or heme-independent conditions has provided ample support for NO-independent routes for cyclic GMP synthesis. Figure 2 shows pathways for cyclic GMP formation following sGC activation by NO synthase (NOS)-derived NO (following L-arginine conversion to L-citrulline in nicotinamide adenine dinucleotide phosphate (NADPH)/oxygen-dependent manner) and HO-derived CO (and biliverdin (Bv)/bilirubin (Br)) from degradation of heme.

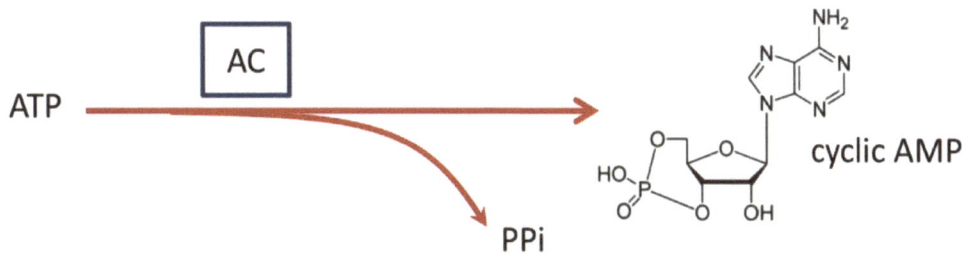

Figure 1: Formation of cyclic AMP

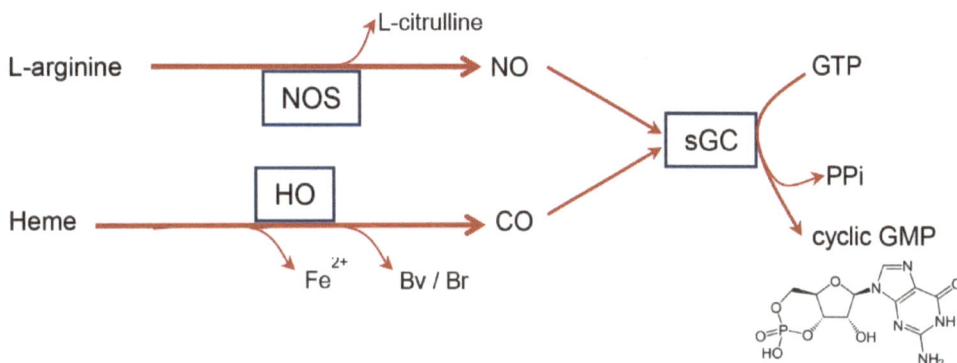

Figure 2: Formation of cyclic GMP

Following syntheses of cyclic AMP and cyclic GMP, these molecules can activate downstream cyclic AMP- and/or cyclic GMP-dependent protein kinases (PKA, PKG, respectively), their canonical signaling pathways in cardiovascular tissues (Francis & Corbin, 1999). New discoveries using selective pharmacology and transgenic models, however, reveal lack of specificity for customary upstream modes of activation as well as promiscuity and crosstalk for traditional downstream targets (Cornwell *et al.*, 1994; Pelligrino & Wang, 1998; Worner *et al.*, 2007; Mendelev *et al.*, 2009; Joshi *et al.*, 2011) including protein kinase C (PKC) (Adderley *et al.*, 2012a) and AMP-activated protein kinase (AMP kinase) (Stone *et al.*, 2012). In addition to signaling through kinase phosphorylative cascades, cyclic AMP and cyclic GMP can operate through kinase-independent processes such as direct ion channel modulation (Yau, 1994) or become dephosphorylated and inactivated by specific members of the phosphodiesterase (PDE) family (Beavo, 1995; Maurice *et al.*, 2003). Again, promiscuity among historically-considered selective PDE isoforms for cyclic AMP versus cyclic GMP degradation adds another level of complexity to the regulation of cyclic nucleotide signaling (Adderley *et al.*, 2012b). Ultimately, these intricate signaling cascades elicit a multitude of growth-regulating effects in cardiac and vascular tissues.

The goal of this chapter is to provide updated discussion of novel capacities of cyclic nucleotide signaling with particular emphasis on cyclic GMP processes to control pathologic VSM growth in the context of CVD. Topics for conversation include the role of abnormal VSM growth in CVD pathogenesis, novel routes for upstream control of cyclic GMP with particular emphasis on newly described sGC activators and stimulators, downstream pathways of cyclic GMP signaling including distinct kinases and PDEs, and novel targets for cyclic GMP signaling including kinase-specific vasodilator-activated serum phosphoprotein (VASP), transforming growth factor (TGF)-β/Smad, and crosstalk with the cyclic AMP/PKA and AMP kinase pathways. Capacities of these intricate systems to control pathologic VSM growth in the context of CVD are clear and highly significant in the basic and clinical medical sciences.

2   VSM Growth in CVD Pathogenesis

Abnormal or uncontrolled growth of VSM is an essential component of CVD pathogenesis. According to latest reports from the World Health Organization (2011) and the American Heart Association (2012), abnormal growth of VSM is considered foundational to coronary and cerebral artery disease and associated vessel disorders which comprise the primary forms of CVD. Aberrant VSM growth is elemental in both primary occlusive vascular disease and complications following balloon angioplasty, bypass grafting or stent deployment (Spyridopoulos & Andres, 1998; Berk, 2001; Marx *et al.*, 2011; American Heart Association, 2012). Abnormal VSM growth is also inherent in remodeling events following alterations in flow-mediated shear stress (Davies, 2009) or elevations in arterial blood pressure (Intengan & Schiffrin, 2001). In atherosclerosis, a primary form of occlusive vascular disease, abnormal growth of VSM constitutes the main element during the evolution of a growing plaque which can then lead to plaque complication, rupture and thrombosis. During plaque evolution and complication, VSM cells undergo de-differentiation into an embryonic, growth-promoting phenotype with establishment of a synthetic and pro-fibrotic character coincident with increased proliferation and migration and extracellular matrix formation and deposition (Spyridopoulos & Andres, 1998; Marx *et al.*, 2011). Concomitantly the affected vessels lose their normal contractile function and suffer from reduced vessel compliance and integrity along with exaggerated medial and oftentimes neointimal growth. These alterations in vessel geometry can result in diminished lumen caliber and vessel stenosis which then impede blood flow to downstream tissues while elevating arterial blood pressures within the local site of occlusion. Moreover, flow disturbances including loss of laminar flow and onset of turbulent flow often result from luminal obstruction which can also lead to focal thickening of the vessel wall (Davies, 2009). Indeed, given the centrality of aberrant VSM growth in cardiovascular disorders, therapeutic targeting of this pathophysiologic process is critical not only to gain advances in our understanding of basic vessel wall biology but also to make inroads into our ability to control and possibly ameliorate these adverse and clinically significant problems.

3   Upstream Control of Cyclic Nucleotide Synthesis

Excellent discussions of the key mechanisms of cyclase activation and cyclic nucleotide formation have been previously published (Kobialka & Gorczyca, 2000; Lucas *et al.*, 2000; Tulis, 2004; Jackson *et al.*, 2007). To date, mechanisms for AC-mediated cyclic AMP synthesis are generally well established (Serezani *et al.*, 2008). Cyclic AMP is synthesized following activation of AC, located on the inner plasma membrane and consisting of two transmembrane domains (M_1 and M_2, each with six α-helices), by a variety of stimuli which can include members of the 7 transmembrane G protein-coupled receptor (GPCR) family, receptors that can stimulate, via $G_{\alpha s}$, or inhibit, via $G_{\alpha i}$, AC catalysis and subsequent cyclic AMP synthesis. Also in the GPCR family, cyclic AMP can be formed by stimulation of adrenergic receptors or adrenoceptors by catecholamines such as epinephrine or norepinephrine. Cyclic AMP can also be produced following treatment with AC-activating ligands such as forskolin or 8-bromo-cyclic AMP or in response to changes in intracellular calcium. Interestingly, photoactivation of AC has been recently described (Schroder-Lang et al., 2007) which may provide a powerful tool for light-induced manipulation of cellular cAMP in animal cells. Nonetheless, synthetic mechanisms for cyclic AMP are generally established and routinely used as therapeutic targets for a variety of pathophysiologic disorders.

In comparison, recent discoveries have clouded traditional theories regarding routes for GC-mediated cyclic GMP formation. Traditional dogma contends that the primary mechanism leading to synthesis of cyclic GMP is by either pGC activation from natriuretic peptides or by sGC activation from NO. Membrane-bound pGC consists of an external N-terminal ligand-binding extracellular domain (ECD), a single transmembrane domain (TMD), and an intracellular C-terminus comprised of kinase-like (KLD), dimerization (DD), and catalytic (CD) domains (see Figure 3, next page) (Kobialka & Gorczyca, 2000). Subunit dimerization is thought to be required for a competent enzyme which can then be activated by peptides such as atrial natriuretic peptide (ANP) or intestinal peptides. Following extracellular ligand binding, phosphorylation of the KLD and intracellular interaction with calcium binding proteins occur, in turn converting GTP to cyclic GMP and pyrophosphate. Interestingly, pGC point mutants lacking the ECD, TMD and KLD regions still retain capacity to dephosphorylate GTP and synthesize cyclic GMP (Rudner et al., 1995; Zhou et al., 2004), suggesting predominantly regulatory roles for these membrane-associated domains.

Cytoplasmic sGC functions as a heterodimer of α (α_1 and α_2) and β (β_1 and β_2) polypeptide chains, each containing a DD and a CD homologous to those found in pGCs (Wedel et al., 1995; Poulos, 2006). Even though four potential heterodimers could be formed from the α and β subunits, only the $\alpha_1\beta_1$ and $\alpha_2\beta_1$ combinations have been reported to be active (Russwurm et al., 1998). The β-subunit contains an N-terminal HNOX (heme/nitric oxide/oxygen binding) site along with a prosthetic heme group that senses the gaseous ligands NO and CO. A PAS regulatory domain, named after first three proteins in which it was identified (period clock protein, ARNT protein, single-minded protein), acts as a sensor that mediates heterodimer formation and that likely serves a role in signal propagation from the HNOX domain to the C-terminal catalytic domain. The 250-residue C-terminal catalytic domain is highly conserved across GCs and is responsible for synthesizing cyclic GMP (and pyrophosphate) from GTP. Biologically existing as a heterodimer in 1:1 stoichiometry, the $\alpha_1\beta_1$ isoform is usually expressed and has the greatest activity of any sGC isoform (Katsuki et al., 1977). The native resting state of sGC is five-coordinate with an iron bound to four nitrogen atoms in the center of a heme porphyrin ring and a histidine bound to an axial fifth-coordinate site. Basal sGC has low activity and contains a prosthetic, high-spin proximal ferrous heme with a histidine[105] as the axial fifth or sixth ligand on the NH_2-terminal region of the β_1 subunit (Wedel et al., 1994; Stone & Marletta, 1998). Intriguingly, some evidence suggests that sGC may be partially membrane-bound, with the α_2 subunit thought to mediate membrane-association of the $\alpha_2\beta_1$ heterodimer, an isoform found in brain tissue, via a PDZ recognition domain and through interaction with the adapter protein PSD95 (Russwurm et al., 2001; Zabel et al., 2002; Mergia et al., 2006). Figure 3 shows a schematic of AC, pGC and sGC subunits responsible for cyclic nucleotide formation including possible membrane-association for sGC via its α_2 subunit.

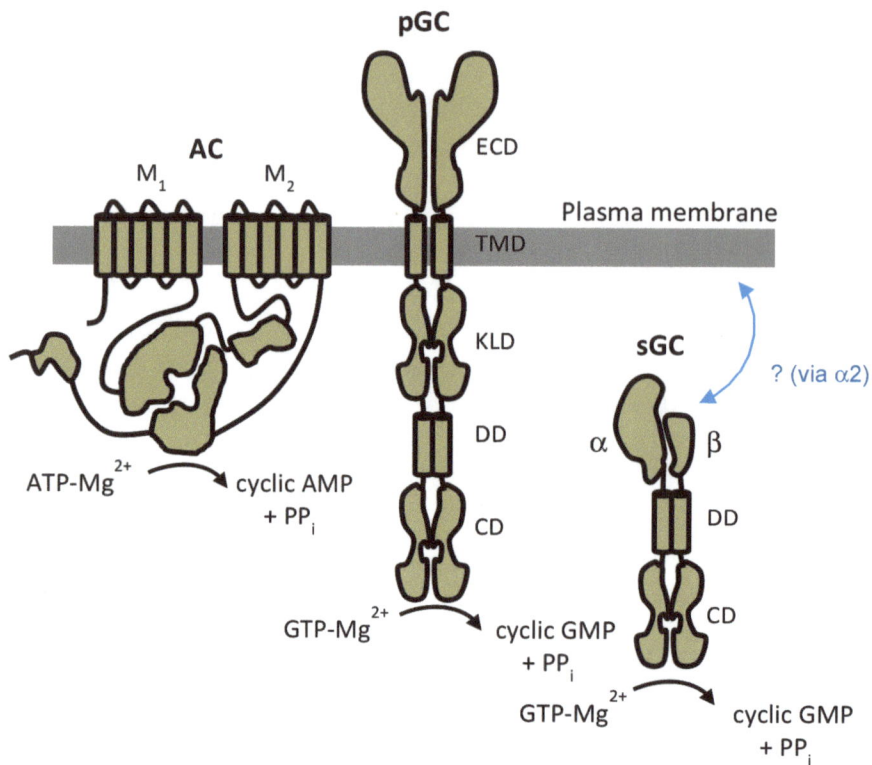

Figure 3: Subunits of adenylate cyclase (AC), particulate guanylate cyclase (pGC), and soluble guanylate cyclase (sGC) in cyclic nucleotide synthesis.

Stimulation of sGC by NO occurs via distinct processes compared to that of CO. Nitric oxide directly stimulates sGC by binding to the sixth position of the heme iron in the ferrous and ferric states, breaking the iron-histidine bond and creating a five-coordinate nitrosyl-heme complex that has capacity to increase sGC activity up to 400-fold (Friebe *et al.* 1996; Sharma & Magde, 1999). In comparison, CO directly stimulates sGC by binding to the reduced ferrous iron in the heme sixth position while keeping the iron-proximal histidine bond intact, thus maintaining a six-coordinate complex (Stone & Marletta, 1998; Sharma & Magde, 1999). Interestingly, dissociation of CO from the activated cyclase is thought to occur via a five-coordinate intermediate, which may be partly responsible for the nominal (~5-fold) magnitude of cyclase stimulation from CO alone (Deinum *et al.*, 1996; Friebe *et al.* 1996). Regardless of these differences between NO- and CO-mediated stimulation of sGC, the activated cyclase mediates cleavage of pyrophosphate from GTP to produce the critical second messenger cyclic GMP.

The intricacies of cyclic nucleotide signaling and in particular sGC-mediated cyclic GMP production provide multiple sites for regulation and thus for potential therapeutic intervention. Upstream control can occur through substrate modulation of L-arginine (for NO) and/or heme (for CO), through competitive pathways such as arginase conversion of L-arginine to L-ornithine as in the final step of the urea cycle (Peyton *et al.*, 2009), through changing the expression and/or activities of NOS or HO (Liu *et al.*, 2009), through provision or removal of key substrates or cofactors, or via use of enzymatic modifiers such as repressors, competitors, or agonists. Pharmacologic modulation can proceed directly at the level of NO and/or CO through use of NO donors or NO mimetics (Artz *et al.*, 2001), through use of saturated gas-containing solutions (Tulis *et al.*, 2005) or CO-releasing molecules (Motterlini *et al.*, 2005; Sawle *et al.*, 2005), or through use of direct cyclic nucleotide analogs such as 8-bromo-cyclic GMP or 8-pCPT-cyclic GMP (Adderley *et al.*, 2012a; Adderley *et al.*, 2012b). As discussed in detail below, upstream control of cyclic nucleotide signaling can also be achieved through use of isoform-specific sGC ablation or via select cyclase agonists such as sGC activators or sGC stimulators. Lastly, cyclic nucleotide content can be significantly altered through modulation of the expression and/or activity of specific PDEs that serve to degrade these signals to inactive 5′-monophosphates (Adderley *et al.*, 2012b). Specific PDE blockade is widely used clinically to treat symptoms of erectile dysfunction, pulmonary arterial hypertension, and high altitude pulmonary edema.

4   Soluble GC Ablation

Considering the critical role of sGC in synthesizing NO/CO-stimulated cyclic GMP and keeping in mind its isoform-specificity, sGC mutants were developed that offer unique genetic models with which to examine sGC-dependency of vascular function. Genetic mutants using α_1- (Mergia *et al.*, 2006; Nimmegeers *et al.*, 2007; Buys *et al.*, 2008; Buys *et al.*, 2012; Sips & Buys, 2013), α_2- (Mergia *et al.*, 2006) and β_1-specific (Rukoyatkina *et al.*, 2011; Groneberg *et al.*, 2010; Zhang *et al.*, 2011) ablation have been developed and characterized, with the most widely used model being the α_1 knockout. The α_1 is the principal subunit found in vascular sGC, and considering that $\alpha_1\beta_1$ has the greatest activity (Katsuki *et al.*, 1977) and is believed to be the most important sGC heterodimer in vascular tissue (Nimmegeers *et al.*, 2007), global knockout of sGC has been achieved primarily through ablation of the α_1 subunit. Intriguing results show that α_1-deficient arteries still retain their capacity to dilate and constrict, suggesting that sGC operates in reserve and only a fractional amount (estimated at 6%) of cyclase (perhaps the $\alpha_2\beta_1$ form) is required to mediate vessel function (Mergia *et al.*, 2006). Using α_1 knockout mice, both $\alpha_1\beta_1$ and $\alpha_2\beta_1$ forms of sGC have been determined to be responsible for VSM relaxation and blood pressure control (Nimmegeers *et al.*, 2007; Buys *et al.*, 2008). In agreement, SM-specific deletion of the β_1 subunit resulted in time-dependent onset of hypertension, supporting a role for the $\alpha_1\beta_1/\alpha_2\beta_1$ forms of sGC in blood pressure regulation (Groneberg *et al.*, 2010). These studies utilizing genetic knockout models verify $\alpha_1\beta_1$ and $\alpha_2\beta_1$ as essential components of a functional sGC in vascular tissues and substantiate criticality of sGC-mediated cyclic GMP in mediating vascular function.

5   Soluble GC Stimulators & Activators

As shown in Figure 2, the traditional route for cyclic GMP synthesis is through NOS-mediated conversion of L-arginine to L-citrulline, in NADPH/oxygen-dependent manner, with side-production of NO. In the cardiovascular system, NO has wide-ranging and powerful effects such as vascular dilation and elevation in blood flow, inhibition of platelet and inflammatory cell function, and reduction of VSM contraction and growth (Davis *et al.*, 2001; Bohl Masters *et al.*, 2005). Thus, NO-based therapies such as amyl nitrate and nitroglycerin have been widely used to treat a wide variety of ischemia- and inflammatory-based disorders. However, major limitations of NO/cyclic GMP signaling and NO-based therapies have been identified such as its reaction with amines, hemes, thiols, radicals, and reactive oxygen species

(ROS) in wide ranging cellular and extracellular proteins, ion channels, and receptors (Davis *et al.*, 2001; Gori & Parker, 2002). Nitric oxide, a paramagnetic free radical gas carrying an unpaired electron in its outer shell, can interact with molecular oxygen and superoxide radicals to generate reactive nitrogen species (RNS), can react with nucleic acids, transition metals and other biological molecules to induce oxidation and exacerbate ROS formation, and can elicit deamination, nitration and/or nitrosylation in turn provoking detrimental cellular and molecular events (Davis *et al.*, 2001; Andrews *et al.*, 2002; Raghaven & Dikshit, 2003; Parker, 2004). Additionally, in the clinical setting sustained NO-based therapy often results in diminished bioactivity, tachyphylaxis, and development of tolerance (LaBlanche *et al.*, 1997; Fung, 2004; Munzel *et al.*, 2005). These limitations of traditional NO/cyclic GMP-based signaling along with the modest ability of solitary CO to stimulate cyclase-mediated events to biologically relevant levels led to the discovery of novel routes for cyclic GMP synthesis that do not suffer from these drawbacks and yet have capacity to produce cyclic GMP at biologically relevant levels.

Thus, over the past ~20 years a family of synthetic sGC agonists have been developed that serve as NO-alternate routes for sGC activation and cyclic GMP control and that lack these aforementioned limitations associated with traditional NO and CO signaling (Friebe *et al.* 1996; Stasch *et al.*, 2001; Straub *et al.*, 2001; Straub *et al.*, 2002; Hobbs, 2002; Tulis, 2004; Evgenov *et al.*, 2006; Jackson *et al.*, 2007; Tulis, 2008; Priviero & Webb, 2010). These agents, which can enhance NO- and/or CO-mediated sGC activation and cyclic GMP synthesis but that can operate in NO-independent fashion, consist of two classes: heme-dependent sGC stimulators and heme-independent sGC activators. Heme-dependent sGC stimulators synergize with upstream NO and/or CO and rely upon a functional prosthetic cyclase heme that is in a reduced (Fe^{2+}) state under normal conditions; thus, under settings whereby the cyclase heme is removed or when it becomes dysfunctional or oxidized (Fe^{3+}) these agents lose their bioactivity and are rendered inactive. In comparison, heme-independent sGC activators maintain functionality under heme-deficient or heme-oxidized conditions and can activate the cyclase even more potently under those settings. These agents are particularly attractive for use under deleterious conditions in disease pathogenesis or following injury when oxidative and/or nitrosative stresses are elevated and oxidation of the core prosthetic cyclase heme (Fe^{3+}) takes place. Under such settings, heme-independent agents stimulate sGC more strongly and operate at higher potencies, thus rendering them therapeutically-selective for diseased or injured tissues. It should be noted that sGC stimulators and activators act preferentially with upstream cyclase-activating ligands (NO, CO) to exacerbate their ability to activate the cyclase and that these agents do not possess enzyme-activating ability when used alone in the absence of upstream activation (Evgenov *et al.*, 2006). Also, although many of these agents remain proprietary in nature, several are commercially available. For example, YC-1 can be purchased from Sigma-Aldrich, Millipore, and several other vendors, BAY 41-2272 can be purchased from Sigma-Aldrich, Enzo Life Sciences, Tocris Bioscience and others, A-350619 can be purchased from Tocris, etc. Some representative members of these two classes of sGC agonists are shown in Figure 4. In this schematic the abilities of heme-dependent sGC stimulators and heme-independent sGC activators to act on normally reduced sGC (Fe^{2+}) and to synthesize cyclic GMP as well as the unique capacity of sGC activators to stimulate cyclic GMP production under abnormal heme-oxidized (Fe^{3+}) or heme-deficient conditions are shown.

In cardiovascular tissues and particularly in VSM, use of sGC stimulators and sGC activators to control pathophysiologic responses to disease or injury has gained popularity among basic scientists and clinicians alike. As mentioned, excellent comprehensive articles are available that provide in-depth discussion of this exciting and broadly valuable family of reagents (Friebe *et al.* 1996; Stasch *et al.*, 2001; Straub *et al.*, 2001; Straub *et al.*, 2002; Hobbs, 2002; Tulis, 2004; Evgenov *et al.*, 2006; Jackson *et al.*,

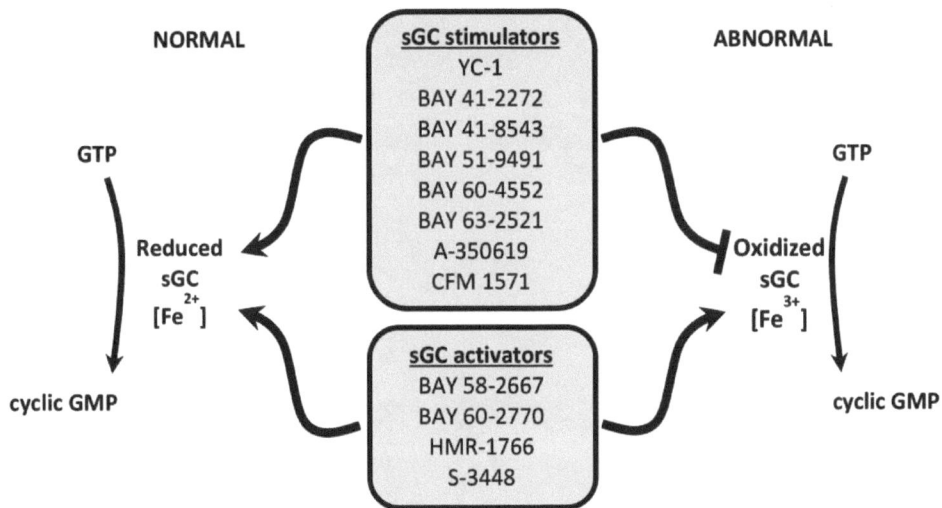

Figure 4: Representative members of heme-dependent sGC stimulators that enhance cyclic GMP synthesis when the cyclase heme is normally reduced (Fe^{2+}) and heme-independent sGC activators that enhance cyclic GMP synthesis under both heme-reduced and heme-oxidized (Fe^{3+}) conditions.

2007; Tulis, 2008; Priviero & Webb, 2010). One specific compound that has gained notoriety as biologically relevant in cardiovascular tissues is YC-1, a benzylindazole derivative originally discovered and characterized in 1994 (Ko *et al.*, 1994) and again in 1995 by the same group (Wu *et al.*, 1995). The chemical structure of YC-1 is shown in Figure 5 (next page). Briefly, YC-1 [3-(5'-hydroxymethyl-2'-furyl)-1-benzyl indazole] operates through redundant mechanisms to enhance cyclic GMP synthesis via augmentation of upstream sGC catalytic activity by stabilizing the active configuration of the enzyme, by increasing the affinity of the enzyme for GTP substrate, and by decreasing dissociation of the activating gaseous ligands NO and/or CO from the active enzyme-ligand complex (Friebe and Koesling, 1998; Lee *et al.*, 2000; Russwurm *et al.*, 2002). Importantly, biologic activity of YC-1 is dependent upon a functional reduced (Fe^{2+}) cyclase heme and perturbation of this heme (via oxidation or ablation) renders YC-1 inactive. YC-1 has ability to modify ion currents by activating large conductance K^+ channels and inducing hyperpolarization in VSM (Seitz *et al.*, 1999) and by reducing L-type calcium currents and elevations in intracellular calcium concentrations in neonatal (Vulcu *et al.*, 2000) but not in adult (Wegener *et al.*, 1997; Vulcu *et al.*, 2000) myocardium. YC-1 also serves to prevent cyclic nucleotide hydrolysis by inhibiting PDE isoforms including cyclic GMP-specific PDE-V (Galle *et al.*, 1999). Thus, through multiple mechanisms using both upstream and downstream actions YC-1 serves to strongly synergize with NO and/or CO to elicit robust and persistent cyclic GMP signaling.

In terms of growth-mitigating properties, we have previously published comprehensive reviews that document wide-ranging growth-retarding effects of YC-1 in cardiovascular and hematological tissues under in vitro, ex vivo and in vivo conditions (Tulis, 2004; Jackson *et al.*, 2007; Tulis, 2008). Supplemental work from our lab has firmly established anti-platelet, anti-proliferative, anti-synthetic and pro-apoptotic actions of YC-1 in VSM (Tulis *et al.*, 2000; Tulis *et al.*, 2002; Keswani *et al.*, 2009). Some of our more recent work discovered that YC-1 has capacity to stimulate upstream activation of both NOS and HO, adding to its appeal for therapeutic utility (Liu *et al.*, 2009).

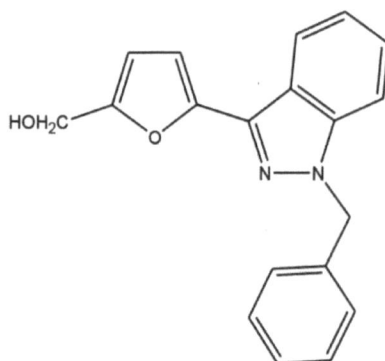

Figure 5: Chemical structure of the sGC stimulator YC-1 (Ko et al., 1994).

Using YC-1 as the prototype, thousands of YC-1-like mimetics have been developed over the years with varying degrees of biological efficacy and clinical relevance. With the discovery of a novel regulatory site on sGC that is unresponsive to NO stimulation yet is still capable of generating ample quantities of cyclic GMP came identification of a new pyrazolopyridine BAY 41-2272 [(5-cyclopropyl-2-[1-(2-fluorobenzyl)-1H-pyrazolo[3,4-b]pyridine-3-yl]-pyrimidin-4-ylamine)] (Becker *et al.*, 2001; Stasch *et al.*, 2001). Mechanistically, BAY 41-2272 operates in similar fashion to YC-1 (but with higher potency) and its function depends on activity of a reduced (Fe^{2+}) cyclase heme. BAY 41-2272 strongly synergizes with upstream NO and/or CO but can also operate irrespective of NO activation. Interestingly, BAY 41-2272, originally characterized as lacking PDE inhibitory action (Stasch *et al.*, 2001), was later suggested to possess PDE-V inhibitory capacity by another team of investigators (Mullershausen *et al.*, 2004), raising speculation for context- and/or intracellular microenvironment-specificity. The chemical structure of BAY 41-2272 is shown in Figure 6.

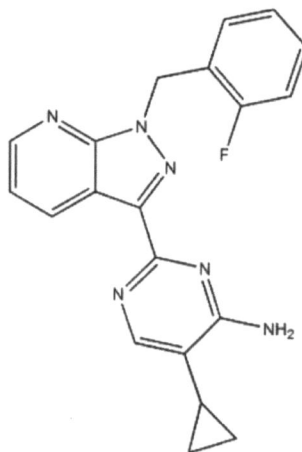

Figure 6: Chemical structure of the sGC stimulator BAY 41-2272 (Stasch et al., 2001).

Regarding the influence of BAY 41-2272 on the cardiovascular system, we have previously reviewed biological actions of BAY 41-2272 including some of its originally documented growth-retarding effects on various cardiovascular and hematological tissues including VSM (Tulis, 2004; Jackson *et al.*,

2007; Tulis, 2008). More recently we examined the impact of BAY 41-2272 on commercial (Mendelev *et al.*, 2009) and primary (Joshi *et al.*, 2011; Adderley *et al.*, 2012a; Adderley *et al.*, 2012b) VSM under both in vitro and in vivo settings. Cumulative results show that BAY 41-2272 operates to significantly elevate cyclic GMP levels (in the presence or absence of broad PDE inhibition) without marked effects on cyclic AMP content, that it stimulates activity of both PKG and PKA (the latter via crosstalk), that it phosphorylates downstream kinase-specific targets including VASP (and does so in both PKG- and PKA-specific fashion), and that it attenuates expression and activities of extracellular matrix (ECM)-degrading gelatinolytic matrix metalloproteinases (MMP)-2 and -9. Functionally, BAY 41-2272 was found to markedly reduce vascular neointimal development after injury in vivo and to significantly inhibit proliferation and migration of VSM cells in vitro. Intriguingly, pharmacologic blockade experiments suggest that BAY 41-2272 possess divergent downstream actions as it inhibits cellular proliferation completely through PKA yet inhibits cellular migration largely via PKG (Joshi *et al.*, 2011; Adderley *et al.*, 2012a).

Lastly, knowing that adverse conditions associated with disease or injury can lead to oxidative and/or nitrosative stresses and given that heme-independent sGC activators maintain their biological efficacy under conditions of oxidation or ablation of the cyclase heme, we have recently investigated the utility of BAY 60-2770 [4-({(4-carboxybutyl)[2-(5-fluoro-2-{[4'-(trifluoromethyl)biphenyl-4yl]methoxy} phenyl) ethyl]amino}methyl)benzoic acid], a heme-independent sGC activator, as a potential therapeutic agent to combat VSM growth. The chemical structure of BAY 60-2770 is shown in Figure 7. Our initial characterization of BAY 60-2770 in primary VSM cells (as a kind gift from Bayer HealthCare, Germany) revealed that it significantly increases cyclic GMP content in dose- and time-dependent fashion (maximum increases observed with 1 and 10 uM after 15 minutes) without appreciable effects on cyclic AMP levels. BAY 60-2770 elevated PKG activity which was reversed with PKG blockade (using DT-2) yet did not markedly alter PKA activity. Interestingly, BAY 60-2770 significantly increased both VASP-Ser239 (PKG marker) and VASP-Ser157 (PKA marker), again arguing for non-selectivity and promiscuity in VASP phosphorylation. In terms of growth, using automatic cell counting and trypan blue exclusion staining BAY 60-2770 significantly and dose-dependently (0.05 - 50 uM) reduced cell numbers after 72 hours without noticeable effects on cell toxicity (unpublished). These new results were complemented with those from an MTT assay as a marker of cellular metabolic activity and mitochondrial function (Peyton *et al.*, 2012).

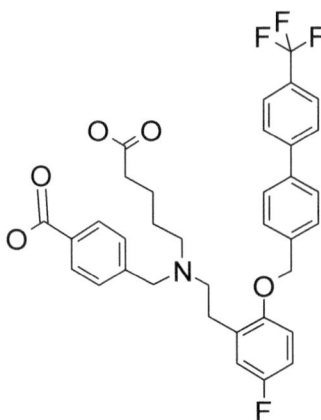

Figure 7: Chemical structure of the sGC activator BAY 60-2770 (Bayer HealthCare, Germany).

Figure 8A shows results of an MTT assay on primary VSM cells treated with BAY 60-2770 over 72 hours (using 3 replicates of an "n" of 5 per group, with one-way ANOVA). Using flow cytometry BAY 60-2770 significantly reduced S-phase cell numbers after 16 hours, and using an in vitro wounding assay and a modified transwell migration system BAY 60-2770 significantly inhibited VSM cell migration in response to serum or PDGF over 16 hours (see Figure 8B). Studies are underway investigating the impact of BAY 60-2770 on PKA, PKG, PKC and AMP kinase, examining key mechanisms of VASP regulation by BAY 60-2770, and characterizing the influence of BAY 60-2770 on associated ECM/focal adhesion/cytoskeletal proteins such as paxillin and focal adhesion kinase as previously reported (Mendelev et al., 2009). Preliminary data in rat VSM cells show upregulation of paxillin expression after 1 and 24 hours of incubation with BAY 60-2770 (see Figure 9, next page). These results suggest that BAY 60-2770 operates at least in part by enhancing cell-to-cell contacts and, in turn, reducing the ability of cells to proliferate and migrate. Certainly, these initial findings suggest BAY 60-2770 as a therapeutically attractive agent with clinical potential for targeting abnormal growth of vascular tissues associated with cardiovascular disorders.

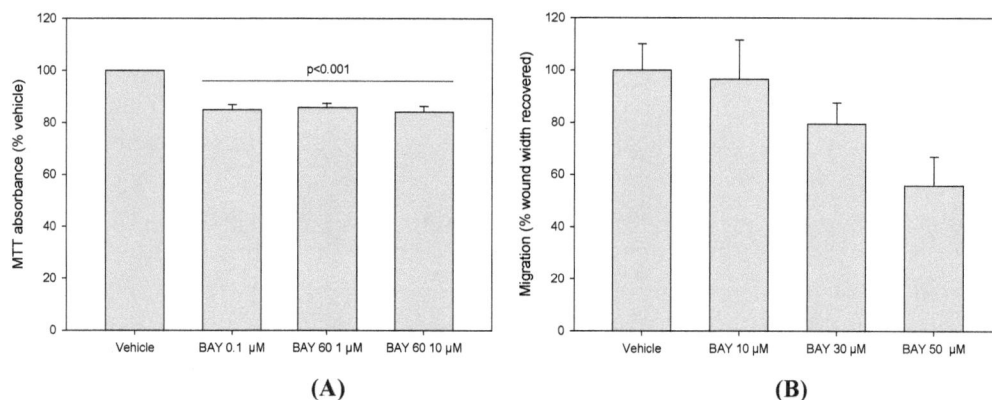

(A)   (B)

Figure 8: **A:** MTT assay as readout for cellular metabolism on primary VSM cells treated with BAY60-2770 (0.1-10 uM, 72 hours). **B:** In vitro wounding assay on VSM cells treated with BAY 60-2770 (10-50 uM, 16 hours). Data suggest that BAY 60-2770 inhibits cellular metabolism and proliferation and cell migration in response to growth (10% FBS) stimulation.

6   Downstream cGMP Signaling

Following synthesis through traditional NO and/or CO signals with/without enhancement from heme-dependent sGC stimulators and/or heme-independent sGC activators, the fate of synthesized cyclic GMP depends on several additional factors. These can include localized intracellular microenvironment, the availability of target proteins and substrates, and the presence and/or activity of cyclic nucleotide-degrading enzymes. Cellular microenvironments and in particular focal regions that contain specific cyclic nucleotide-targeted kinases and/or cyclic nucleotide-hydrolyzing PDEs largely dictate the magnitude and duration and thus, biological significance, of cyclic GMP signaling. In VSM, promiscuity and cross-talk among cyclic AMP and cyclic GMP signals, heretofore considered discrete signaling pathways, have been revealed which clouds the traditional viewpoint of distinct cyclic AMP/PKA and cyclic GMP/PKG cascades (Pelligrino & Wang, 1998; Mendelev et al., 2009; Joshi et al., 2011; Adderley et al., 2012a; Stone et al., 2012).

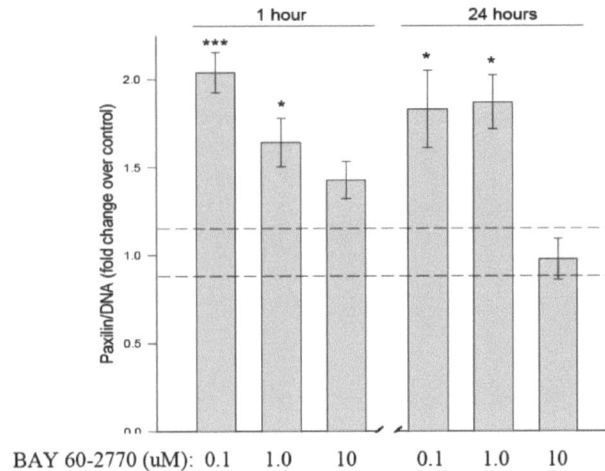

Figure 9: In VSM cells, BAY 60-2770 (0.1-10 uM) Bayer HealthCare, Germany) increases expression of the focal adhesion protein paxillin after 1 and 24 hours incubation compared to vehicle controls (control range shown by dotted lines). Results suggest that BAY 60-2770 reduces capacity of cells to proliferate and migrate by stabilizing their cell-to-cell contacts. *p<0.05, ***p<0.001 versus controls.

Availability of target proteins to cyclic nucleotide activation are of particular importance as well as those associated with cell-to-cell contact and extracellular-to-intracellular communication such as gap junction and focal adhesion proteins. Lastly, cyclic AMP and cyclic GMP can also operate through non-kinase/non-PDE processes including direct binding to ion channels or multi-drug transporters (Yau, 1994; Francis *et al.*, 2005). Following stimulation, cyclic GMP can affect multiple discrete downstream signaling pathways which are largely dependent upon localization of specific targets such as kinases and PDEs in precise intracellular domains. Intracellular compartmentalization of proteins and in particular, cytosolic- versus membrane-association of those elements including kinases and PDEs, is considered to be critical in cellular and biomolecular signaling in order to ensure specificity of responses to a particular stimulus (Xiang, 2011; Adderley *et al.*, 2012a; Adderley *et al.*, 2012b). Regarding cyclic nucleotide-directed protein kinases, the serine/threonine family of kinases including PKA, PKG and protein kinase C (PKC) operates through phosphorylation events of downstream substrates to moderate a wide variety of homeostatic events (Francis & Corbin, 1999); however, abnormal and uncontrolled activation or inhibition of these kinases with subsequent modification of phosphorylation events on downstream targets is implicated in the dysregulation of cell growth as either a cause or a consequence of a particular disorder. Figure 10 depicts some of the downstream targets of cyclic GMP signaling.

7   TGF-β1/Smad

In terms of targeted proteins for cyclic GMP in VSM, our latest heretofore unpublished findings suggest that cyclic GMP possesses ability to regulate signaling of the fibrotic, highly synthetic and growth-promoting TGF-β/Smad system. Among elements capable of controlling growth is TGF-β1, a multifunctional member of the TGF superfamily with widespread yet often opposite effects in cardiovascular tissues (Bertolino *et al.*, 2005; Bobik, 2006; Tang *et al.*, 2011).

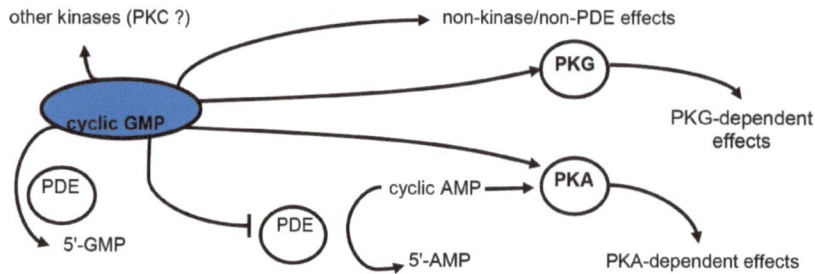

Figure 10: Possible downstream targets of cyclic GMP signaling in VSM.

Following a complicated mechanism of activation, TGF-β1 can phosphorylate receptor-activated Smad2 and Smad3, which then bind to the common Smad4 to form an activated complex which moves into the nucleus to activate or repress transcription of growth-regulatory target genes (depending on cellular context). Concomitantly, Smad3 activates inhibitory Smad7 in negative feedback to antagonize TGF-β signaling (Yan & Chen, 2011). Of note, even though the majority of TGF-β1 effects occur via canonical Smad signaling in VSM, TGF-β1 can also activate Smad-independent processes involving small GTPases, Erk, JNK, and p38 MAPK (Derynck & Zhang, 2003; Wrighton & Feng, 2008). Functionally, TGF-β1/Smad3 is generally considered anti-inflammatory but pro-fibrotic leading to ECM fibrosis with accumulation of fibronectin and collagen (Wang *et al.*, 2006; Ruiz-Ortega *et al.*, 2007). TGF-β1/Smad3 has also been implicated as a regulator of apoptosis (Kim *et al.*, 2009) and migration (Mao *et al.*, 2012) during VSM cell growth yet the influence of TGF-β1/Smad3 on vascular cell proliferation is complex and controversial and often conflicting. Some investigators found TGF-β1/Smad3 to be inhibitory for VSM proliferation (Berk, 2001; Kobayashi *et al.*, 2005; Akhurst & Hata, 2012), while others observed that TGF-β1/Smad3 stimulates VSM proliferation (Tsai *et al.*, 2009; Suwanabol *et al.*, 2012a; Suwanabol *et al.*, 2012b; Li *et al.*, 2013). In fact, in cultured vascular cells TGF-β1 is suggested to switch between growth stimulation and suppression depending on concentration and cell density (Ruiz-Ortega *et al.*, 2007; Hneino *et al.*, 2009).

Given these discordant findings in the literature on the role of TGF-β1/Smad signaling in VSM growth, we sought to determine the impact of induced TGF-β1 signaling on indices of VSM growth. Using a paired t-tests (with experimental "n" = 4-6/cohort), preliminary studies in primary VSM cells verified that recombinant TGF-β1 (10 ng/ml, 24 hours in 10% serum) significantly induced phosphorylated Smad2-Thr8 (normalized to total Smad2) and phosphorylated Smad3-Ser423/425 (normalized to total Smad3), markers of activated TGF-β1 signaling, and concurrently decreased (albeit not statistically significantly) inhibitory Smad7 levels compared to vehicle controls (see Figure 11).

Following verification of our approach to induce TGF-β1/Smad signaling (via increases in pSmad2-Thr8 and pSmad3-Ser423/425 as shown in Figure 11), we analyzed the influence of TGF-β1 on VSM growth. Using fluorescent flow cytometry and Western blotting on cellular homogenates after 24 hours, recombinant TGF-β1 (10 ng/ml, 10% serum) significantly increased cells in the G_2/M phase of the cell cycle, increased expression of cell cycle regulatory cyclins D and E and cyclin-dependent kinase (Cdk)-2 and Cdk4, and decreased expression of cell cycle inhibitory p21 and p27 compared to vehicle controls. Using automatic cell counting, recombinant TGF-β1 (10 ng/ml) significantly increased cell numbers compared to controls after 48 and 72 hours. These findings verified ability to experimentally induce TGF-β1/Smad signaling and that it possesses potent growth-promoting capacities in primary VSM cells.

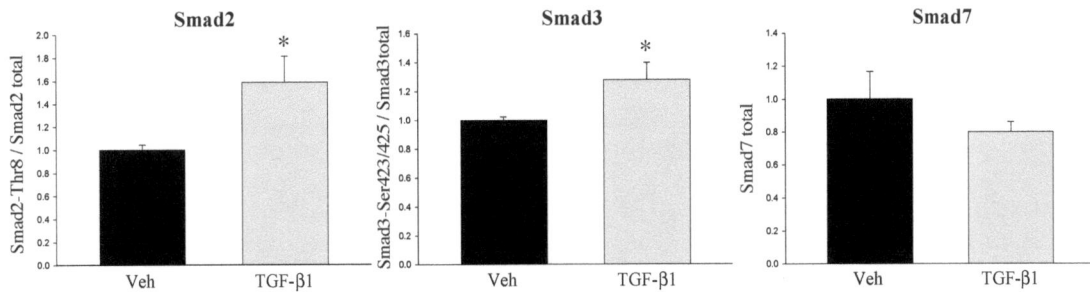

Figure 11: Recombinant TGF-β1 (10 ng/ml, 10% serum, 24 hours) induces activation of Smad2 and Smad3 and reduces inhibitory Smad7 compared to vehicle (Veh) controls in primary VSM cells. *$p<0.05$ versus Veh per paired t-test.

In subsequent preliminary efforts we tested the potential regulatory impact of cyclic GMP on TGF-β1 signaling. In rat commercial (A7R5, ATCC) and rat primary VSM cells treated with YC-1 or BAY 41-2272, using In-Cell Western blotting on intact, non-permeabilized cells and ECL-based Western blotting on VSM cell homogenates, results showed significantly reduced expression of total and active TGF-β1 as well as significantly reduced total and phosphorylated Smad3-Ser423/425 after cyclic GMP induction for 24 and 48 hours. Confirmatory results were obtained using double-sandwich ELISA (eBiosciences) for total and active TGF-β1 in cell homogenates and conditioned media in 0.5% or 10% serum. Figure 12 shows early results using one-way ANOVA with Bonferroni posthoc tests for multiple comparisons (with "n" = 3-4/cohort). Following double-sandwich ELISA on cell lysates after 1 hour (12A) or in conditioned media from treated cells after 12 hours (12B), results show that cyclic GMP (from BAY 41-2272 or YC-1) significantly inhibits TGF-β1 content. Data are normalized to total protein for each sample.

Figure 13 illustrates preliminary data showing significantly reduced total and phosphorylated (Ser423/425) Smad3 after cyclic GMP induction with BAY 41-2272 or YC-1 for 1 hour in primary VSM cells (using one-way ANOVA with Bonferroni tests and "n" = 3-4/cohort). In agreement with previously published in vivo observations (Tulis *et al.*, 2005), these intriguing preliminary findings in cultured VSM cells and conditioned media provide evidence that cyclic GMP operates at least partly through a TGF-β1/Smad3-dependent mechanism in its growth retardation of VSM.

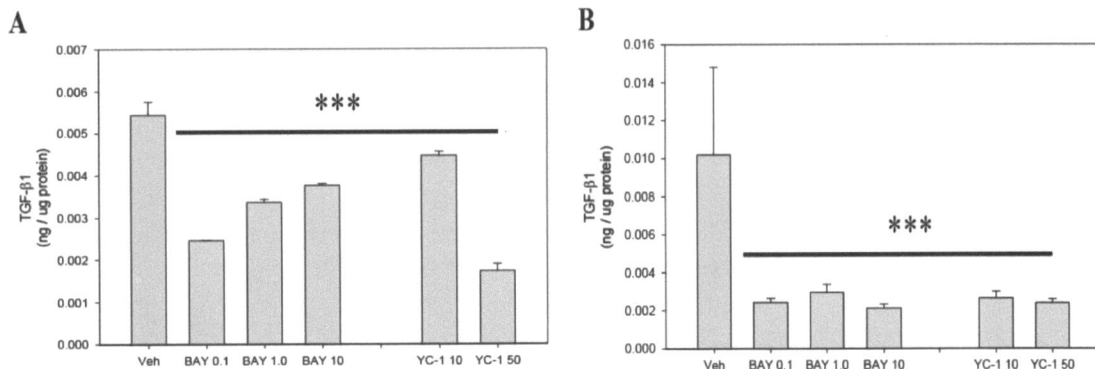

Figure 12: Cyclic GMP, induced with BAY 41-2272 (0.1-10 uM) or YC-1 (10, 50 uM), significantly reduces total TGF-β1 content in cell lysates after 1 hour (**A**) and in conditioned media from treated cells after 12 hours (**B**) compared to vehicle (Veh) controls in primary VSM cells. ***$p<0.001$ versus Veh per one-way ANOVA.

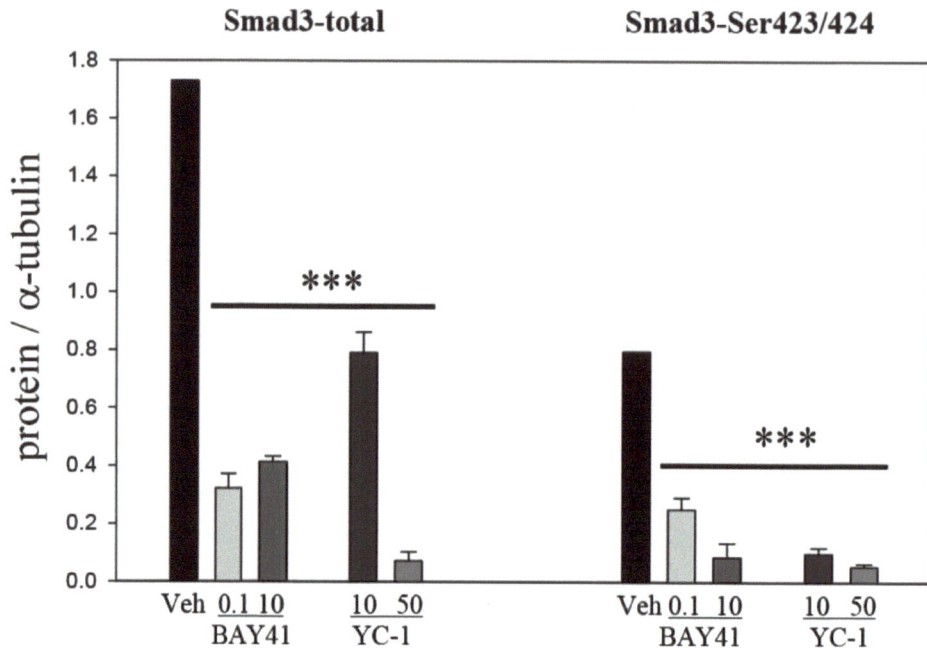

Figure 13: Cyclic GMP, induced with BAY 41-2272 (0.1, 10 uM) or YC-1 (10, 50 uM), significantly reduces total and phosphorylated (Ser423/425) Smad3 in primary VSM cell lysates after 1 hour compared to vehicle (Veh) controls. ***p<0.001 versus Veh per one-way ANOVA.

8   Cell-to-cell and ECM-based Signals

Given the critical roles for TGF-β1 in modulating cellular growth and fibrosis and ECM biology including that associated with cell-to-cell contact and cellular communication, in an associated study (Joshi *et al.*, 2012) we discovered that cyclic GMP (and cyclic AMP) increased expression of connexin 43 (Cx43), an essential gap junction protein involved in cellular integrity and intracellular communication (Chadjichristos *et al.*, 2006; Remo *et al.*, 2012). In this project we observed that cyclic GMP (induced directly via 8-bromo-cyclic GMP and indirectly via BAY 41-2272) and cyclic AMP (induced directly with 8-bromo-cyclic AMP) independently reduced VSM cell growth which we believe is due partly to the ability of these cyclic nucleotides to regulate intracellular communication via gap junction control. Interestingly, using fluorescent recovery after photobleaching (FRAP) as an indicator of gap junction intracellular communication, we observed increases in FRAP only following cyclic AMP induction and failed to detect changes in FRAP following cyclic GMP stimulation (Joshi *et al.*, 2012). Also considering ECM biology and cell-to-cell contacts including focal adhesions, a major emphasis in our lab now is investigation into possible interaction between cyclic GMP/cyclic AMP and VASP, a cytoskeletal focal adhesion-associated protein that belongs to the Ena/VASP family (Bear & Gertler, 2009). VASP plays important roles in regulating cytoskeletal dynamics and processes such as cell adhesion, migration and proliferation (Zhao *et al.*, 2008; Kim *et al.* 2010; Adderley *et al.*, 2012b; Joshi *et al.*, 2012). Originally characterized as a substrate for cyclic nucleotide-dependent PKA and PKG (Reinhard *et al.*, 2001; Krause *et al.*, 2002), VASP has been suggested to be important in control of cellular growth. Currently at least four distinct phosphorylation sites on VASP have been characterized: Ser157, Ser239, Thr278, Ser322 (Butt *et al.*,

1994; Chitaley *et al.*, 2004; Thomson *et al.*, 2011), with VASP-Ser157 the reported site for PKA activation and VASP-Ser239 the site for PKG activation (Reinhard *et al.*, 2001; Krause *et al.*, 2002). Despite this accepted site-specificity for kinase activation of VASP (and thus, its use as a readout for kinase activity), our recent work has identified promiscuity and crosstalk among these phosphorylation sites on VASP in terms of PKA and PKG stimulation (Joshi *et al.*, 2011; Adderley *et al.*, 2012a; Adderley *et al.*, 2012b; Stone *et al.*, 2012). Moreover, we recently characterized a role for PKC (Adderley *et al.*, 2012a) and AMP kinase (Stone *et al.*, 2012; Stone *et al.*, 2013) in mediating site-specific VASP phosphorylation in the context of aberrant vascular growth. Given its role in mediating cellular integrity and growth and its regulation by cyclic nucleotides, we believe that VASP is a key contributor in the control of vascular growth and are currently in the process of examining specificity of key phosphorylation sites on VASP for their regulatory capacity in VSM migration, proliferation and ECM/cellular stability. We are also interested in examining dual-regulation between VASP and TGF-β1/Smad in vascular growth control.

9   AMP Kinase

Considering the apparent 'non-selectivity' of kinase activation following cyclic GMP induction, a new line of work in our lab has recently identified AMP kinase as another potential regulator of VSM growth downstream of cyclic nucleotide stimulation (Stone *et al.*, 2012; Stone *et al.*, 2013). AMP kinase serves as a metabolic gauge that responds to cellular energy depletion and stress by inhibiting ATP-reducing processes, in turn promoting ATP-synthesizing processes within the cell (Rubin *et al.*, 2005). Thus, AMP kinase responds to elevations in the AMP:ATP ratio. Novel results show that AMP kinase has capacity to control proliferation and migration of primary VSM cells and that these events are at least partially regulated by cyclic AMP-mediated PKA (Stone *et al.*, 2012). Interestingly, using an arterial injury model and primary cell culture we also observed AMP kinase to have the ability to promote ECM/focal adhesion/cytoskeleton stability as part of its growth-inhibitory actions (Stone *et al.*, 2013). Unpublished findings from our lab suggest that AMP kinase, in conjunction with cyclic AMP/PKA, also moderates TGF-β1/Smad3 signaling and TGF-β1/Smad3-induced VSM growth (data not shown). Studies are underway using genetically-deficient AMP kinase mouse models to further clarify this exciting new area of cell signaling underlying VSM growth.

10   Pulmonary, Cardiac & Erectile SM

Given the basic science and clinical significance of pulmonary, cardiac and erectile disorders, brief discussion is warranted regarding the influence of these sGC/cyclic GMP signaling processes in VSM in these systems. Pulmonary arterial hypertension (PAH) is a morbid and progressive disease characterized by acute vascular constriction and subsequent vessel remodeling and for which fully effective therapies are not currently available (Belik, 2009; Lasker *et al.*, 2011). Although BAY 41-2272 and another heme-dependent sGC stimulator, BAY 41-8543, have shown promise based on their vasodilatory and anti-platelet actions in pulmonary vasculature (Lasker *et al.*, 2011), limitations in their metabolic and pharmacokinetic properties (Mittendorf *et al.*, 2009) warrant continued investigation. YC-1 (Huh *et al.*, 2011) and BAY 60-2770 (Pankey *et al.*, 2011) have been shown to reduce PAH in experimental rodent models in response to hypoxia or monocrotaline, respectively. Also, BAY 63-2521, otherwise known as Riociguat, is an orally-active, heme-dependent sGC stimulator that has shown promise as a treatment against induced PAH in rats (Lang *et al.*, 2012) and in humans with PAH secondary to ventricular dysfunction (Bonderman, *et al.*, 2013). Several excellent reviews are available that provide comprehensive evaluation of sGC/cyclic GMP-specific approaches aimed at controlling PAH in animal studies and human clinical trials (Belik, 2009; Ghofrani & Grimminger, 2009; Ghofrani *et al.*, 2010; Lasker *et al.*, 2011). Following induction of chronic hypoxia in the neonatal rat heart, BAY 41-2272 was shown to reduce right ventricular hypertrophy and to minimize arterial wall hypertrophy (Deruelle *et al.*, 2006). In an induced myocardial infarction rat model, oral BAY 58-2667 (Cinaciguat) reduced injury-induced oxidative stresses and improved myocardial performance (Korkmaz *et al.*, 2009). Several sGC modulators including BAY 58-2667 and BAY 63-2521 have been utilized to retard the effects of heart failure, notably in patients with acute decompensated heart failure (Lapp *et al.*, 2009), and these have been recently reviewed (Mitrovic *et al.*, 2011). In pharmacotherapy for erectile dysfunction (ED), selective PDE inhibitors have been widely used; however, in greater than 30% of ED cases PDE inhibitors are ineffective (Gur *et al.*, 2010), arguing that basal production of cyclic GMP may be deficient in these patients. Under such conditions, enhancement of sGC-mediated cyclic GMP may be a plausible approach, and use of sGC activators or stimulators, either individually or in combination with PDE blockade, to treat ED has gained wide interest (Brioni *et al.*, 2002; Albersen *et al.*, 2010; Gur *et al.*, 2010; Decaluwe *et al.*, 2011).

11   Summary & Conclusions

The highly significant impact of CVD on morbidity and mortality in the United States and worldwide is staggering. Unfortunately, failure in the translation of findings from basic science and clinical investigation into clinical practice shows that the causes of CVD and associated cardiovascular complications remain incompletely characterized and in turn, fully effective therapies to control or mitigate CVD are lacking. The role of abnormal growth of VSM underlying cardiovascular disorders is clear and critical and presents an essential target for our attention. In this light, over the years we and others have examined important regulatory roles for cyclic nucleotide signaling and in particular, cyclic GMP and its downstream effectors, in controlling aberrant vascular growth. As briefly summarized herein, compelling in vitro and in vivo research findings obtained by our lab and others and lend strong support for cyclic GMP signals in the control of unabated VSM growth. In particular, recent observations using novel sGC activators and stimulators are highly promising and may offer novel approaches for use in the clinical arena to combat not only cardiovascular but also pulmonary and sexual disorders. Ample support is presented for key targets of cyclic GMP signaling that may include PKG and crosstalk with PKA, AMP kinase, VASP and the TGF-β/Smad pathways. Indeed, this highly promising field of study warrants further characterization and continued attention in the basic and clinical sciences.

Acknowledgement

I would like to enthusiastically thank all of the individuals with whom I have worked over the years in this complicated yet exciting field of scientific inquiry. I would also like to acknowledge investigators who have contributed significantly to the field of cyclic nucleotide signaling as related to cardiovascular biology and pathophysiology but whose works were not cited in this chapter due to formatting limitations. I would also like to acknowledge Bayer HealthCare in Germany for their kind contribution of BAY 60-2770. Work in the preparation of this chapter was supported by grants from the American Heart Association (AHA), the National Institutes of Health (NIH) National Heart, Lung, and Blood Institute (NHLBI) Award Number HL-81720, and the Brody School of Medicine Seed/Bridge Grant Program. This content is solely the responsibility of the authors and does not necessarily represent the official views of the AHA, NIH or NHLBI.

References

Adderley, S.P., Joshi, C.N., Martin, D.N., Mooney, S., Tulis, D.A. (2012a). Multiple Kinase Involvement in the Regulation of Vascular Growth, Advances in Protein Kinases, Chapter 6, pp. 131-150, Ed. G. Da Silva Xavier, InTech Open Access Publishers ISBN 978-953-51-0633-3.

Adderley, S.P., Joshi, C.N., Martin, D.N., Tulis, D.A. (2012b). Phosphodiesterases regulate BAY 41-2272-induced VASP phosphorylation in vascular smooth muscle cells. Front. Pharmacol., 3, 10; doi:10.3389/fphar.2012.00010.

Akhurst, R.J., Hata, A. (2012). Targeting the TGFβ signaling pathway in disease. Nat. Rev. Drug Discov. 11: 790-811.

Albersen, M., Shindel, A.W., Mwamukonda, K.B., Lue, T.F. (2010). The future is today: emerging drugs for the treatment of erectile dysfunction. Expert Opin. Emerg. Drugs 15: 467-480.

American Heart Association, on behalf of the American Heart Association Statistics Committee and Stroke Statistics Subcommittee. (2012). Heart Disease and Stroke Statistics – 2012 Update. A Report from the American Heart Association. Circulation 125: 188-197.

Andrews, K.L., Triggle, C.R., Ellis, A. (2002). NO and the vasculature: where does it come from and what does it do? Heart Fail. Rev. 7: 423-45.

Artz, J.D., Toader, V., Zavorin, S.I., Bennett, B.M., Thatcher, G.R.J. (2001). In vitro activation of soluble guanylyl cyclase and nitric oxide release: a comparison of NO donors and NO mimetics. Biochemistry 40: 9256-9264.

Bear, J.E., Gertler, F.B. (2009). Ena/VASP: towards resolving a pointed controversy at the barbed end. J. Cell Sci. 122: 1947-1953.

Beavo, J.A. (1995). Cyclic nucleotide phosphodiesterases: functional implications of multiple isoforms. Physiol. Rev. 75: 725-748.

Beavo, J.A., Brunton, L.L. (2002). Cyclic nucleotide research – still expanding after half a century. Nat. Rev. Mol. Cell Biol. 3: 710-718.

Beavo, J., Francis, S., Houslay, M. (2010). Cyclic nucleotide phosphodiesterases in health and disease. CRC Press, Boca Raton, FL. ISBN: 9780849396687.

Becker, E.M., Alonso-Alija, C., Apeler, H., Gerzer, R., Minuth, T., Pleib, U., Schmidt, P., Schramm, M., Schroder, H., Schroeder, W., Steinke, W., Straub, A., Stasch, J-P. (2001). NO-independent regulatory site of direct sGC stimulators like YC-1 and BAY 41-2272. BMC Pharmacol. 1: 13-24.

Belik, J. (2009). Riociguat, an oral soluble guanylate cyclase stimulator for the treatment of pulmonary hypertension. Curr. Opin. Investig. Drugs 10: 971-979.

Berk, B.C. (2001). Vascular smooth muscle growth: autocrine growth mechanisms. Physiol. Rev. 81: 999-1030.

Bertolino, P., Deckers, M., Lebrin, F., ten Dijke, P. (2005). Transforming growth factor-beta signal transduction in angiogenesis and vascular disorders. Chest 128: 585S-590S.

Bobik, A. (2006). Transforming growth factor-βs and vascular disorders. Arterioscler. Thromb. Vasc. Biol. 26: 1712-1720.

Bohl Masters, K.S., Lipke, E.A., Rice, E.E.H., Liel, M.S., Myler, H.A., Zygourakis, C., Tulis, D.A., West, J.L. (2005). Nitric oxide-generating hydrogels inhibit neointima formation. J. Biomater. Sci. Polym. Ed. 16: 659-672.

Brioni, J.D., Nakane, M., Hsieh, G.C., Moreland, R.B., Kolasa, T., Sulluvan, J.P. (2002). Activators of soluble guanylate cyclase for the treatment of male erectile dysfunction. Int. J. Impot. Res. 14: 8-14.

Butt, E., Abel, K., Krieger, M., Palm, D., Hoppe, V., Hoppe, J., Walter, U. (1994). cAMP- and cGMP-dependent protein kinase phosphorylation sites of the focal adhesion vasodilator-stimulated phosphoprotein (VASP) in vitro and in intact human platelets. J. Biol. Chem. 269: 14509-14517.

Buys, E.S., Raher, M.J., Kirby, A., Mohd, S., Baron, D.M., Hayton, S.R., Tainsh, L.T., Sips, P.Y., Rauwerdink, K.M., Yan, Q., Tainsh, R.E.T., Shakartzi, H.R., Stevens, C., Decaluwe, K., da Gloria Rodrigues-Machado, M., Malhotra, R., Van de Voorde, J., Wang, T., Brouckaert, P., Daly, M.J., Bloch, K.D. (2012). Genetic modifiers of hypertension in soluble guanylate cyclase α1-deficient mice. J. Clin. Invest. 122: 2316-2325.

Buys, E.S., Sips, P., Vermeersch, P., Raher, M.J., Rogge, E., Ichinose, F., Dewerchin, M., Bloch, K.D., Janssens, S., Brouckaert, P. (2008). Gender-specific hypertension and responsiveness to nitric oxide in sGCα1 knockout mice. Cardiovasc. Res. 79: 179-186.

Chadjichristos, C.E., Derouette, J.P., Kwak, B.R. (2006). Connexins in atherosclerosis. Adv. Cariol. 42: 255-267.

Chitaley, K., Chen, L., Galler, A., Walter, U., Daum, G., Clowes, A.W. (2004). Vasodilator-stimulated phosphoprotein is a substrate for protein kinase C. FEBS Lett. 556: 211-215.

Cornwell, T.L., Arnold, E., Boerth, N.J., Lincoln, T.M. (1994). Inhibition of smooth muscle cell growth by nitric oxide and activation of cAMP-dependent protein kinase by cGMP. Am. J. Physiol., 267, C1405-C1413.

Davies, P.F. (2009). Hemodynamic shear stress and the endothelium in cardiovascular pathophysiology. Nat. Clin. Pract. Cardiovasc. Med. 6: 16-26.

Davis, K.L., Martin, E., Turko, I.V., Murad, F. (2001). Novel effects of nitric oxide. Annu. Rev. Pharmacol. Toxicol. 41: 203-36.

Decaluwe, K., Pauwels, B., Verpoest, S., Van de Voorde, J. (2011). New therapeutic targets for the treatment of erectile dysfunction. J. Sex. Med. 8: 3271-3290.

Deinum, G., Stone, J.R., Babcock, G.T., Marletta, M.A. (1996). Binding of nitric oxide and carbon monoxide to soluble guanylate cyclase as observed with Resonance raman spectroscopy. Biochem. 35: 1540-47.

Deruelle, P., Balasubramaniam, V., Kunig, A.M., Seedorf, G.J., Markham, N.E., Abman, S.H. (2006). BAY 41-2272, a direct activator of soluble guanylate cyclase, reduces right ventricular hypertrophy and prevents pulmonary vascular remodeling during chronic hypoxia in neonatal rats. Biol. Neonate 90: 135-144.

Derynck, R., Zhang, Y.E. (2003). Smad-dependent and Smad-independent pathways in TGF-β family signaling. Nature 425: 577-584.

Evgenov, O.V., Pacher, P., Schmidt, P.M., Hasko, G., Schmidt, H.H.H.W., Stasch, J-P. (2006). NO-independent stimulators and activators of soluble guanylate cyclase: discovery and therapeutic potential. Nat. Rev. Drug Disc. 5: 755-768.

Francis, S.H., Blount, M.A., Zoraghi, R., Corbin, J.D. (2005). Molecular properties of mammalian proteins that interact with cGMP: protein kinases, cation channels, phosphodiesterases, and multi-drug anion transporters. Front. Biosci. 10: 2097-17.

Francis, S.H., Corbin, J.D. (1999). Cyclic nucleotide-dependent protein kinases: intracellular receptors for cAMP and cGMP action. Crit. Rev. Clin. Lab Sci. 36: 275-328.

Friebe, A., Koesling, D. (1998). Mechanism of YC-1-induced activation of soluble guanylyl cyclase. Mol. Pharmacol. 53: 123-127.

Friebe, A., Schultz, G., Koesling, D. (1996). Sensitizing soluble guanylyl cyclase to become a highly CO-sensitive enzyme. EMBO J. 15: 6863-68.

Fung, H.L. (2004). Biochemical mechanism of nitroglycerin action and tolerance: is this old mystery solved? Annu. Rev. Pharmacol. Toxicol. 44: 67-85.

Galle, J., Zabel, U., Hubner, U., Hatzelmann, A., Wagner, B., Wanner, C., Schmidt, H.H.H.W. (1999). Effects of the soluble guanylate cyclase activator, YC-1, on vascular tone, cyclic GMP levels and phosphodiesterase activity. Br. J. Pharmacol. 127: 195-203.

Ghofrani, H.A., Grimminger, F. (2009). Soluble guanylate cyclase stimulation: an emerging option in pulmonary hypertension therapy. Eur. Respir. Rev. 18: 35-41.

Ghofrani, H.A., Voswinckel, R., Gall, H., Schermuly, R., Weissmann, N., Seeger, W., Grimminger, F. (2010). Riociguat for pulmonary hypertension. Future Cardiol. 6: 155-166.

Gori, T., Parker, J.D. (2002). The puzzle of nitrate tolerance: pieces smaller than we thought? Circulation 106: 2404-2408.

Groneberg, D., Konig, P., Wirth, A., Offermanns, S., Koesling, D., Friebe, A. (2010). Smooth muscle-specific deletion of nitric oxide-sensitive guanylyl cyclase is sufficient to induce hypertension in mice. Circulation 121: 401-409.

Gur, S., Kadowitz, P.J., Hellstrom, W.J. (2010). Exploring the potential of NO-independent stimulators and activators of soluble guanylate cyclase for the medical treatment of erectile dysfunction. Curr. Pharm. Des. 16: 1619-1633.

Heart Disease and Stroke Statistics – 2012 Update. A Report from the American Heart Association. On behalf of the American Heart Association Statistics Committee and Stroke Statistics Subcommittee. (2012). Circulation 125: 188-197.

Hneino, M., Bouazza, L., Bricca, G., Li, J.Y., Langlois, D. (2009). Density-dependent shift of transforming growth factor-beta-1 from inhibition to stimulation of vascular smooth muscle cell growth is based on unconventional regulation of proliferation, apoptosis and contact inhibition. J. Vasc. Res. 46: 85-97.

Hobbs, A.J. (2002). Soluble guanylate cyclase: an old therapeutic target re-visited. Br. J. Pharmacol. 136: 637-40.

Huh, J.W., Kim, S.Y., Lee, J.H., Lee, Y.S. (2011). YC-1 attenuates hypoxia-induced pulmonary arterial hypertension in mice. Pulm. Pharmacol. Ther. 24: 638-646.

Intengan, H.D., Schiffrin, E.L. (2001). Vascular remodeling in hypertension: roles of apoptosis, inflammation, and fibrosis. Hypertension 38: 581-587.

Jackson, Jr., E.B., Mukhopadhyay, S., Tulis, D.A. (2007). Pharmacologic modulators of soluble guanylate cyclase/cyclic guanosine monophosphate in the vascular system – from bench top to bedside. Curr. Vasc. Pharmacol. 5: 1-14.

Joshi, C.N., Martin, D.N., Fox, J.C., Mendelev, N.N., Brown, T.A., Tulis, D.A. (2011). The soluble guanylate cyclase stimulator BAY 41-2272 inhibits vascular smooth muscle growth through the cAMP-dependent protein kinase and cGMP-dependent protein kinase pathways. J. Pharm. Exp. Ther., 339, 394-402.

Joshi, C.N., Martin, D.N., Shaver, P., Madamanchi, C., Muller-Borer, B.J., Tulis, D.A. (2012). Control of vascular smooth muscle cell growth by connexin 43. Front. Physiol. 3:220; doi: 10.3389/fphys.2012.00220.

Katsuki S., Arnold, W., Mittal, C., Murad, F. (1977). Stimulation of guanylate cyclase by sodium nitroprusside, nitroglycerin and nitric oxide in various tissue preparations and comparison to the effects of sodium azide and hydroxylamine. J. Cyclic Nucleotide Res. 3: 23-35.

Keswani, A.N., Peyton, K.J., Durante, W., Schafer, A.I., Tulis, D.A. (2009). The cyclic GMP modulators YC-1 and zaprinast reduce vessel remodeling through anti-proliferative and pro-apoptotic effects. J. Cardiovasc. Pharm. Ther. 14: 116-124.

Kim, H.J., Kim, M.Y., Jin, H., Kim, H.J., Kang, S.S., Kim, H.J., Lee, J.H., Chang, K.C., Hwang, J.Y., Yabe-Nishimura, C., Kim, J.H., Seo, H.G. (2009). Peroxisome proliferator-activated receptor {delta} regulates extracellular matrix and apoptosis of vascular smooth muscle cells through the activation of transforming growth factor-{beta}1/Smad3. Circ. Res. 105: 16-24.

Kim, H.R., Graceffa, P., Ferron, F., Gallant, C., Boczkowska, M., Dominquez, R., Morgan, K.G. (2010). Actin polymerization in differentiated vascular smooth muscle cells requires vasodilator-stimulated phosphoprotein. Am. J. Physiol. Cell Physiol. 298: C559-C571.

Ko, F.N., Wu, C.C., Kuo, S.C., Lee, F.Y., Teng, C.M. (1994). YC-1, a novel activator of platelet guanylate cyclase. Blood 84: 4226-4233.

Kobayashi, K., Yokote, K., Fujimoto, M., Yamashita, K., Sakamoto, A., Kitahara, M., Kawamura, H., Maezawa, Y., Asaumi, S., Tokuhisa, T., Mori, S., Saito, Y. (2005). Targeted disruption of TGF-beta-Smad3 signaling leads to enhanced neointimal hyperplasia with diminished matrix deposition in response to vascular injury. Circ. Res. 96: 904-912.

Kobialka, M., Gorczyca, W.A. (2000). Particulate guanylyl cyclases: multiple mechanisms of activation. Acta Biochim. Pol., 47, 517-528.

Korkmaz, S., Radovits, T., Barnucz, E., Hirschberg, K., Neugebauer, P., Loganathan, S., Veres, G., Pali, S., Seidel, B., Zollner, S., Karck, M., Szabo, G. (2009). Pharmacological activation of soluble guanylate cyclase protects the heart against ischemic injury. Circulation 120: 677-686.

Krause, M., Bear, J.E., Loureiro, J.J., Gertler, F.B. (2002). The Ena/VASP enigma. J. Cell Sci. 115: 4721-4726.

LaBlanche, J-M., Grollier, G., Lusson, J.R., Bassand, J-P., Drobinski, G., Bertrand, B., Battaglia, S., Desveaux, B., Juillie`re, Y., Juliard, J-M., Metzger, J-P., Coste, P., Quiret, J-C., Dubois-Rande´, J-L., Crochet, P.D., Letac, B., Boschat, J., Virot, P., Finet, G., Le Breton, H., Livarek, B., Leclercq, F., Be´ard, T., Giraud, T., McFadden, E.P., Bertrand, M.E. (1997). Effect of the direct nitric oxide donors linsidomine and molsidomine on angiographic restenosis after coronary balloon angioplasty. The ACCORD Study. Angioplastic Coronaire Corvasal Diltiazem. Circulation 95: 83-89, 1997.

Lang, M., Kojonazarov, B., Tian, X., Kalymbetov, A., Weissmann, N., Grimminger, F., Kretschmer, A., Stasch, J.P., Seeger, W., Ghofrani, H.A., Schermuly, R.T. (2012). The soluble guanylate cyclase stimulator Riociguat ameliorates pulmonary hypertension induced by hypoxia and SU5416 in rats. PLoS ONE 7: e43433, doi:10.1371/journal.pone.0043433.

Lapp, H., Mitrovic, V., Franz, N., Heuer, H., Buerke, M., Wolfertz, J., Mueck, W., Unger, S., Wensing, G., Frey, R. (2009). Cinaciguat (BAY 58-2667) improves cardiopulmonary hemodynamics in patients with acute decompensated heart failure. Circulation 119: 2781-2788.

Lasker, G.F., Maley, J.H., Pankey, E.A., Kadowitz, P.J. (2011). Targeting soluble guanylate cyclase for the treatment of pulmonary hypertension. Expert Rev. Respir. Med. 5: 153-161.

Lee, Y.C., Martin, F., Murad, F. (2000). Human recombinant soluble guanylyl cyclase: expression, purification, and regulation. Proc. Natl. Acad. Sci. USA 97: 10763-10768.

Li, J., Li, P., Zhang, Y., Li, G.B., Zhou, Y.G., Yang, K., Dai, S.S. (2013). c-Ski inhibits the proliferation of vascular smooth muscle cells via suppressing Smad3 signaling but stimulating p38 pathway. Cell Signal. 25: 159-167.

Liu, X.M., Peyton, K.J., Mendelev, N.N., Wang, H., Tulis, D.A., Durante, W. (2009). YC-1 stimulates the expression of gaseous monoxide-generating enzymes in vascular smooth muscle cells. Mol. Pharmacol. 75: 1-10.

Lucas, K.A., Pitari, G.M., Kazerounian, S., Ruiz-Stewart, I., Park, J., Schulz, S., Chepenik, K.P., Waldman, S.A. (2000). Guanylyl cyclases and signaling by cyclic GMP. Pharmacol. Rev., 52, 375-413.

Mao, X., Debenedittis, P., Sun, Y., Chen, J., Yuan, K., Jiao, K., Chen, Y. (2012). Vascular smooth muscle cell Smad4 gene is important for mouse vascular development. Arterioscler. Thromb. Vasc. Biol. 32: 2171-2177.

Marx, S.O., Totary-Jain, H., Marks, A.R. (2011). Vascular smooth muscle cell proliferation in restenosis. Circ. Cardiovasc. Interv. 4: 104-111.

Maurice, D.H., Palmer, D., Tilley, D.G., Dunkerley, H.A., Netherton, S.J., Raymond, D.R., Elbatarny, H.S., Jimmo, S.L. (2003). Cyclic nucleotide phosphodiesterase activity, expression, and targeting in cells of the cardiovascular system. Mol. Pharmacol. 64: 533-546.

Mendelev, N.N., Williams, V.S., Tulis, D.A. (2009). Anti-growth properties of BAY 41-2272 in vascular smooth muscle cells. J. Cardiovasc. Pharmacol., 53, 121-131.

Mergia, E., Friebe, A., Dangel, O., Russwurm, M., Koesling, D. (2006). Spare guanylyl cyclase NO receptors ensure high NO sensitivity in the vascular system. J. Clin. Invest. 116: 1731-1737.

Mitrovic, V., Jovanovic, A., Lehinant, S. (2011). Soluble guanylate cyclase modulators in heart failure. Curr. Heart Fail. Rep. 8: 38-44.

Mittendorf, J., Weigand, S., Alonso-Alija, C., Bischoff, E., Feurer, A., Gerisch, M., Kern, A., Knorr, A., Lang, D., Muenter, K., Radtke, M., Schirok, H., Schlemmer, K.H., Stahl, E., Straub, A., Wunder, F., Stasch, J.P. (2009). Discovery of riociguat (BAY 63-2521): a potent, oral stimulator of soluble guanylate cyclase for the treatment of pulmonary hypertension. Chem. Med. Chem. 4: 853-865.

Motterlini, R., Sawle, P., Hammad, J., Bains, S., Alberto, R., Foresti, R., Green, C.J. (2005). CORM-A1: a new pharmacologically active carbon monoxide-releasing molecule. FASEB J. 19: 284-286.

Mullershausen, F., Russwurm, M., Friebe, A., Koesling, D. (2004). Inhibition of phosphodiesterase type 5 by the activator of nitric oxide-sensitive guanylyl cyclase BAY 41-2272. Circulation 109: 1711-1713.

Munzel, T., Daiber, A., Mulsch, A. (2005). Explaining the phenomenon on nitrate tolerance. Circ. Res. 97: 618-28.

Nimmegeers, S., Sips, P., Buys, E., Brouckaert, P., Van de Voorde, J. (2007). Functional role of the soluble guanylyl cyclase $\alpha 1$ subunit in vascular smooth muscle relaxation. Cardiovasc. Res. 76: 149-159.

Nossaman, B., Pankey, E., Kadowitz, P. (2012). Stimulators and activators of soluble guanylate cyclase: review and potential therapeutic indications. Crit. Care Res. Practice, Article ID 290805, 12 pages, doi:10.1155/2012/290805.

Pankey, E.A., Bhartiya, M., Badejo, Jr., A.M., Haider, U., Stasch, J.P., Murthy, S.N., Nossaman, B.D., Kadowitz, P.J. (2011). Pulmonary and systemic vasodilator responses to the soluble guanylyl cyclase activator, BAY 60-2770, are not dependent on endogenous nitric oxide or reduced heme. Am. J. Physiol. Heart Circ. Physiol. 300: H792-H802.

Parker, J.D. (2004). Nitrate tolerance, oxidative stress, and mitochondrial function: another worrisome chapter on the effects of organic nitrates. J. Clin. Invest. 113: 352-54.

Pelligrino, D.A., Wang, Q. (1998). Cyclic nucleotide crosstalk and the regulation of cerebral vasodilation. Prog. Neurobiol., 56, 1-18.

Peyton, K.J., Ensenat, D., Azam, M.A., Keswani, A.N., Sankaranaryanan, K., Liu, X.M., Wang, H., Tulis, D.A., Durante, W. (2009). Arginase promotes neointima formation in rat injured carotid arteries. Arterioscler. Thromb. Vasc. Biol. 29: 488-494.

Peyton, K.J., Shebib, A.R., Azam, M.A., Liu, X-M., Tulis, D.A., Durante, W. (2012). Bilirubin inhibits neointima formation and vascular smooth muscle cell proliferation and migration. Front. Pharmacol. 3:48, doi:10.3389/fphar. 2012.00048.

Poulos, T.L. (2006). Soluble guanylate cyclase. Curr. Opin. Struct. Biol. 16: 736-743.

Priviero, F.B.M., Webb, R.C. (2010). Heme-dependent and independent soluble guanylate cyclase activators and stimulators. J. Cardiovasc. Pharmacol. 56: 229-233.

Raghavan, S.A.V., Dikshit, M. (2004). Vascular regulation by the L-arginine metabolites, nitric oxide and agmatine. Pharmacol. Res. 49: 397-414.

Reinhard, M., Jarchau, T., Walter, U. (2001). Actin-based motility: stop and go with Ena/VASP proteins. Trends Biochem. Sci. 26: 243-249.

Remo, B.F., Giovannone, S., Fishman, G.I. (2012). Connexin43 cardiac gap junction remodeling: lessons from genetically engineered murine models. J. Membr. Biol. 245: 275-281.

Rubin, L.J., Magliola, L., Feng, X., Jones, A.W., Hale, C.C. (2005). Metabolic activation of AMP kinase in vascular smooth muscle. J. Appl. Physiol. 98: 296-306.

Rudner, X.L., Mandal, K.K., De Sauvage, F.J., Kindman, L.A., Almenoff, J.S. (1995). *Regulation of cell signaling by the cytoplasmic domains of the heat-stable enterotoxin receptor: identification of autoinhibitory and activating motifs. Proc. Natl. Acad. Sci. USA 92: 5169-5173.*

Ruiz-Ortega, M., Rodriguez-Vita, J., Sanchez-Lopez, E., Carvajal, G., Egido, J. (2007). *TGF-β signaling in vascular fibrosis. Cardiovasc. Res. 74: 196-206.*

Rukoyatkina, N., Walter, U., Friebe, A., Gambaryan, S. (2011). *Differentiation of cGMP-dependent and –independent nitric oxide effects on platelet apoptosis and reactive oxygen species production using platelets lacking soluble guanylyl cyclase. Thromb. Haemost. 106: 922-933.*

Russwurm, M., Behrends, S., Harteneck, C., Koesling, D. (1998). *Functional properties of a naturally occurring isoform of soluble guanylyl cyclase. Biochem. J. 335: 125-130.*

Russwurm, M., Mergia, E., Mullershausen, F., Koesling, D. (2002). *Inhibition of deactivation of NO-sensitive guanylyl cyclase accounts for the sensitizing effect of YC-1. J. Biol. Chem. 277: 24883-24888.*

Russwurm, M., Wittau, N., Koesling, D. (2001). *Guanylyl cyclase/PSD-95 interaction: targeting of the nitric oxide-sensitive alpha2beta1 guanylyl cyclase to synaptic membranes. J. Biol. Chem. 276: 44647-52.*

Sawle, P., Foresti, R., Mann, B.E., Johnson, T.R., Green, C.J., Motterlini, R. (2005). *Carbon monoxide-releasing molecules (CO-RMs) attenuate the inflammatory response elicited by lipopolysaccharide in RAW264.7 murine macrophages. Br. J. Pharmacol. 1-11.*

Schroder-Lang, S., Schwarzel, M., Seifert, R., Strunker, T., Kateriya, S., Looser, J., Watanabe, M., Kaupp, U.B., Hegemann, P., Nagel, G. (2007). *Fast manipulation of cellular cAMP level by light in vivo. Nat. Methods, 4, 39-42.*

Seitz, S., Wegener, J.W., Rupp, J., Watanabe, M., Jost, A., Gerhard, R., Shainberg, A., Ochi, R., Nawrath, H. (1999). *Involvement of K^+ channels in the relaxant effects of YC-1 in vascular smooth muscle. Eur. J. Pharmacol. 382:11–18.*

Serezani, C.H., Ballinger, M.N., Aronoff, D.M., Peters-Golden, M. (2008). *Cyclic AMP: Master regulator of innate immune cell function. Am. J. Respir. Cell Mol. Biol. 39: 127-132.*

Sharma, V.S., Magde, D. (1999). *Activation of soluble guanylate cyclase by carbon monoxide and nitric oxide: a mechanistic model. Methods 19: 494-505.*

Sips, P.Y., Buys, E.S. (2013). *Genetic modification of hypertension by sGCα1. Trends Cardiovasc. Med. 23:312-318,doi: 10.1016/j.tcm.2013.05.001.*

Spyridopoulos, I., Andres, V. (1998). *Control of vascular smooth muscle and endothelial cell proliferation and its implication in cardiovascular disease. Front. Biosci. 3:d269-287.*

Stasch, J.P., Becker, E.M., Alonso-Alija, C., Apeler, H., Dembowsky, K., Feurer, A., Gerzer,, R., Minuth, T., Perzborn, E., Pleib, U., Schroder, H., Schroeder, W., Stahl, E., Steinke, W., Straub, A., Schramm, M. (2001). *NO-independent regulatory site on soluble guanylate cyclase. Nature 410: 212-215.*

Stone, J.D., Narine, A., Tulis, D.A. (2012). *Inhibition of vascular smooth muscle growth via signaling crosstalk between AMP-activated protein kinase and cAMP-dependent protein kinase. Front. Physiol., 3, 409. doi: 10.3389/fphys.2012. 00409.*

Stone, J.D., Narine, A., Shaver, P.R., Fox, J.C., Vuncannon, J.R., Tulis, D.A. (2013). *AMP-activated protein kinase inhibits vascular smooth muscle cell proliferation and migration and vascular remodeling following injury. Am. J. Physiol. Heart Circ. Physiol. 304: H369-H381.*

Stone, J.R., Marletta, M.A. (1998). *Synergistic activation of soluble guanylate cyclase by YC-1 and carbon monoxide: implications for the role of cleavage of the iron-histidine bond during activation by nitric oxide. Chem. Biol. 5: 255-61.*

Straub, A., Stasch, J.P., Alonso-Alija, C., Benet-Buckholz, J., Ducke, B., Feurer, A., Furstner, C. (2001). *NO-independent stimulators of soluble guanylate cyclase. Bioorg. Med. Chem. Lett. 11: 781-784.*

Straub, A., Benet-Buckholz, J., Frode, R., Kern, A., Kohlsdorfer, C., Schmitt, P., Schwarz, T., Siefert, H.M., Stasch, J.P. (2002). Metabolites of orally active NO-independent pyrazolopyridine stimulators of soluble guanylate cyclase, Bioorg. Med. Chem. 10: 1711-1717.

Suwanabol, P.A., Seedial, S.M., Shi, X., Zhang, F., Yamanouchi D., Roenneburg, D., Liu, B., Kent, K.C. (2012a). TGF-β increases vascular smooth muscle cell proliferation through the Smad3 and ERK MAPK pathways. J. Vasc. Surg. 56: 446-454.

Suwanabol, P.A., Seedial, S.M., Zhang, F., Shi, X., Si, Y., Liu, B., Kent, K.C. (2012b). TGF-β and Smad3 modulate PI3K/Akt signaling pathway in vascular smooth muscle cells. Am. J. Physiol. Heart Circ. Physiol. 302: J2211-H2219.

Tang, Y., Yang, X., Friesel, R.E., Vary, C.P.H., Liaw, L. (2011). Mechanisms of TGF-β-induced differentiation in human vascular smooth muscle cells. J. Vasc. Res. 48: 485-494.

Thomson, D.M., Ascione, M.P., Grange, J., Nelson, C., Hansen, M.D. (2011). Phosphorylation of VASP by AMPK alters actin binding and occurs at a novel site. Biochem. Biophys. Res. Commun. 414: 215-219.

Tsai, E.J., Kass, D.A. (2009). Cyclic GMP signaling in cardiovascular pathophysiology and therapeutics. Pharmacol. Ther. 122: 216-238.

Tsai, S., Hollenbeck, S.T., Ryer, E.J., Edlin, R., Yamanouchi, D., Kundi, R., Wang, C., Liu, B., Kent, K.C. (2009). TGF-beta through Smad3 signaling stimulates vascular smooth muscle cell proliferation and neointimal formation. Am. J. Physiol. Heart Circ. Physiol. 297: H540-H549.

Tulis, D.A. (2004). Salutary properties of YC-1 in the cardiovascular and hematological systems. Curr. Med. Chem. 2: 343-359.

Tulis, D.A. (2008). Novel therapies for cyclic GMP control of vascular smooth muscle growth. American J. Therapeutics 15: 551-564.

Tulis, D.A., Bohl Masters, K.S., Lipke, E.A., Schiesser, R.L., Evans, A.J., Peyton, K.J., Durante, W., West, J.L., Schafer, A.I. (2002). YC-1-mediated vascular protection through inhibition of smooth muscle cell proliferation and platelet function. Biochem. Biophys. Res. Comm. 291: 1014-1021.

Tulis, D.A., Durante, W., Peyton, K.J., Chapman, G.B., Evans, A.J., Schafer, A.I. (2000). YC-1, a benzyl indazole derivative, stimulates vascular cGMP and inhibits neointima formation. Biochem. Biophys. Res. Comm. 279: 646-652.

Tulis, D.A., Keswani, A.N., Peyton, K.J., Wang, H., Schafer, A.I., Durante, W. (2005). Local administration of carbon monoxide inhibits neointima formation in balloon injured rat carotid arteries. Cell Mol. Biol. 51: 441-446.

Vulcu, S.D., Wegener, J.W., Nawrath, H. (2000). Differences in the nitric oxide/soluble guanylyl cyclase signalling pathway in the myocardium of neonatal and adult rats. Eur. J. Pharmacol. 406:247–255.

Waldman, S.A., Murad, F. (1987). Cyclic GMP synthesis and function. Pharmacol. Rev. 39: 163-196.

Wang, W., Huang, X.R., Canlas, E., Oka, K., Truong, L.D., Deng, C., Bhowmick, N.A., Ju, W., Bottinger, E.P., Lan, H.Y. (2006). Essential role of Smad3 in Angiotensin II-induced vascular fibrosis. Circ. Res. 98: 1032-1039.

Wedel, B., Harteneck, C., Foerster, J., Friebe, A., Schultz, G., Koesling, D. (1995). Functional domains of soluble guanylyl cyclase. J. Biol. Chem. 270: 24871-24875.

Wedel, B., Humbert, P., Harteneck, C., Foerster, J., Malkewitz, J., Bohme, E., Schultz, G., Koesling, D. (1994). Mutation of His-105 in the beta 1 subunit yields a nitric oxide-insensitive form of soluble guanylyl cyclase. Proc. Natl. Acad. Sci. USA 91: 2592-96.

Wegener, J.W., Gath, I., Forstermann, U., Nawrath, H. (1997). Activation of soluble guanylyl cyclase by YC-1 in aortic smooth muscle but not in ventricular myocardium from rat. Br. J. Pharmacol. 122: 1523-1529.

World Health Organization; World Heart Federation; World Stroke Organization. (2011). Global atlas on cardiovascular disease prevention and control: Policies, strategies and interventions. ISBN: 978 92 4 156437 3.

Worner R, Lukowski R, Hofmann F, Wegener JW. (2007). cGMP signals mainly through cAMP kinase in permeabilized murine aorta. Am. J. Physiol. Heart Circ. Physiol., 292, H237-H244.

Wrighton, K.H., Feng, X.-H. (2008). To (TGF)β or not to (TGF)β: Fine tuning of Smad signaling via post-translational modifications. Cell Signal. 20: 1579-1591.

Wu, C.C., Ko, F.N., Kuo, S.C., Lee, F.Y., Teng, C.M. (1995). YC-1 inhibited human platelet aggregation through NO-independent activation of soluble guanylate cyclase. Br. J. Pharmacol. 116: 1973-1978.

Xiang, Y.K. (2011). Compartmentalization of beta-adrenergic signals in cardiomyocytes. Circ. Res. 109: 231-244.

Yan, X., Chen, Y-G. (2011). Smad7: not only a regulator, but also a cross-talk mediator of TGF-β signaling. Biochem. J. 434: 1-10.

Yau, K.W. (1994). Cyclic nucleotide gated ion channels: an expanding new family of ion channels. Proc. Natl. Acad. Sci. USA 91: 3481-3483.

Zabel, U., Kleinshnitz, C., Oh, P., Nedvestky, P., Smolenski, A., Muller, H., Kronich, P., Kugler, P., Walter, U., Schnitzer, J.E., Schmidt, H.H. (2002). Calcium-dependent membrane association sensitizes soluble guanylyl cyclase to nitric oxide. Nat. Cell Biol. 4: 307-11.

Zhang, G., Xiang, B., Dong, A., Skoda, R.C., Daugherty, A., Smyth, S.S., Du, X., Li, X. (2011). Biphasic roles for soluble guanylyl cyclase (sGC) in platelet activation. Blood 118: 3670-3679.

Zhao, H., Guan, Q., Smith, C.J., Quilley, J. (2008). Increased phosphodiesterase 3A/4B expression after angioplasty and the effect of VASP phosphorylation. Eur. J. Pharmacol. 590: 29-35.

Zhou, Z., Gross, S., Roussos, C., Meurer, S., Muller-Ester, W., Papapetropoulos, A. (2004). Structural and functional characterization of the dimerization region of soluble guanylyl cyclase. J. Biol. Chem. 279: 24935-24943.

Esophageal Injury Following Radiofrequency Ablation for Atrial Fibrillation

Jonathan Keshishian

Division of Digestive Diseases and Nutrition
University of South Florida Morsani College of Medicine, Tampa, Florida, USA

Yasser Saloum

Division of Digestive Diseases and Nutrition
University of South Florida Morsani College of Medicine, Tampa, Florida, USA

Patrick G. Brady

Division of Digestive Diseases and Nutrition
University of South Florida Morsani College of Medicine, Tampa, Florida, USA

1   Introduction

Atrial fibrillation is the most common clinically significant arrhythmia, with a prevalence of 3.8% in persons 60 years or older and 9.0% in persons over the age of 80, and is a major cause of stroke. Due to the rapidly growing elderly population, it has been projected that there would be a 2.5 fold increase in the prevalence of atrial fibrillation by 2050.(Go *et al.*, 2001) In an attempt to surgically correct the arrhythmia, the maze procedure was developed and described by Cox *et al* in 1991; this procedure involved creating incisions within the left atrium in order to interrupt the reentrant circuits responsible for atrial fibrillation.(Cox, 1991; Cox, Schuessler, Lappas, & Boineau, 1996) The subsequent development of percutaneous radiofrequency ablation (RFA) to create transmural lines of electrically inactive scar within the left atrium (LA) endocardially and the right atrium epicardially significantly shortened procedure time.(Raman, Seevanayagam, Storer, & Power, 2001)

The approach to RFA changed dramatically in 1998 with the discovery by Haïssaguerre *et al*(Haissaguerre *et al.*, 1998) demonstrating that the majority of ectopic atrial beats originate somewhere within one or more of the four pulmonary veins (PVs) along the course of muscular bands extending from the LA into the PVs. Following this, mapping and ablation of arrhythmogenic foci of both the PVs and the LA have been evaluated and have shown success rates of 60 to 90%.(Lin *et al.*, 2003; Marrouche *et al.*, 2002; Oral *et al.*, 2003; Pappone *et al.*, 2004; Pappone *et al.*, 2001) Although RFA has been effective in treating atrial fibrillation, esophageal injury is a known complication that can occur, and, in certain circumstances, cause fatal injury.

2   Anatomic Proximity of Esophagus to Pulmonary Veins

In order to establish a better understanding of the anatomic relationship between the esophagus and the posterior LA wall, Sanchez-Quintana *et al.*(Sanchez-Quintana *et al.*, 2005) found in 40% of cadaveric specimens there was less than 5 mm between the esophagus and LA endocardium. In addition to these findings, Tsao *et al*(Tsao *et al.*, 2005) described two variations of the esophageal course in relation to the PVs: Type 1, which is the most common, in which the esophagus passes along the left-sided PVs with the shortest distances being 10.1 ± 3.4 mm from the left superior PV and 2.8 ± 2.5 mm from the left inferior PV, and Type 2 in which the esophagus passes along the right-sided PVs with distances measuring 10.5 ± 5.7 mm from the right superior PV and 3.7 ± 3.4 mm from the right inferior PV. The wide variability in distance has been attributed to a thin discontinuous layer of fat pad between the adventitia of the esophagus and epicardium of the posterior LA. The thinnest layer of the fat pad has consistently been seen at the level of the inferior PVs, explaining the close proximity of the esophagus and the inferior PVs. Furthermore, anterior to the esophageal adventitia are the esophageal arteries and vagus nerve plexus, which can easily be injured with transmural ablation of the LA or PVs. Extensive RFA to the posterior PV or posterior LA could lead to damage of these structures and cause neurovascular compromise of the esophagus, which if left unchecked could cause esophageal necrosis and perforation.

3   Endoscopic Esophageal Injury Classification

Esophageal injury secondary to radiofrequency ablation was first described in 2001 following intraoperative ablation for atrial fibrillation. The patient presented 9 days following RFA with an elevated white count and odynophagia, and was found to have a transmural esophageal perforation of the anterior wall that proved to be fatal (Gillinov, Pettersson, & Rice, 2001). Doll *et al* (Doll *et al.*, 2003) later reported finding 4 (1%) out of 387 patients undergoing intraoperative RFA developed left atrial-esophageal fistulas, which were diagnosed secondary to neurologic defects from air emboli, massive hematemesis, or septic shock. Although all of these patients had unremarkable early postoperative courses, they began to develop signs of perforation 6 to 12 days following RFA.

Following these initial reports of esophageal injury with intraoperative RFA, the first report of atrial-esophageal fistula formation following percutaneous RFA were reported by Scanavacca and Pappone in 2004(Pappone *et al.*, 2004; Scanavacca, D'Avila, Parga, & Sosa, 2004) in which 3 patients presented with nonspecific signs and symptoms including persistent fever, dysphagia, odynophagia, sepsis, endocarditis, and neurologic ischemia. These patients presented to their physicians 10 days to 3 weeks following the ablation procedure, but esophageal injury was not initially considered in the differential diagnosis. Cummings *et al* (Cummings *et al.*, 2006) reported 9 fatal cases of atrial-esophageal fistula formation in a retrospective case series based on anonymous identification in 2006. These nine patients presented 10 to 16 days post-operatively with a similar constellation of symptoms reported previously; however, only 4 patients received the correct diagnosis before death. The remaining patients were diagnosed at autopsy. Due to the considerable delay in diagnosis, Dagres *et al* (Dagres *et al.*, 2006) attempted to identify criteria for rapid detection of esophageal perforation. They concluded that although the symptoms are generally non-specific, patients presented with two distinct symptoms, fever and severe chest or epigastric pain, which occurred 1 to 4 weeks following procedure.

Atrial-esophageal fistula formation appears to take at least 1 week to develop in most cases, which allows esophagogastroduodenoscopy (EGD) to be performed within 24 to 72 hours following the procedure with low likelihood of inducing air embolization. Due to the nature of RFA injury to the esophagus, only transmural lesions are visible on endoscopy. In an attempt to classify these lesions further, Keshishian *et al* developed an injury classification in 2012 to help risk stratify these patients.(Keshishian, Young, Hill, Saloum, & Brady, 2012) This divides esophageal thermal injury into three classes based on endoscopic appearance. These classes are illustrated in the figures below and summarized in Table 1.

3.1 Class I Thermal Injury

These patients have erythema or discoloration of the anterior esophageal wall with minimal mucosal disruption. These lesions should be shallow erosions without vessel involvement and should be less than 5 mm in diameter. These patients seem to have a low risk of progressing into frank perforation. They can be medically managed with proton-pump inhibitor (PPI) and sucralfate with clinical follow-up to assess for any worsening of symptoms.

3.2 Class II Thermal Injury

These patients have ulcers of the anterior esophageal wall with or without exudate. These lesions tend to penetrate further into the esophageal wall without extension into the muscularis externa. There should not be overlying clot or vessel involvement with these lesions. These patients appear to be at an intermediate risk for progression. In addition to medical management with PPI and sucralfate, these patients require close follow-up and repeat endoscopy to ensure lesion improvement.

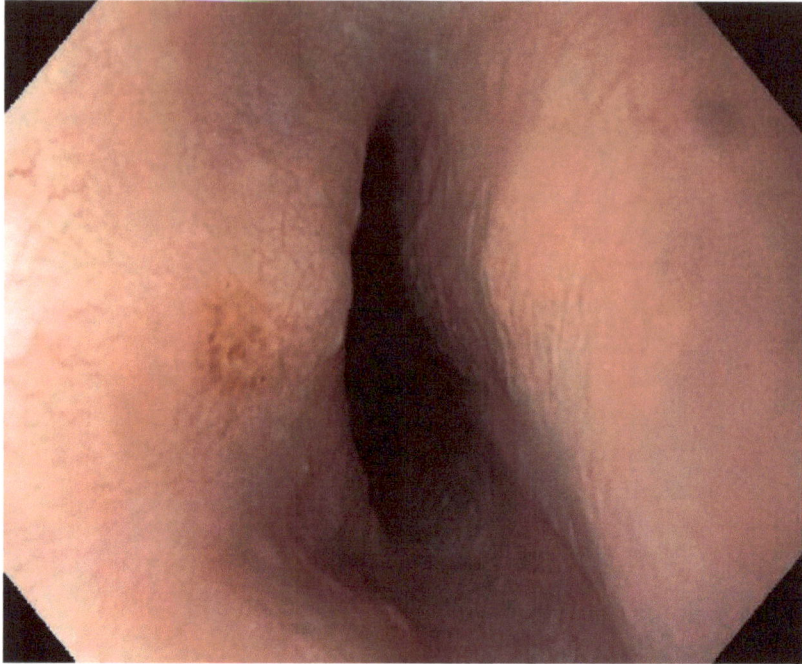

Figure 1: Class I thermal injury.

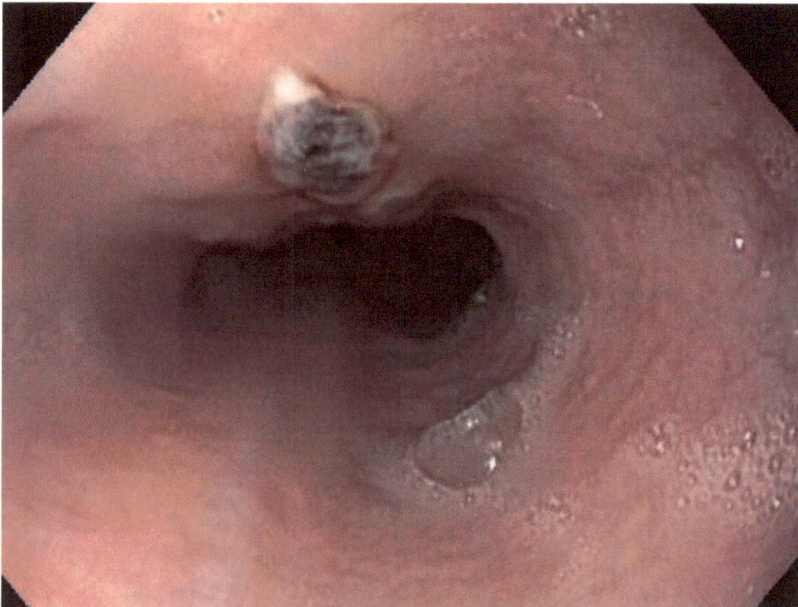

Figure 2: Class II thermal injury.

3.3   Class III Thermal Injury

These patients have deep ulceration that extends into and beyond the muscularis. These lesions can have evidence of eschar formation, overlying clot, or necrosis. As a result, there is an increased probability of compromising tissue blood flow and worsening the injury. These patients are at high risk of esophageal perforation and atrial-esophageal fistula formation. They should be made nil per os (NPO) and started on medical management. Cardiothoracic surgery consultation is warranted with CT of the chest. If findings do not require an emergent operation, then repeat imaging and endoscopy can be considered to reassess healing of ulcer.

This injury classification has not been tested in large prospective trials and thus it should only be viewed as a proposed means for risk assessment and follow-up pending further verification.

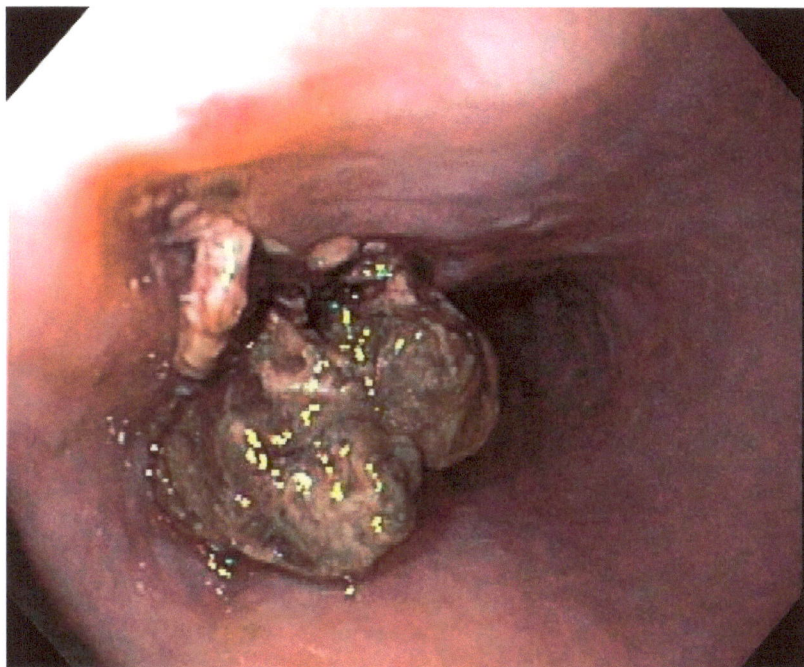

Figure 3: Class III thermal injury

Thermal Injury	Endoscopic Appearance	Treatment	Recommended Follow-up	Perforation Risk
Class I	Lesion less than 5 mm in diameter with minimal mucosal disruption	Oral PPI with sucralfate	Clinical follow-up to assess for worsening symptoms	Low
Class II	Ulcers that do not extend beyond the muscularis externa with no overlying clot or visible vessel.	PPI and sucralfate	Repeat endoscopy in 2 weeks	Intermediate
Class III	Deep ulceration extending into and beyond the muscularis with eschar formation, overlying clot, or necrosis.	NPO IV PPI Chest CT scan Cardiothoracic surgery consultation	Repeat imaging and endoscopy based on findings	High

Table 1: Esophageal Injury Classification

4   Endoscopic Injury Progression

Below we document serial images of a patient with Class II Thermal Injury with subsequent endoscopy performed 10 days (Figure 4) and 17 days (Figure 5) following diagnosis. No further endoscopy was performed after day 17. Initial endoscopy image was documented in Figure 2.

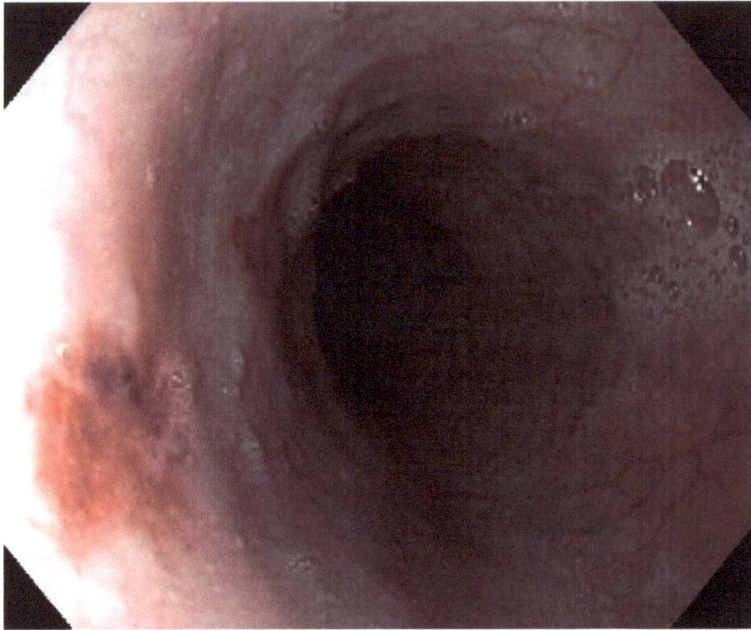

Figure 4: Class II thermal injury 10 days following RFA

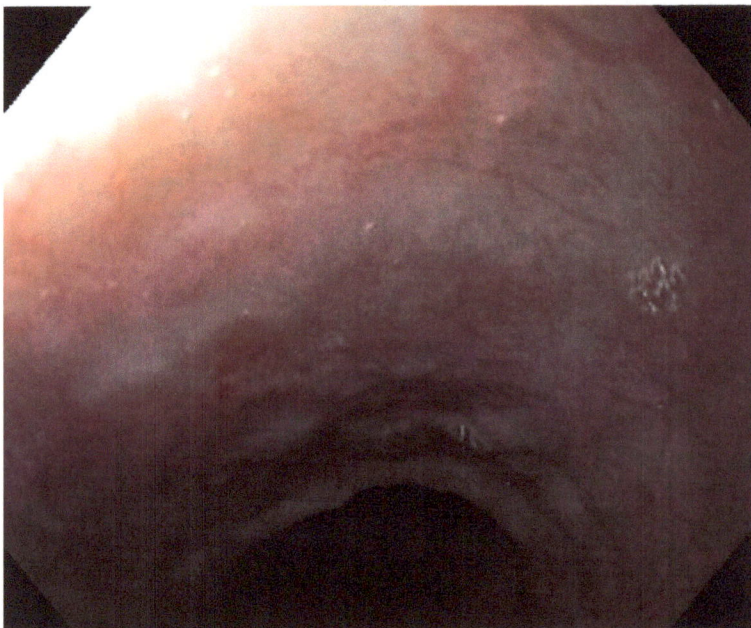

Figure 5: Class II thermal injury 17 days following RFA

5   Incidence of Esophageal Injury

Esophageal injury is a known complication of RFA of the PVs and LA for treatment of atrial fibrillation. The etiology of the injury is multifactorial. As stated by Gillinov *et al.* (Gillinov *et al.*, 2001) the goal of RFA is to achieve a series of transmural lesions in the LA, however, only the temperature and duration of energy delivered can be controlled. There is no means of controlling the lesion depth; thus it is possible to create a non-transmural lesion resulting in an unsuccessful operation, or a lesion that is too deep with consequent injury to adjacent structures. Additionally, it has been shown that intestinal tissue is far more susceptible to radiofrequency-induced thermal injury than muscle tissue, and that the convection of heat generated within the LA by the ablation probe can result in esophageal injury without direct contact of the probe to the esophagus.(Doll *et al.*, 2003)

In order to determine the incidence of esophageal injury following RFA, Schmidt *et al.* (Schmidt *et al.*, 2008) conducted the first observational study evaluating 28 patients following RFA for symptomatic and refractory atrial fibrillation. All patients underwent endoscopy within 24 hours following RFA. Esophageal wall changes were described as no change, erythema, necrosis, or atrio-esophageal fistula. If changes were seen, then patients were started on PPI and had repeat endoscopy 2 weeks later. They noted that within 24 hours of ablation 13 patients (47%) had esophageal changes with recovery seen in all patients after 2 weeks.

Following this, Halm *et al.* (Halm *et al.*, 2010) performed a prospective study with 185 consecutive patients who had received RFA for symptomatic atrial fibrillation. The esophagus was intubated with a temperature probe in order to obtain intraluminal temperature monitoring in three-dimensions. All patients had endoscopy performed 1-4 days following ablation. Localized ulcer-like lesions of the esophagus were found in 27 of 185 patients (14.6%). Of these, 15 patients (8%) had lesions larger than 5 mm. In all patients with lesions, the intraluminal temperature reached at least 41°C. Maximal intraluminal temperature was significantly higher in patients with esophageal damage than in those without esophageal lesions (42.6±1.7°C vs 41.4±1.7°C) with $P=0.003$. The study concluded that for every 1 °C increase in endoluminal temperature, the odds of an esophageal lesion increased by a factor of 1.36 (95% CI 1.07-1.74, $P=0.012$). No atrio-esophageal fistula or symptoms suggestive of this occurred during study.

6   Mediastinal and Submucosal Changes in Esophagus

A recent study by Zellerhoff *et al.* (Zellerhoff *et al.*, 2010) demonstrated that mucosal injury of the esophagus was only the "tip of the iceberg" in terms of the thermal injury dealt to the surrounding region following RFA. This study evaluated 29 patients with both EGD as well as endosonography before and after RFA in order to detect both esophageal mucosal injury as well as injury to the esophageal submucosa and mediastinum. The study showed that 8 patients (27%) demonstrated new disruption of the regular esophageal wall layer pattern with edema and periesophageal accumulation of fluid, swelling of the posterior wall of the LA beyond site of ablation, and mediastinal adenopathy. All patients had resolution of these findings one week after RFA. Interestingly, none of these patients had mucosal injury in the form of ulcers or erythema on EGD, nor was there the development of any atrioesophageal fistulas. This study implies that the absence of esophageal lesions seen on EGD does not indicate that indirect thermal injury has not occurred to surrounding structures within the mediastinum.

7   Prevention of Esophageal Injury: Temperature Monitoring

The most commonly implemented strategy utilized to minimize esophageal injury is to limit the magnitude of power and duration the catheter is in contact with the PV or posterior wall of LA. As mentioned earlier, there is a wide variability in the distance between the adventitia of the esophagus and the epicardium of the posterior LA. For this reason, additional measures other than simply lower the magnitude of power is required because esophageal injury may still occur despite keeping the power lower in a patient whose esophagus is in close proximity to the LA. Real-time luminal esophageal temperature (LET) monitoring has been developed in order to monitor esophageal luminal temperatures. A prospective study conducted by Rillig *et al.* (Rillig *et al.*, 2010) demonstrated that LET monitoring led to a reduction in esophageal injury. LET does confer three limitations however: (1) The accuracy of LET is dependent on adequate contact between the probe and esophageal wall during RFA; (2) Suboptimal orientation and positioning of the LET probe may show only a slow rise in temperature, allowing esophageal injury to occur at while showing acceptable temperatures; (3) the LET probe may fix the esophagus in a position where it may enhance contact to the LA posterior wall (Liu *et al.*, 2012). Esophageal injury has been reported in patients following RFA in combination with LET in 6% to 26% of cases (Liu *et al.*, 2012; Rillig *et al.*, 2010; Singh *et al.*, 2008) (Table 2).

Study	Study type	No. of patients	Incidence	Lesions	Injury assessment tool	Recovery
Schmidt et al(Schmidt et al., 2008)	Observational	28	47% (24 hours)	Not reported	Endoscopy alone	100% (2 weeks)
Halm et al(Halm et al., 2010)	Prospective	185	14.6% (1-4 days)	Ulcer-like	LET 41°C	Not reported
Zellerhoff et al(Zellerhoff et al., 2010)	Before and after study	29	0% (mucosal) 27% (mural and mediastinal injury)	No mucosal lesions	EGD (mucosal) EUS (mural/mediastinal)	100% (1 week)
Rillig et al(Rillig et al., 2010)	Prospective	42	14.3% (24 hours)	Mucosal lesions	LET EGD	100% (2 weeks)
Sing et al[24]	Prospective	81	11% (1-3 days)	Ulcers	LET EGD	100% (1 week)
Berjano et al(Berjano & Hornero, 2005)	Case control	8	0%	None	LET IECB	Not reported

LET – luminal esophageal temperature
EGD – esophagogastroduodenoscopy
EUS – Endoscopic ultrasound
IECB – Intraesophageal cooling balloon

Table 2: Incidence of Esophageal Injury with RFA

8 Prevention of Esophageal Injury: Esophageal Cooling Technique

Berjano *et al.* (Berjano & Hornero, 2005) reported the feasibility of a cooled intraesophageal balloon reducing esophageal injury using a three-dimensional finite element model computer simulation. Their simulation demonstrated that chilling the esophagus minimizes the lesion in the esophageal wall compared to cases in which no balloon, or a non-cooled balloon was used. Following this, a pilot study was conducted on eight patients who underwent RFA for refractory atrial fibrillation using a 9-Fr esophageal balloon in combination with LET. These study patients were compared to controls that only had LET. In the control, the LET increased from 36.4 ± 0.8 °C to 40.5 ± 1.7 °C within 26.1 ± 8.2 seconds, whereas the patients who received the esophageal cooling balloon went from a lower baseline of 30.2 ± 2.9 °C to 33.5 ± 2.9 °C within 30 seconds. No study patients were found to have esophageal injury throughout the follow-up period; thus, the authors concluded that the placement of an intraesophageal cooling balloon may help to minimize esophageal injury.

9 Prevention of Esophageal Injury: Cryoablation

RFA with temperatures exceeding 40°C has been implicated with esophageal injury; for this reason, it was believed that cryoablation may be a less damaging means of ablating patients with atrial fibrillation. Ahmed *et al.* (Ahmed *et al.*, 2009) performed 67 cryoablations on patients with atrial fibrillation with concurrent LET. There were significant LET decreases noted in 62 of 67 patients, which was defined as greater than 1 °C. LET continued to decrease after termination of cryoablation, and was more pronounced in the inferior than in the superior pulmonary veins with the lowest observed temperature of 0°C. Post-cryoablation endoscopy revealed esophageal ulceration in 17% of patients, all of which healed on subsequent endoscopy. There were no patients who developed atrio-esophageal fistulas; however, the presence of esophageal ulceration in a significant percentage of these patients treated with cryoablation indicates that the potential for esophageal perforation exists. More data on esophageal injury with cryoablation is needed before it can be recommended as a safer alternative to radiofrequency ablation.

10 Conclusion

Esophageal injury following ablation for atrial fibrillation is relatively frequent, although perforation of the esophagus is uncommon. Mucosal injury and esophageal perforation as a result of ablation therapy for atrial fibrillation are important complications to be aware of. It appears that the primary risk factor for post-ablation esophageal injury is close proximity of the esophageal wall to the posterior wall of the LA and inferior pulmonary veins. Esophageal thermal injury has been noted to occur despite several interventions to monitor intraluminal temperature, decrease maximum threshold power, and use of cryotherapy. Esophageal cooling technique has proven, on a small scale, to be an effective means of preventing esophageal injury from RFA, and if not available, early upper endoscopy should be considered even in asymptomatic patients based on high incidence of esophageal injury of up to 47%. Patients who develop symptoms of odynophagia, dysphagia, heartburn, or substernal chest pain following ablation therapy should be evaluated with EGD and those with mucosal injury require close monitoring and follow up as detailed in the algorithm in Figure 6.

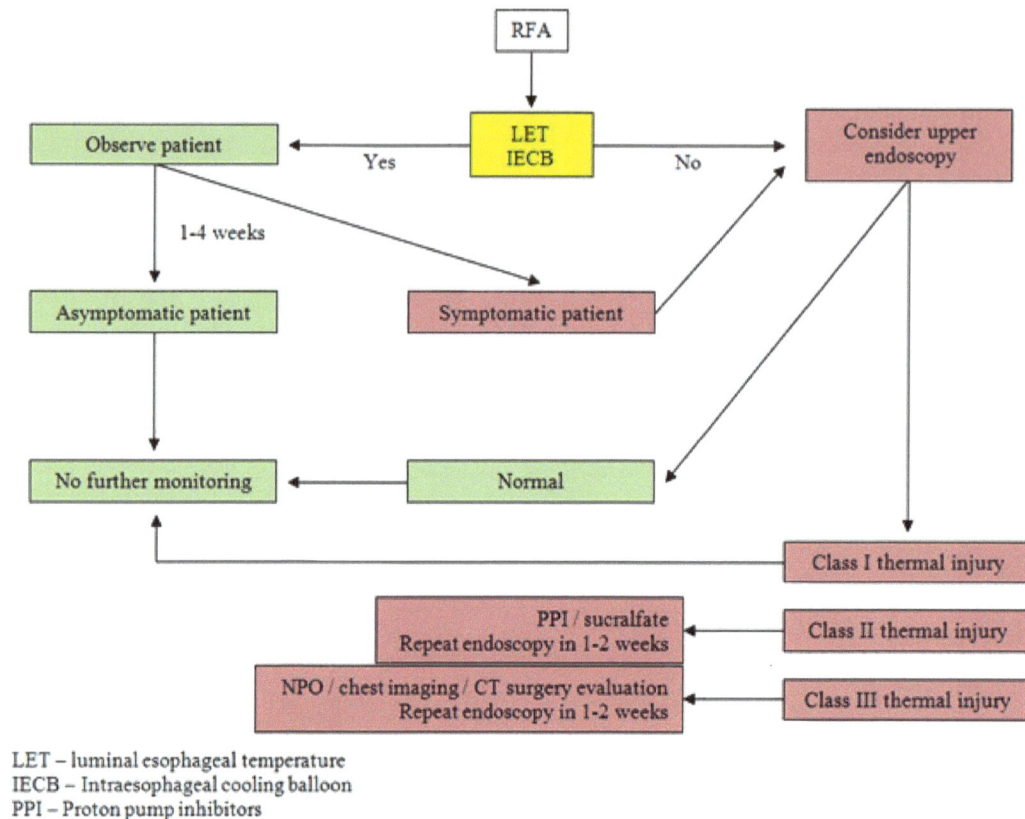

Figure 6: Diagnosis and proposed management of RFA-induced esophageal injury

References

Ahmed, H., Neuzil, P., d'Avila, A., Cha, Y. M., Laragy, M., Mares, K., . . . Reddy, V. Y. (2009). The esophageal effects of cryoenergy during cryoablation for atrial fibrillation. Heart Rhythm, 6(7), 962-969. doi: 10.1016/j.hrthm.2009.03.051.

Berjano, E. J., & Hornero, F. (2005). A cooled intraesophageal balloon to prevent thermal injury during endocardial surgical radiofrequency ablation of the left atrium: a finite element study. Phys Med Biol, 50(20), N269-279. doi: 10.1088/0031-9155/50/20/n03.

Cox, J. L. (1991). The surgical treatment of atrial fibrillation. IV. Surgical technique. J Thorac Cardiovasc Surg, 101(4), 584-592.

Cox, J. L., Schuessler, R. B., Lappas, D. G., & Boineau, J. P. (1996). An 8 1/2-year clinical experience with surgery for atrial fibrillation. Ann Surg, 224(3), 267-273; discussion 273-265.

Cummings, J. E., Schweikert, R. A., Saliba, W. I., Burkhardt, J. D., Kilikaslan, F., Saad, E., & Natale, A. (2006). Brief communication: atrial-esophageal fistulas after radiofrequency ablation. Ann Intern Med, 144(8), 572-574.

Dagres, N., Kottkamp, H., Piorkowski, C., Doll, N., Mohr, F., Horlitz, M., . . . Hindricks, G. (2006). Rapid detection and successful treatment of esophageal perforation after radiofrequency ablation of atrial fibrillation: lessons from five cases. J Cardiovasc Electrophysiol, 17(11), 1213-1215. doi: 10.1111/j.1540-8167.2006.00611.x

Doll, N., Borger, M. A., Fabricius, A., Stephan, S., Gummert, J., Mohr, F. W., . . . Hindricks, G. (2003). Esophageal perforation during left atrial radiofrequency ablation: Is the risk too high? J Thorac Cardiovasc Surg, 125(4), 836-842. doi: 10.1067/mtc.2003.165.

Gillinov, A. M., Pettersson, G., & Rice, T. W. (2001). Esophageal injury during radiofrequency ablation for atrial fibrillation. J Thorac Cardiovasc Surg, 122(6), 1239-1240. doi: 10.1067/mtc.2001.118041.

Go, A. S., Hylek, E. M., Phillips, K. A., Chang, Y., Henault, L. E., Selby, J. V., & Singer, D. E. (2001). Prevalence of diagnosed atrial fibrillation in adults: national implications for rhythm management and stroke prevention: the AnTicoagulation and Risk Factors in Atrial Fibrillation (ATRIA) Study. JAMA, 285(18), 2370-2375.

Haissaguerre, M., Jais, P., Shah, D. C., Takahashi, A., Hocini, M., Quiniou, G., . . . Clementy, J. (1998). Spontaneous initiation of atrial fibrillation by ectopic beats originating in the pulmonary veins. N Engl J Med, 339(10), 659-666.

Halm, U., Gaspar, T., Zachaus, M., Sack, S., Arya, A., Piorkowski, C., . . . Husser, D. (2010). Thermal esophageal lesions after radiofrequency catheter ablation of left atrial arrhythmias. Am J Gastroenterol, 105(3), 551-556. doi: 10.1038/ajg.2009.625.

Keshishian, J., Young, J., Hill, E., Saloum, Y., & Brady, P. G. (2012). Esophageal Injury Following Radiofrequency Ablation for Atrial Fibrillation: Injury Classification. Gastroenterol Hepatol (N Y), 8(6), 411-414.

Lin, W. S., Tai, C. T., Hsieh, M. H., Tsai, C. F., Lin, Y. K., Tsao, H. M., . . . Chen, S. A. (2003). Catheter ablation of paroxysmal atrial fibrillation initiated by non-pulmonary vein ectopy. Circulation, 107(25), 3176-3183. doi: 10.1161/01.cir.0000074206.52056.2d.

Liu, E., Shehata, M., Liu, T., Amorn, A., Cingolani, E., Kannarkat, V., . . . Wang, X. (2012). Prevention of esophageal thermal injury during radiofrequency ablation for atrial fibrillation. J Interv Card Electrophysiol, 35(1), 35-44. doi: 10.1007/s10840-011-9655-0.

Marrouche, N. F., Dresing, T., Cole, C., Bash, D., Saad, E., Balaban, K., . . . Natale, A. (2002). Circular mapping and ablation of the pulmonary vein for treatment of atrial fibrillation: impact of different catheter technologies. J Am Coll Cardiol, 40(3), 464-474. doi: S0735109702019721 [pii]

Oral, H., Scharf, C., Chugh, A., Hall, B., Cheung, P., Good, E., . . . Morady, F. (2003). Catheter ablation for paroxysmal atrial fibrillation: segmental pulmonary vein ostial ablation versus left atrial ablation. Circulation, 108(19), 2355-2360. doi: 10.1161/01.cir.0000095796.45180.88.

Pappone, C., Manguso, F., Vicedomini, G., Gugliotta, F., Santinelli, O., Ferro, A., . . . Santinelli, V. (2004). Prevention of iatrogenic atrial tachycardia after ablation of atrial fibrillation: a prospective randomized study comparing circumferential pulmonary vein ablation with a modified approach. Circulation, 110(19), 3036-3042. doi: 10.1161/01.cir.0000147186.83715.95.

Pappone, C., Oreto, G., Rosanio, S., Vicedomini, G., Tocchi, M., Gugliotta, F., . . . Alfieri, O. (2001). Atrial electroanatomic remodeling after circumferential radiofrequency pulmonary vein ablation: efficacy of an anatomic approach in a large cohort of patients with atrial fibrillation. Circulation, 104(21), 2539-2544.

Raman, J. S., Seevanayagam, S., Storer, M., & Power, J. M. (2001). Combined endocardial and epicardial radiofrequency ablation of right and left atria in the treatment of atrial fibrillation. Ann Thorac Surg, 72(3), S1096-1099.

Rillig, A., Meyerfeldt, U., Birkemeyer, R., Wiest, S., Sauer, B. M., Staritz, M., & Jung, W. (2010). Oesophageal temperature monitoring and incidence of oesophageal lesions after pulmonary vein isolation using a remote robotic navigation system. Europace, 12(5), 655-661. doi: 10.1093/europace/euq061.

Sanchez-Quintana, D., Cabrera, J. A., Climent, V., Farre, J., Mendonca, M. C., & Ho, S. Y. (2005). Anatomic relations between the esophagus and left atrium and relevance for ablation of atrial fibrillation. Circulation, 112(10), 1400-1405. doi: 10.1161/circulationaha.105.551291.

Scanavacca, M. I., D'Avila, A., Parga, J., & Sosa, E. (2004). Left atrial-esophageal fistula following radiofrequency catheter ablation of atrial fibrillation. J Cardiovasc Electrophysiol, 15(8), 960-962. doi: 10.1046/j.1540-8167.2004.04083.x

Schmidt, M., Nolker, G., Marschang, H., Gutleben, K. J., Schibgilla, V., Rittger, H., . . . Marrouche, N. F. (2008). Incidence of oesophageal wall injury post-pulmonary vein antrum isolation for treatment of patients with atrial fibrillation. Europace, 10(2), 205-209. doi: 10.1093/europace/eun001.

Singh, S. M., d'Avila, A., Doshi, S. K., Brugge, W. R., Bedford, R. A., Mela, T., . . . Reddy, V. Y. (2008). Esophageal injury and temperature monitoring during atrial fibrillation ablation. Circ Arrhythm Electrophysiol, 1(3), 162-168. doi: 10.1161/circep.107.789552.

Tsao, H. M., Wu, M. H., Higa, S., Lee, K. T., Tai, C. T., Hsu, N. W., . . . Chen, S. A. (2005). Anatomic relationship of the esophagus and left atrium: implication for catheter ablation of atrial fibrillation. Chest, 128(4), 2581-2587. doi: 10.1378/chest.128.4.2581.

Zellerhoff, S., Ullerich, H., Lenze, F., Meister, T., Wasmer, K., Monnig, G., . . . Eckardt, L. (2010). Damage to the esophagus after atrial fibrillation ablation: Just the tip of the iceberg? High prevalence of mediastinal changes diagnosed by endosonography. Circ Arrhythm Electrophysiol, 3(2), 155-159. doi: 10.1161/circep.109.915918.

The Role of Autonomic Neural System in Atrial Fibrillation

Shaohua Zheng, Yong Zhang

Department of Cardiology
Shandong Provincial Qianfoshan Hospital, Shandong University, China

Jianying Sun

Department of Health Care
Shandong Provincial Qianfoshan Hospital, Shandong University, China

Yujiao Zhang

Department of Cardiology
Shandong Provincial Qianfoshan Hospital, Shandong University, China

Wenchang Duan

Department of Health Care
Shandong Provincial Qianfoshan Hospital, Shandong University, China

Yinglong Hou

Department of Cardiology
Shandong Provincial Qianfoshan Hospital, Shandong University, China

1   The Introduction of Cardiac Autonomic Nervous System

Autonomic innervation of the heart involves extrinsic and intrinsic cardiac ANS. The former includes the ganglias in the brain or along the spinal cord and their axons en route to the heart, while the latter consists of the autonomic ganglias and axons located on the heart itself or along the great vessels in the thorax (Scherlag & Po, 2006), and is affected by extrinsic ANS (Hou, Scherlag, Lin, Zhang, *et al.*, 2007) and composed of a neural network formed by axons and autonomic ganglia concentrated at the ganglionated plexi (GP) embedded within epicardial fat pads on the heart itself and the ligament of Marshall.

The detailed map of the ANS of human heart has been provided in the study performed by Armour (Armour *et al.*, 1997), which indicated that the autonomic nerves often gather at certain positions of the surface of atrium and pulmonary vein (PV) to form GP. Then axons extending from those GPs cross to form an ANS network. There are 4 chief GPs that participate in the neuroelectrical activity of the atria, which are the anterior right GP, inferior right GP, superior left GP and inferior left GP (Figure 1) (Nakagawa *et al.*, 2009; Scherlag, Nakagawa, *et al.*, 2005).

Both sympathetic and parasympathetic nerves could affect the electrophysiological activity of cardiac cells, such as action potential duration, effective refractory period (ERP) and conduction velocity, which play an important role in the initiation and maintenance of AF (Patterson *et al.*, 2005; Schauerte, *et al.*, 2001; Takahashi *et al.*, 2006; Zipes *et al.*, 1974). Sympathetic activation allows an increasing calcium entry and the spontaneous release of calcium from the sarcoplasmic reticulum (Bers, 2002; Ter Keurs & Boyden, 2007), which triggers ectopic excitement or form reentrant cycle. Parasympathetic stimulation could shorten action potential duration and atrial ERP, and increase dispersion of atrial ERP, which could cause hyperpolarization of cell and tend to form reentrant cycle (Coumel, 1994).

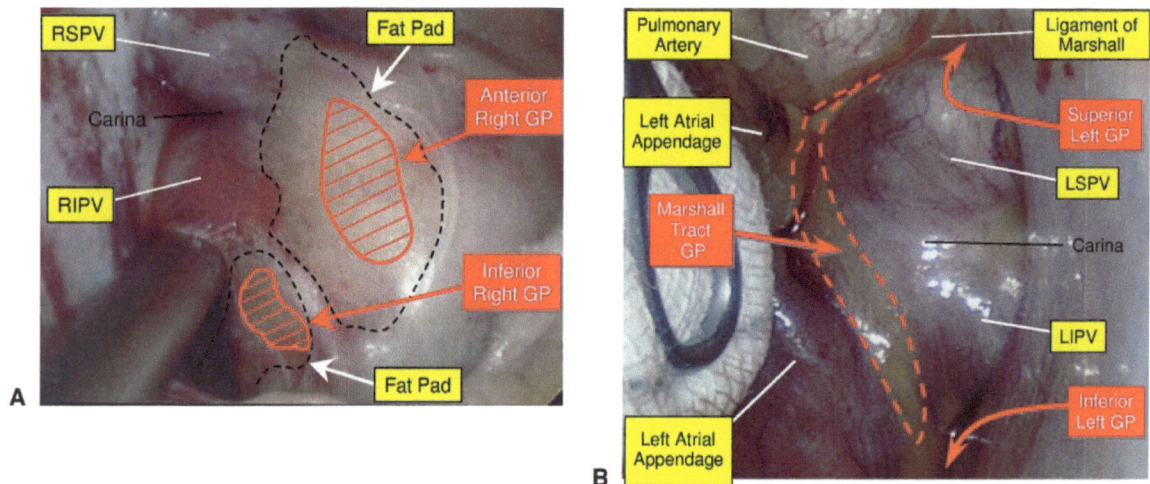

Figure 1: Locations of major left atrial autonomic GP in patients undergoing surgical ablation of AF. A: Thoracoscopic photograph in the right side of the chest during minimally invasive surgical ablation in a patient with persistent AF. An epicardial left atrial fat pad is located anterior to the right superior PV (RSPV) and another epicardial fat pad is located inferoposterior to the right inferior PV (RIPV). B: Thoracoscopic photograph in the left side of the chest in the same patient showing the left superior PV (LSPV), left inferior PV (LIPV) (Nakagawa, *et al.*, 2009).

2   The Imbalance and Remodeling of Autonomic Nervous System in Atrial Fibrillation

In the early ninety's of the last century, the relationship between ANS and AF had got a lot of attention. In 1994, Coumel (Coumel, 1994) referred that vagal AF (vagal drive as the determinant factor of AF episodes) was more common in young people with non-structural heart disease. In contrast, the sympathetic (sympathetic drive as the determinant factor of AF episodes) AF often occurred in patients with structural heart disease. Similar result was also got by Huang (Huang, *et al.*, 1998). In their research, AF could be divided into vagal type, sympathetic type and non-related type according to the heart rate variability of patients, and it was found that most of idiopathic paroxysmal AF was parasympathetic dependent, while organic paroxysmal AF was more sympathetic dependent (Figure 2). Coumel also found the vagal type AF often occurred at night, while the sympathetic type AF usually happened in daytime. This phenomenon was described as circadian variation of AF, and several clinical follow-up studies could also confirm the circadian variation (Deguchi *et al.*, 2009; Herweg *et al.*, 1998). With more in-depth study, the important role of ANS on AF began to emerge. Either the adrenergic or vagal arm of the ANS may be involved in atrial electrical instability. Vagal activation shortens atrial ERP and increases their dispersion, and adrenergic stimulation enhances atrial myocardial automaticity.

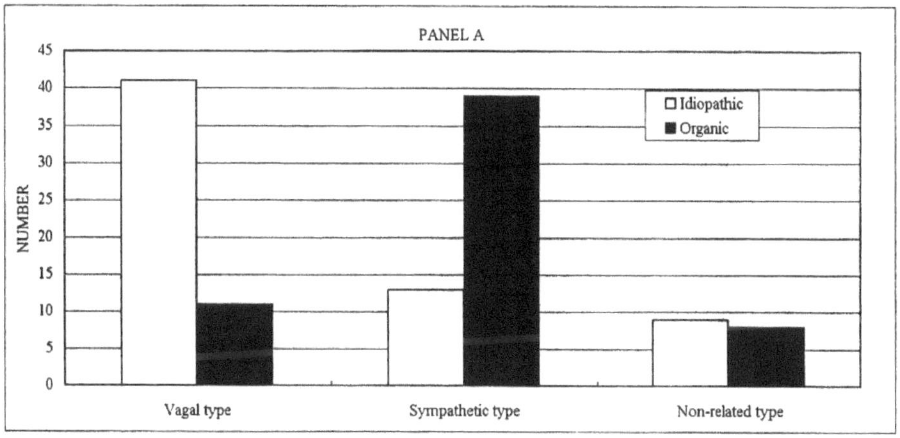

Figure 2: It shows that vagal type is predominant in idiopathic group and sympathetic type is predominant in organic group (Huang, et al., 1998).

2.1   The Role of Autonomic Nervous System Locating at Pulmonary Vein in the Occurrence of Atrial Fibrillation

Cardiac muscle of left atrium (LA) extends 1-2cm into PVs to form sleeves, which is considered to be the most common ectopic trigger of AF according to the previous research (Hocini *et al.*, 1999). Because of the special nerve distribution and electrophysiological characteristics different from LA, PVs have a stronger potential to initiate and perpetuate AF.

The nerve distribution at PVs was quite complicated. A quantitative study on the innervation of PVs in adult hearts was performed by Chevalier (Chevalier *et al.*, 2005). They found that the nerve density at the ostia of PVs was significantly higher than that in the distal part, and gradually decreasing gradients were found from left to right and from epicardium to endocardium. Similarly, according to another neurohistological study performed by Tan *et al.* (Tan *et al.*, 2006), it was found that longitudinally, the density of adrenergic and cholinergic nerve was highest in LA within 5 mm of the LA-PV junction than either the rest of LA or distal part of PV, and circumferentially, nerve density was higher in the anterosuperior segments of both superior veins and inferior segments of both inferior veins, and higher in epicardium than endocardium (Figure 3). However, there was no significant advantage of regional distribution of either sympathetic or parasympathetic nerve, because over 90% of ganglion cells expressed dual adrenocholinergic phenotypes at PVs. Consequently, the high density and heterogeneous distribution of autonomic nerves at PVs may provide an anatomic basis for the initiation and perpetuation of AF.

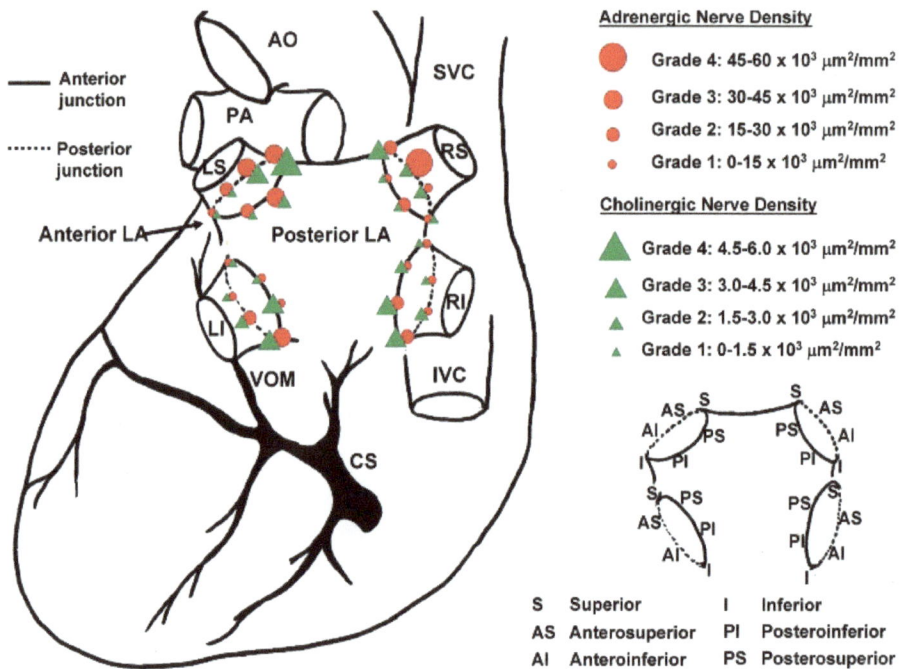

Figure 3: It shows circumferential distribution of autonomic nerves at the PV-LA junction. AO= aorta; CS= coronary sinus; IVC= inferior vena cava; LIPV= left inferior PV; LSPV= left superior PV; PA= pulmonary artery; RIPV= right inferior PV; RSPV= right superior PV; SVC= superior vena cava; VOM= vein of marshall (Tan, *et al.*, 2006).

The electrical characteristics between proximal and distal part of PV are different. Compared with the distal part of PV, the proximal part possesses longer ERP, which results it could inhibit the ectopic trigger originating from distal part and then decrease AF inducibility (Kumagai, 2007). However, this difference of ERP could be attenuated by isoprenaline, suggesting that isoprenaline could weaken the protective effect of proximal PV. This makes spontaneous ectopic activation from distal PV easier to conduct to proximal PV and the atrium, resulting formation of AF. Patterson (Patterson, *et al.*, 2005) recorded the action potential of PV sleeve cells after stimulating autonomic nerve innervating PV and found that action potential duration and ERP are much shorter and early-afterdepolarization is induced. Atropine could normalize action potential. β-blocker could also inhibit the abnormal discharge of PV induced by early-afterdepolarization. Meanwhile, the atrium was not triggered even though atrial ERP shortened.

2.2   The Imbalance of Autonomic Nervous System in Atrial Fibrillation

As raised by Huang (Huang *et al.*, 1998), heart rate variability is a valuable noninvasive tool for assessment of autonomic status and could be used to assess whether there was an alteration of autonomic tone immediately before the onset of AF. According to Huang, spectral heart rate variability could be expressed as low and high frequency (LF and HF) components. The HF component mainly reflects changes in vagal tension, while the LF component mainly gives a measure of sympathetic activity. Thus, the LF/HF ratio could be used as an index of the sympathovagal balance of the heart.

Several studies confirmed that the occurrence of paroxysmal AF greatly depends on variations of autonomic tone based on heart rate variability analysis. A research performed by Bettoni (Bettoni & Zimmermann, 2002) was designed to analyze dynamic changes in autonomic tone preceding the onset of paroxysmal AF. In the frequency-domain analyses, a significant increase in HF component was observed before paroxysmal AF, together with a progressive decrease in LF component. The LF/HF ratio showed a linear increase until 10 minutes before AF, followed by a sharp decrease immediately before the onset of AF, suggesting a primary increase in adrenergic tone followed by a marked modulation toward vagal predominance. In canine model, researchers (Lu *et al.*, 2013) found that in the first 30min of hypoxia, the LF and HF components of heart rate variability increased equivalently, resulting in the LF/HF ratio staying unchanged, as well as ERP, ERP dispersion and the window of vulnerability (a quantitative measure of AF inducibility). However, in the second 30min, the HF component increased significantly, resulting in the decrease of LF/HF ratio, which means the increase of parasympathetic activity and the imbalance of ANS, and at the same time, the ERPs detected were shortened significantly, and ERP dispersion and window of vulnerability increased obviously. Those changes of ERP and window of vulnerability were regarded as the index of AF inducibility, which were observed parallel with LF/HF ratio in this study. Thus they concluded that there may be close relationship between autonomic imbalance and the initiation of AF.

In another study performed by Oligin (Olgin *et al.*, 1998), heterogeneous sympathetic denervation was established with phenol in canine model. It was observed that compared with the sham group, the dispersion of ERP and AF cycle length was significantly increased in the phenol group, as well as the sustained AF inducibility. Thus the imbalance of ANS caused by regional sympathetic denervation could also contribute to the initiation and perpetuation of AF.

Otherwise, during imbalance of ANS, sympathetic and parasympathetic nerves may act alone, or together. In the study performed by Tan (Tan *et al.*, 2008) choosing ambulatory canine as animal model, the nerve activity of left stellate ganglion and vagus was recorded directly by implanted radio transmitter after intermittent rapid atrial pacing using pacemaker. Finally it was found that simultaneous sympathovagal discharge was the most common trigger of paroxysmal AF and atrial tachycardia. Similarly, according to the study conducted by Shen (Shen *et al.*, 2011), the AF inducibility of dog was analyzed in states of different correlations between nerve activity of the stellate ganglion and vagus, and it was showed that AF was more easily induced in dogs with high sympathetic-vagus correlation by rapid atrial pacing. Therefore, although sympathetic and vagus nerves promote the occurrence of AF through different mechanisms, these mechanisms do not attenuate each other but even are synergistic.

2.3   The Remodeling of Autonomic Nervous System in Atrial Fibrillation

According to the study performed by Jayachandran (Jayachandran, *et al.*, 2000) using 11C-hydroxyephedrine to label sympathetic nerve endings, it was found that the heterogeneous atrial sympathetic hyperinnervation occurred in persistent AF canine and the degree of uneven distribution of atrial autonomic nerves kept increasing as rapid atrial rates continued (Figure 4). Besides 11C-hydroxyephedrine, growth-associated protein 43 (GAP43) and tyrosine hydroxylase (TH) were always used as markers of autonomic nerves. GAP43 is a kind of protein that widely distributes in neurons of ANS and is supposed to be an intrinsic factor in the progression of neural development and regeneration, while TH is located in the cytoplasm of adrenergic nerve fibers and works as the limiting velocity enzyme for noradrenalin synthesis, which makes it a relatively stable marker for the sympathetic innervation. Chang (Chang, *et al.*, 2001) observed significant nerve sprouting and heterogeneous sympathetic hyperinnervation of atria by labeling GAP43 and TH in sustained AF canine model, which confirmed Jayachandran's results (Figure 5 and Figure 6).

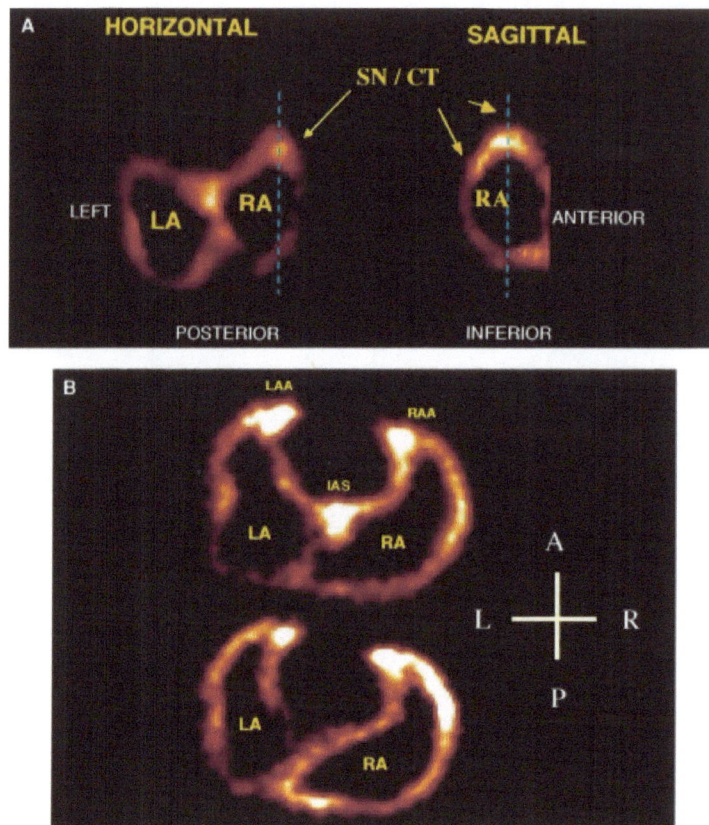

Figure 4: A. PET image of atrium of control animal. HED uptake is represented in red-white color scale with white representing maximal HED uptake. On left is an axial tomographic section in plane of AV rings. On right is a parasagittal section through crista terminalis that shows increased HED retention in area of sinus node. B. PET images of axial tomographic sections from 2 dogs in AF group. Several areas in both atria had increased and heterogeneous distribution of HED (sympathetic innervation). SN indicates sinus node; LA, left atrium; RA, right atrium; RAA, right atrial appendage; LAA, left atrial appendage; IAS, interatrial septum; CT, crista terminalis; A, anterior; P, posterior; L, left; and R, right; HED, hydroxyephedrine (Jayachandran, *et al.*, 2000).

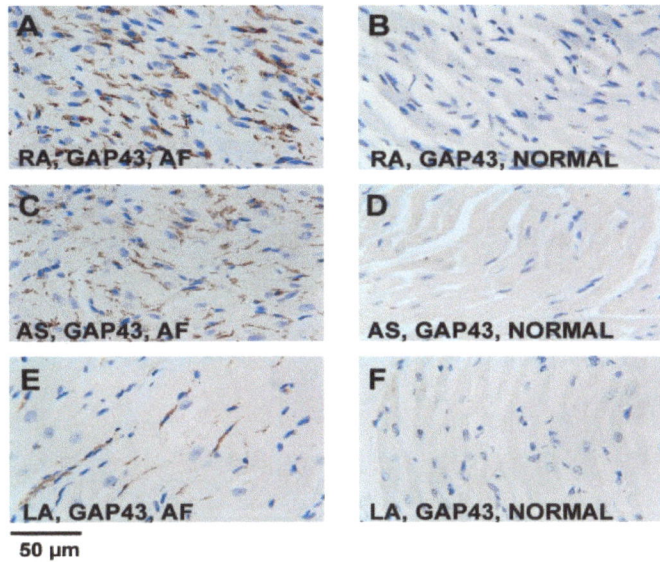

Figure 5: GAP43 staining of cardiac nerves (brown twigs) in control dogs and dogs with AF. AS indicates atrial septum (40×) . GAP43 indicates growth-associated protein 43; RA, right atrium; AS, atrial septum; LA, left atrium; AF, atrial fibrillation (Chang, *et al.*, 2001).

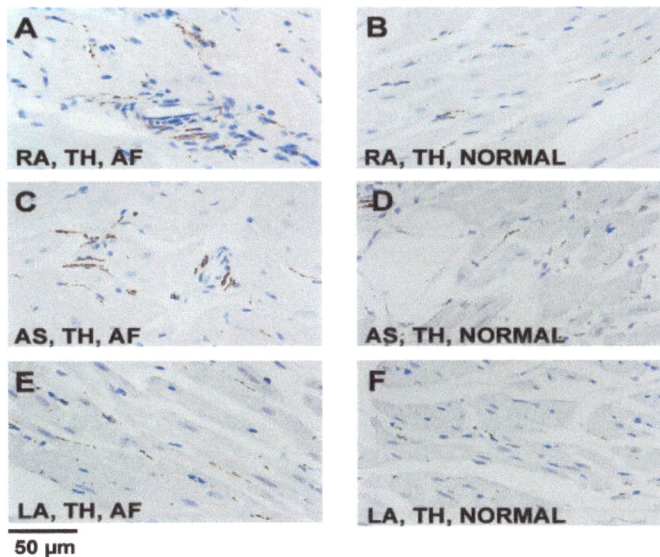

Figure 6: TH staining of cardiac nerves in control dogs and dogs with AF. AS indicates atrial septum. Magnification, (40×). TH indicates tyrosine hydroxylase; RA, right atrium; AS, atrial septum; LA, left atrium; AF, atrial fibrillation (Chang, *et al.*, 2001).

Parasympathetic remodeling was also supposed to occur in AF. Choline acetyltransferase (ChAT) is the synthetase of acetylcholine, which is supposed to be the specific marker of cholinergic neurons and could reflect distribution and regeneration of vagus. A study (Yu, *et al.*, 2010) in which paroxysmal AF canine model was established through 48-hour rapid right atrial pacing showed that GAP43 and ChAT expression in bilateral atria and atrial appendages was significantly higher than the control group, suggesting that vagal nerve sprouting was obvious in AF animals.

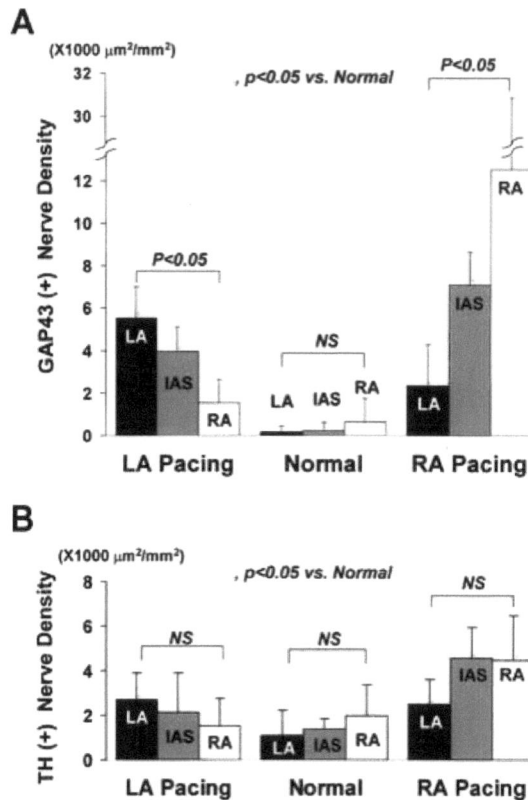

Figure 7: Cardiac nerve density and pacing sites. GAP43 indicates growth-associated protein 43; TH, tyrosine hydroxylase; SN, sinus node; LA, left atrium; RA, right atrium; IAS, interatrial septum (Hamabe, *et al.*, 2003).

ANR was also researched in other animal models without rapid atrial pacing. Swissa (Swissa, *et al.*, 2005) researched acute myocardial infarction (AMI), atria-ventricular block (AVB) and sympathetic hyperinnervation canine models. They found that paroxysmal AF or paroxysmal atrial tachycardia onset significantly increased in those groups, and the circadian variation was also apparent, with the peak incidence in the morning (about 4:00 am to 12:00 am) and a low one in late evening or midnight (Figure 8). Meanwhile, immunostaining showed nerve densities at both atria were all significantly higher in those groups than control canine.

In the study performed by Miyaochi (Miyauchi *et al.*, 2003), AMI canine model was established, and after 8 weeks, compared with the control group, the incidence of AF was higher and the duration of AF was longer. Moreover, it was also found that the density of GAP43 and TH positive nerve fibers in the sinoatrial node and PV tissue of AMI group was 5-8 times higher than that of control group, and the distribution was more heterogeneous (Figure 9). It suggests that there should be close relationship between ANR and AF initiation. The possible reason may lie in that AMI first induced local NGF release, followed by NGF production at the infarcted sites and retrograde transport of NGF to the LSG, which subsequently triggered cardiac nerve sprouting (Zhou *et al.*, 2004).

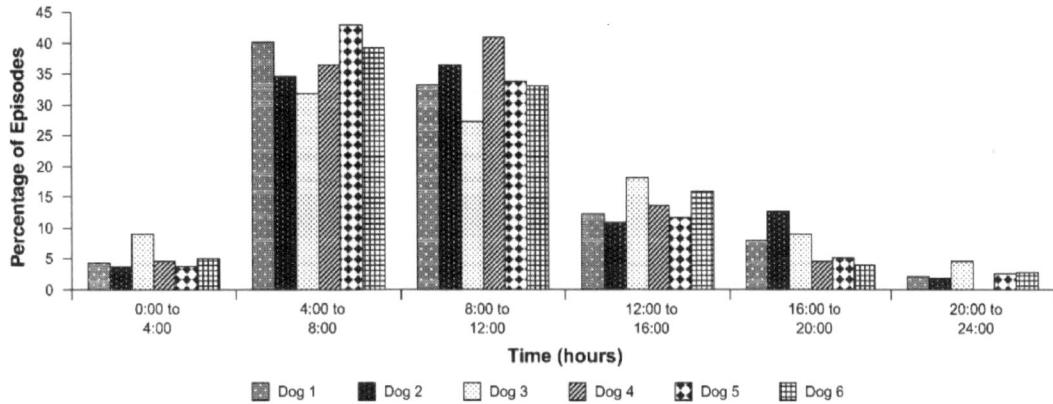

Figure 8: Frequencies of PAF and PAT over 24-h period in 6 canines with AMI, AVB and sympathetic hyperinnervation. We divided the events into 4-h periods and computed percentage of events for each dog in each time period. There is a circadian pattern of arrhythmia frequencies (*P*<0.01), with the peak incidence in early morning (Swissa, *et al.*, 2005).

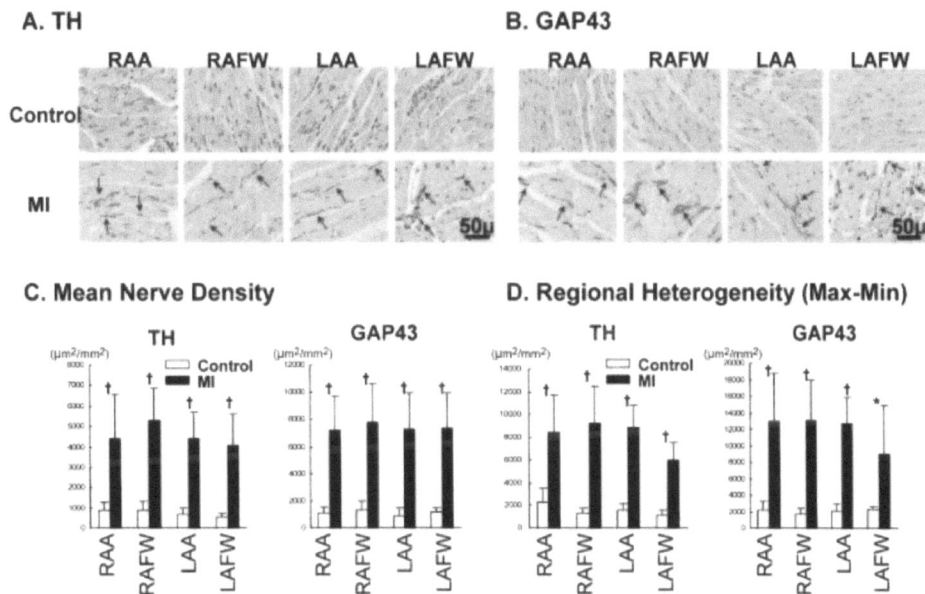

Figure 9: Atrial immunostaining of TH-positive (A) and GAP43-positive nerves (B) at different atrial sites. Increased TH- and GAP43- positive nerves at the 4 atrial sites are evident in the dogs with AMI. C. Histograms of mean TH- and GAP43-positive nerve density at all 4 atrial sites. D. Graphs show regional atrial heterogeneity (ie, the difference between maximum and minimum nerve density) (Miyauchi, *et al.*, 2003).

There is also close relationship between ANR after chronic heart failure and AF. Ng *et al.* (Ng *et al.*, 2011) found that both sympathetic and parasympathetic nerves of the left atrium remodeled in chronic heart failure dogs, and the innervation increased over time. The remodeling was more significant in posterior left atrial wall and PV than other parts of atrium. It was found that parasympathetic blockade could significantly shorten the duration of AF, and double autonomic blockade had no addition affect on AF duration. Thus they supposed that parasympathetic nervous system was the dominant autonomic limb contributing to AF in chronic heart failure, while the sympathetic system played a more modulatory role.

3   Autonomic Neural Remodeling after Ganglionated Plexi Ablation

GP is a component of intrinsic cardiac ANS, which has certain effects on the atrial electrophysiological activity and AF inducibility. High-frequency electrical stimulation to GP (Scherlag, Yamanashi, et al., 2005) or injection of parasympathomimetics into GP (Po et al., 2006) showed its critical role on the initiation and maintenance of AF. As a result, the GP ablation has emerged as a novel treatment of AF. However, though GP ablation has proven to be an effective way to treat AF, especially during a short-term follow-up after procedure (Pokushalov et al., 2008), its long-term success rate is quite variable (40%~90%, approximately), and the reasons remain under investigation (Mikhaylov et al., 2011; Pokushalov et al., 2010).

In the experiment performed by Oh (Oh et al., 2006), reactivity of sinoatrial node and atrioventricular node towards VNS and AF inducibility was observed significantly decreased immediately after GP ablation in canine. However, these phenomenons disappeared after 4 weeks, which led to the conclusion that GP ablation could not achieve long-term suppression of AF induction. Sakamoto (Sakamoto et al., 2010) and Pokushalov (Pokushalov et al., 2009) also reported vagal effects recovery after GP ablation in 4 weeks and 6 months respectively. These all supported the existence of nerve regeneration after GP ablation. Zhao (Zhao et al., 2010) supposed that ANR may be the mechanism of AF recurrence after GP ablation. They randomly divided 13 canines into GP ablation group and sham-operated group, and in the former group, anterior right GP and inferior right GP were selectively ablated. Eight weeks later, it was found that AF was easily induced in ablation animals, but not in sham-operated ones. Although the nerve density of ablation group was still lower than sham group, the researchers held that the reconstruction of atrial autonomic nerves might be the mechanism of AF reoccurrence after GP ablation. And irregular nerve regeneration may result in the imbalance between sympathetic and parasympathetic intensity.

References

Armour, J. A., Murphy, D. A., Yuan, B. X., Macdonald, S., & Hopkins, D. A. (1997). Gross and microscopic anatomy of the human intrinsic cardiac nervous system. Anat Rec, 247(2), 289-298.

Bers, D. M. (2002). Cardiac excitation-contraction coupling. Nature, 415(6868), 198-205.

Bettoni, M., & Zimmermann, M. (2002). Autonomic tone variations before the onset of paroxysmal atrial fibrillation. Circulation, 105(23), 2753-2759.

Chang, C. M., Wu, T. J., Zhou, S., Doshi, R. N., Lee, M. H., Ohara, T., et al. (2001). Nerve sprouting and sympathetic hyperinnervation in a canine model of atrial fibrillation produced by prolonged right atrial pacing. Circulation, 103(1), 22-25.

Chevalier, P., Tabib, A., Meyronnet, D., Chalabreysse, L., Restier, L., Ludman, V., et al. (2005). Quantitative study of nerves of the human left atrium. Heart Rhythm, 2(5), 518-522.

Coumel, P. (1994). Paroxysmal atrial fibrillation: a disorder of autonomic tone? Eur Heart J, 15 Suppl A, 9-16.

Deguchi, Y., Amino, M., Adachi, K., Matsuzaki, A., Iwata, O., Yoshioka, K., et al. (2009). Circadian distribution of paroxysmal atrial fibrillation in patients with and without structural heart disease in untreated state. Ann Noninvasive Electrocardiol, 14(3), 280-289.

Gong, Y. T., Li, W. M., Li, Y., Yang, S. S., Sheng, L., Yang, N., et al. (2009). Probucol attenuates atrial autonomic remodeling in a canine model of atrial fibrillation produced by prolonged atrial pacing. Chin Med J (Engl), 122(1), 74-82.

Hamabe, A., Chang, C. M., Zhou, S., Chou, C. C., Yi, J., Miyauchi, Y., et al. (2003). Induction of atrial fibrillation and nerve sprouting by prolonged left atrial pacing in dogs. Pacing Clin Electrophysiol, 26(12), 2247-2252.

Herweg, B., Dalal, P., Nagy, B., & Schweitzer, P. (1998). Power spectral analysis of heart period variability of preceding sinus rhythm before initiation of paroxysmal atrial fibrillation. Am J Cardiol, 82(7), 869-874.

Hocini, M., Haissaguerre, M., & Jais, P. (1999). Predominant origin of ectopic triggering atrial fibrillation from the pulmonary veins: mapping and ablation in 100 patients. Pacing Clin Electrophysiol, 22, 75.

Hou, Y., Scherlag, B. J., Lin, J., Zhang, Y., Lu, Z., Truong, K., et al. (2007). Ganglionated plexi modulate extrinsic cardiac autonomic nerve input: effects on sinus rate, atrioventricular conduction, refractoriness, and inducibility of atrial fibrillation. J Am Coll Cardiol, 50(1), 61-68.

Hou, Y., Scherlag, B. J., Lin, J., Zhou, J., Song, J., Zhang, Y., et al. (2007). Interactive atrial neural network: Determining the connections between ganglionated plexi. Heart Rhythm, 4(1), 56-63.

Huang, J. L., Wen, Z. C., Lee, W. L., Chang, M. S., & Chen, S. A. (1998). Changes of autonomic tone before the onset of paroxysmal atrial fibrillation. Int J Cardiol, 66(3), 275-283.

Jayachandran, J. V., Sih, H. J., Winkle, W., Zipes, D. P., Hutchins, G. D., & Olgin, J. E. (2000). Atrial fibrillation produced by prolonged rapid atrial pacing is associated with heterogeneous changes in atrial sympathetic innervation. Circulation, 101(10), 1185-1191.

Kumagai, K. (2007). Patterns of activation in human atrial fibrillation. Heart Rhythm, 4(3 Suppl), S7-S12.

Lu, Z., Nie, L., He, B., Yu, L., Salim, M., Huang, B., et al. (2013). Increase in vulnerability of atrial fibrillation in an acute intermittent hypoxia model: Importance of autonomic imbalance. Auton Neurosci.

Mikhaylov, E., Kanidieva, A., Sviridova, N., Abramov, M., Gureev, S., Szili-Torok, T., et al. (2011). Outcome of anatomic ganglionated plexi ablation to treat paroxysmal atrial fibrillation: a 3-year follow-up study. Europace, 13(3), 362-370.

Miyauchi, Y., Zhou, S., Okuyama, Y., Miyauchi, M., Hayashi, H., Hamabe, A., et al. (2003). Altered atrial electrical restitution and heterogeneous sympathetic hyperinnervation in hearts with chronic left ventricular myocardial infarction: implications for atrial fibrillation. Circulation, 108(3), 360-366.

Nakagawa, H., Scherlag, B. J., Patterson, E., Ikeda, A., Lockwood, D., & Jackman, W. M. (2009). Pathophysiologic basis of autonomic ganglionated plexus ablation in patients with atrial fibrillation. Heart Rhythm, 6(12 Suppl), S26-34.

Ng, J., Villuendas, R., Cokic, I., Schliamser, J. E., Gordon, D., Koduri, H., et al. (2011). Autonomic remodeling in the left atrium and pulmonary veins in heart failure: creation of a dynamic substrate for atrial fibrillation. Circ Arrhythm Electrophysiol, 4(3), 388-396.

Oh, S., Zhang, Y., Bibevski, S., Marrouche, N. F., Natale, A., & Mazgalev, T. N. (2006). Vagal denervation and atrial fibrillation inducibility: epicardial fat pad ablation does not have long-term effects. Heart Rhythm, 3(6), 701-708.

Olgin, J. E., Sih, H. J., Hanish, S., Jayachandran, J. V., Wu, J., Zheng, Q. H., et al. (1998). Heterogeneous atrial denervation creates substrate for sustained atrial fibrillation. Circulation, 98(23), 2608-2614.

Patterson, E., Po, S. S., Scherlag, B. J., & Lazzara, R. (2005). Triggered firing in pulmonary veins initiated by in vitro autonomic nerve stimulation. Heart Rhythm, 2(6), 624-631.

Po, S. S., Scherlag, B. J., Yamanashi, W. S., Edwards, J., Zhou, J., Wu, R., et al. (2006). Experimental model for paroxysmal atrial fibrillation arising at the pulmonary vein-atrial junctions. Heart Rhythm, 3(2), 201-208.

Pokushalov, E., Romanov, A., Artyomenko, S., Turov, A., Shugayev, P., Shirokova, N., et al. (2010). Ganglionated plexi ablation for longstanding persistent atrial fibrillation. Europace, 12(3), 342-346.

Pokushalov, E., Romanov, A., Shugayev, P., Artyomenko, S., Shirokova, N., Turov, A., et al. (2009). Selective ganglionated plexi ablation for paroxysmal atrial fibrillation. Heart Rhythm, 6(9), 1257-1264.

Pokushalov, E., Turov, A., Shugayev, P., Artyomenko, S., Romanov, A., & Shirokova, N. (2008). Catheter ablation of left atrial ganglionated plexi for atrial fibrillation. Asian Cardiovasc Thorac Ann, 16(3), 194-201.

Qu, X., Yu, Y., Jiang, J., Bai, B., Guo, H., & Song, Y. (2008). Variance of peptidic nerve innervation in a canine model of atrial fibrillation produced by prolonged atrial pacing. Pacing Clin Electrophysiol, 31(2), 207-213.

Sakamoto, S., Schuessler, R. B., Lee, A. M., Aziz, A., Lall, S. C., & Damiano, R. J., Jr. (2010). Vagal denervation and reinnervation after ablation of ganglionated plexi. J Thorac Cardiovasc Surg, 139(2), 444-452.

Schauerte, P., Scherlag, B. J., Patterson, E., Scherlag, M. A., Matsudaria, K., Nakagawa, H., et al. (2001). Focal atrial fibrillation: experimental evidence for a pathophysiologic role of the autonomic nervous system. J Cardiovasc Electrophysiol, 12(5), 592-599.

Scherlag, B. J., Nakagawa, H., Jackman, W. M., Yamanashi, W. S., Patterson, E., Po, S., et al. (2005). Electrical stimulation to identify neural elements on the heart: their role in atrial fibrillation. J Interv Card Electrophysiol, 13 Suppl 1, 37-42.

Scherlag, B. J., & Po, S. (2006). The intrinsic cardiac nervous system and atrial fibrillation. Curr Opin Cardiol, 21(1), 51-54.

Scherlag, B. J., Yamanashi, W., Patel, U., Lazzara, R., & Jackman, W. M. (2005). Autonomically induced conversion of pulmonary vein focal firing into atrial fibrillation. J Am Coll Cardiol, 45(11), 1878-1886.

Shen, M. J., Choi, E. K., Tan, A. Y., Han, S., Shinohara, T., Maruyama, M., et al. (2011). Patterns of baseline autonomic nerve activity and the development of pacing-induced sustained atrial fibrillation. Heart Rhythm, 8(4), 583-589.

Swissa, M., Zhou, S., Paz, O., Fishbein, M. C., Chen, L. S., & Chen, P. S. (2005). Canine model of paroxysmal atrial fibrillation and paroxysmal atrial tachycardia. Am J Physiol Heart Circ Physiol, 289(5), H1851-1857.

Takahashi, Y., Jais, P., Hocini, M., Sanders, P., Rotter, M., Rostock, T., et al. (2006). Shortening of fibrillatory cycle length in the pulmonary vein during vagal excitation. J Am Coll Cardiol, 47(4), 774-780.

Tan, A. Y., Li, H., Wachsmann-Hogiu, S., Chen, L. S., Chen, P. S., & Fishbein, M. C. (2006). Autonomic innervation and segmental muscular disconnections at the human pulmonary vein-atrial junction: implications for catheter ablation of atrial-pulmonary vein junction. J Am Coll Cardiol, 48(1), 132-143.

Tan, A. Y., Zhou, S., Ogawa, M., Song, J., Chu, M., Li, H., et al. (2008). Neural mechanisms of paroxysmal atrial fibrillation and paroxysmal atrial tachycardia in ambulatory canines. Circulation, 118(9), 916-925.

Ter Keurs, H. E., & Boyden, P. A. (2007). Calcium and arrhythmogenesis. Physiol Rev, 87(2), 457-506.

Yu, F. S., Zhang, Y., Feng, Y., Zhang, L., Ma, Y. H., Song, W., et al. (2010). Nerve remodeling in a canine model of atrial fibrillation induced by 48 hours right atrial pacing. Zhonghua Xin Xue Guan Bing Za Zhi, 38(7), 644-647.

Zhao, Q. Y., Huang, H., Zhang, S. D., Tang, Y. H., Wang, X., Zhang, Y. G., et al. (2010). Atrial autonomic innervation remodelling and atrial fibrillation inducibility after epicardial ganglionic plexi ablation. Europace, 12(6), 805-810.

Zhou, S., Chen, L. S., Miyauchi, Y., Miyauchi, M., Kar, S., Kangavari, S., et al. (2004). Mechanisms of cardiac nerve sprouting after myocardial infarction in dogs. Circ Res, 95(1), 76-83.

Zipes, D. P., Mihalick, M. J., & Robbins, G. T. (1974). Effects of selective vagal and stellate ganglion stimulation of atrial refractoriness. Cardiovasc Res, 8(5), 647-655.

Automatic Analysis of Vectorcardiogram Signal for Detection of Cardiovascular Diseases

Alireza Mehri-Dehnavi, Niloufar Salehpour
Biomedical Engineering Department, School of Medicine
Isfahan University of Medical Sciences, Iran

Hossein Rabbani
Biomedical Engineering Department, Medical Image & Signal Processing Research Center
Isfahan University of Medical Sciences, Iran

Amin Farahabadi, Eiman Farahabadi
Biomedical Engineering Department, School of Medicine
Isfahan University of Medical Sciences, Iran

1 Introduction

Electrocardiography (ECG) is a transthoracic (across the thorax or chest) interpretation of the electrical activity of the heart over a period of time, as detected by electrodes attached to the surface of the skin and recorded by a device external to the body. This signal is used to measure the rate and regularity of heart-beats, as well as the size and position of the chambers and presence of any damage to the heart. Using of computer processing in ECG analysis was one of the first times in medicine that computer based analysis was applied (Karsikasthe, 2011).

Although ECG signal is used as a general method in cardiac performance evaluation due to some advantages such as availability in most medical centers, it has a main problem which is lack of accurate and detailed information representation of cardiac electrical activity. An alternative signal that could pro-vide more information without high amount of electrodes and any hardware complication is Vectorcardi-ogram (VCG) signal. Actually, VCG determines the direction and magnitude of the heart dipole and can be obtained using the same hardware used for ECG recording in some devices such as Cardiax which only needs a new electrode placement for VCG recording.

To measure the VCG signal there are many lead systems, but orthogonal Frank lead system is one the most common ways. This method is based on the torso model and introduced in 1954 (Frank, 1954; 1956). According to Figure 1, using 4 front leads named as A, C, E, I from right to left respectively and 2 back leads named as H and M from up to down respectively, XYZ information in a Cartesian coordinate system would be:

$$X = 0.78 \, (0.78A + 0.22C - I) \tag{1}$$

$$Y = 0.35M + 0.65F - H \tag{2}$$

$$Z = 0.78 \, (-0.15A + 0.85M - 0.30I - 0.43E - 0.27C) \tag{3}$$

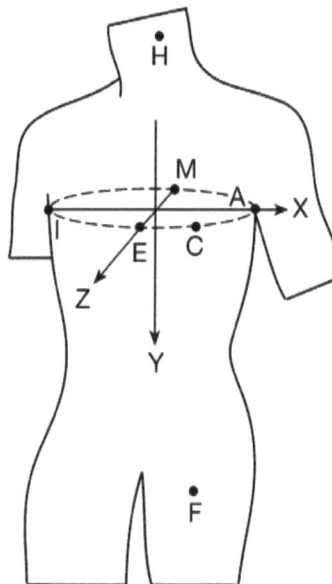

Figure1: VCG electrode placement in Cardiax system.

Since in VCG electrodes are placed in X, Y, Z directions, it can provide total information from all sides of the heart, especially the posterior orientation in Z direction. During the last decade in result of improvement of software and hardware medical signal processing, the capabilities of VCG signal was more recognized (Karsikasthe, 2011). For example in recognizing of some cardiac diseases like ventricular hypertrophy, combined left and right ventricular hypertrophy, right bundle branch block and myocardial infarction (MI) (Hurd *et al.*, 1981) VCG signal had a impressing role. So in many clinical situations VCG signal was really useful, but still 12-lead ECG system remained more common because interpretation of that was much easier for cardiologists. In other words it could be said that recording of VCG was not possible in the past before development of 3D processing tools and VCG just synthesized from standard 12-leads ECG. However synthesized VCG was a great step to improve detection of some cardiac abnormalities so it would be more and more common day by day (Karsikasthe, 2011).

On the other hand, with the recent advances in wireless and microelectromechanical systems (MEMS) sensor technologies, there has been a renewed interest in advancing ambulatory heart monitoring systems that uses these technologies. Bandwidth constraint has been the chief limitation of the wireless technologies for on-patient heart monitoring and advanced clinical diagnostic applications. ECGs that use fewer leads without affecting diagnosis was critical for minimizing bandwidth requirements, thus, leading to practical on-patient diagnostic systems. In such scenarios, VCGs can be preferred over conventional 12-leads ECG systems. Since the standard 12-lead ECG is the most common way to measure electrical function of the heart, the main question is the possibility of using VCG instead of ECG in order to get more accurate results. When standard 12-lead ECG is measured, all the chest leads are on the front side of the body, compared to Frank lead systems, where one of the chest lead locates on the back. Therefore the measurement by Frank lead system is more volumetric comparing to standard 12-lead ECG. As a result, 3-lead VCG provides 3D information of the heart, by showing the 3D vector of the heart. Some projections of this vector in 2D-pages will prepare the information about all sides of the heart. One reason for the slow progress in clinical application of VCG might be attributed to the 3D nature of VCG which was developed too early without any comparable methods to understand its meaning. Lack of powerful computational and 3D monitoring devices in that time has also been suggested for such slow progression. Since the VCG signals are less popular than the ECG signals amongst cardiologists, and it is hard to analyze by them, therefore, introducing methods to convert real VCG to ECG signals has been also investigated.

In addition, the 12-lead ECG which is the preferred lead system in the clinical environments doesn't provide appropriate information from the back of the heart. So, in some special cardiac disorders like atrial fibrillation (AF) and posterior MI, 12-lead ECG is often misjudged and this may be the reason for under treatment because the lack of information of posterior side of the heart. In search of faster and more reliable methods in identifying AF and posterior MI, the extra posterior leads V7 to V9 significantly increase the detection of posterior injury patterns compared with the standard 12-leads ECG. Lead V7 should be placed at the level of lead V6 at the posterior axillary line, lead V8 on the left side of the back at the tip of the scapula and lead V9 is placed halfway between lead V9 and the left paraspinal muscles. In usual trend if cardiologists doubted about AF or posterior MI, receiving the 15-lead ECG from the patient by using right-posterior method in locating ECG leads is ordered. In this trend, the recognition of AF and posterior MI could not be prepared at the primary 12-lead ECG test and after the result of the test observed by the cardiologist, he/she recommends to get the 15-lead ECG from those cases. So, the time is waist and recognition of exact problem of patient postpones. Since in recording VCG in Frank lead system two chest leads are located on the back, the essential question is: "Is it better to use VCG instead of

ECG to get more accurate results?" Actually VCG provides 3D information of the heart, by showing the 3D vector of the heart. Some projections of this vector in 2D pages will prepare the information about posterior side of the heart. However, because using of VCG signals is not usual for cardiologist and it is a bit hard to interpretation, so by using mathematical methods for converting VCG signal to ECG, the information about posterior wall (V7, V8, V9) would be prepared without using 15-lead ECG signals.

In this chapter, an application of VCG for detection of cardiac ischemia is explained in Section 2. For this reason, 22 features are extracted from VCG signals. Feature dimensionalities are reduced by the use of independent components analysis (ICA) and principal component analysis (PCA) tools and fed to a neural network for ischemia detection. The final results show the superiority of VCG-based ischemia detection comparing to ECG-based method. In Section 3, we try to construct synthesized VCG from standard 12-lead ECG signal and show that synthesized VCG would have contribution to improved detection of certain electrocardiographic abnormalities. In this base Dower and least square value (LSV) methods and singular value decomposition (SVD) are investigated. Finally a new method to convert a VCG to ECG signals by using partial linear transformation is introduced in Section 4. In this trend for each part of VCG and ECG signals like P, QRS or ST segments, new conversion coefficients are obtained using least square (LS) method. Also to improve our method and compensate some errors like changing R-R intervals during the time of signal registration, generalized estimation methods like iterative generalized least square (IGLS), non-linear recursive extended least square (NL-RELS) and weighted least square (WLS) methods are also investigated.

2   Application of VCG for Ischemia Detection Using Neural Networks

In this section we explain about the application of VCG for detection of cardiac ischemia and show the superiority of this signal in comparison with ECG for distinguishing between healthy and ischemic subjects based on VCG signal analysis by preprocessing, dimensionality reduction and classification by neural networks (Bishop 1995).

After preprocessing of VCG data using a sixth order Butterworth low pass filter with cut-off frequency of 50HZ for noise reduction, appropriate features have to be extracted from VCG for classification VCG data to healthy and ischemic subjects. For this reason 22 features of the VCG (described in Table 1) are used. In order to reduce the computational complexity, data dimensionality reduction methods including PCA (Jolliffe, 2002) and ICA (Comon, 1994) are employed. In PCA method by removing less significant coordinates the data dimensionality is reduced by choosing 5 biggest eigenvalues. In spite of PCA in which the resulted coordinates are orthogonal to each other, in ICA new data coordinates are not necessarily orthogonal. In ICA we try to find a transfer function which converts a random vector to linear components which are as independent as possible to each other.

After data dimensionality reduction, data is classified using a neural network. For this reason a two layer neural network with an input layer with 5 input nodes, a hidden layer with 2 hidden nodes and an output layer with 2 output nodes is used. The first output node is related to healthy people and the second one is related to patients whose exercise test response was positive.

In this study, totally 60 patients with chest pain, who were suspected to have ischemia and referred to emergency department were examined. Patients were in average age of 55 ± 3 years old. 32 patients were male. At the first stage of admission, 12-lead ECG and VCG signals of all subjects were obtained in rest state. Patients were treated by drug and hospitalization to gain a stable condition. All subjects performed exercise test 6 weeks after releasing from hospital, and results of 12-lead ECG and VCG signals were compared with results of exercise test (according to the Bruce protocol accompanied with heart rate and blood pressure monitoring). Finally, patient's records including 12-lead ECG, VCG and exercise test's results were analyzed by cardiologists. Exclusion criteria were having non-sinus rhythm, bundle branch block, use of anti-ischemic medication and disability to perform exercise tests.

VCG (Ischemic)	VCG (Healthy)	Description	Feature
1.23±0.0039	-1.52±0.0041	Azimuth Angle	$VCG_{azimuth}$
-0.59±0.0017	1.12±0.0028	Elevation Angle	$VCG_{elevation}$
78.68±3.128	46.65±2.146	QRS angle in frontal	QRS_{AF}
-53.15±3.605	79.50±4.012	QRS angle in sagittal	QRS_{AS}
-18.67±1.023	32.10±1.209	QRS angle in horizontal	QRS_{AH}
-86.56±2.45	-86.12±2.87	Angle of The Loop in frontal	T_{AF}
35.65±3.301	61.19±3.125	Angle of The Loop in sagittal	T_{AS}
-2.64±1.084	-23.50±2.13	Angle of The Loop in horizontal	T_{AH}
-0.90±0.0042	-0.54±0.0036	Ratio of QRS_T angle in frontal	$QRS\_T_{ratioAF}$
1.49±0.0041	1.29±0.0036	Ratio of QRS_T angle in sagittal	$QRS\_T_{ratioAS}$
7.07±0.042	-1.36±0.0047	Ratio of QRS_T angle in horizontal	$QRS\_T_{ratioAH}$
0.66±0.0035	104.15±3.27	Differentiation of max QRS_T angle in frontal	Max QRS_T_{AF}
28.66±3.013	62.97±2.65	Differentiation of max QRS_T angle in sagittal	Max QRS_T_{AS}
69.28±4.029	2.21±0.71	Differentiation of max QRS_T angle in horizontal	Max QRS_T_{AH}
69.28±3.16	104.15±4.72	Maximum Angle between QRS and T Loop axes	MA
2.35±0.0021	1.68±0.0067	Ratio of Maximum to Mean T Vector Magnitudes	RMMV
3.45±0.0712	4.69±0.083	Differentiation of angle in azimuth and elevation	DEA
148±1.98	131±2.903	Length of T Loop	$T_{Loop\ Length}$
50±2.019	45±2.701	Length of QRS Loop	$QRS_{Loop\ Length}$
7.72e-04±0.00302	4.03e-04±0.0064	Area of T Loop	$T_{Loop\ area}$
-0.0011±0.000204	0.0012±0.000102	Area of QRS Loop	$QRS_{Loop\ area}$
1.4313±0.0028	2.9854±0.0046	Ratio of Area	$QRS\_T_{ratio\ area}$

Table 1: Extracted features from VCG signal and mean±std values of these features for all healthy and patients.

The mean±std values of extracted features from VCG data of all healthy and patients are listed in Table 1. As explained before the dimensionality of data can be reduced from 22 to 5 by means of the PCA and ICA. Their mean values for both healthy and ischemia subjects are shown in Table 2. Finally 5 extracted features are fed to the mentioned neural network. In the training set, 23 samples including 20 data of suspect persons and 3 data of healthy person were chosen and the remaining 47 cases were used as test data. The training of the network was stopped on base of minimal training root mean square (RMS) error. (Note that for small dataset a k-fold cross-validation / leave one out approach would be lead to more reliable results.)

PCA Output					
Healthy	-215.054	-3.881	71.156	-74.823	57.675
Patient	-355.620	28.373	-110.182	3.511	-24.893
ICA Output					
Healthy	0.5672	2.7662	2.5273	-0.3598	-0.3187
Patient	0.4196	0.6253	-1.0559	-1.0791	-0.3486

Table 2: Output of PCA and ICA algorithms for healthy and ischemic subjects

	sensitivity	specificity	kapa	P value	NPV	PPV	FNR	FPR
ECG	60%	70%	0.208	0.069	89.7%	28.6%	40%	30%
VCG	70%	80%	0.483	0.001	93.5%	50%	30%	14%

Table 3: The statistical analysis of VCG and ECG for ischemia detection

Ischemia can be also detected in ECG signal based on ST segment downward deviation or changes of T wave in the form of negative (greater than 3 mm in depth) or biphasic T wave. The examination results of ECG signals showed that 21 patients had ischemic symptoms and the rest of them were normal while in examining VCG signal only 14 patients showed signs of ischemia and other patients showed normal signs. During exercise test it was determined that 50 patient had negative test and 10 had positive test, which confirmed ischemic heart disease. ECG and VCG analytical results were compared with exercise test results and the sensitivity, specificity and other statistical parameters were obtained (Table 3).

The sensitivity is defined as TP/(TP+FN) which TP shows the number of true positives, i.e., the number of cases that our algorithm detect the ischemic case and the result is in accordance with the exercise test, while FN shows the number of false negatives, i.e., the number of cases that our algorithm detect the ischemic case but the exercise test shows healthy. Similarly specificity is defined as TN/(TN+FP) which TN indicates the number of true negatives, i.e., the number of detected healthy case by our algorithm which their stress test is also negative, while FP indicates the number of false positives, i.e., the number of detected healthy case by our algorithm with positive stress test. The ECG sensitivities and specificities for the ischemia evaluation are 60 and 70 percent and for VCG are 70 and 86 respectively. Kappa coefficient index and p value for VCG is 0.483 and 0.001 and for ECG is 0.208 and 0.069 respectively. Negative predictive value (NPV=TN/(TN+FN)) and positive predictive value (PPV=TP/(TP+FP)) for ECG is 89.7 and 28.6 percent and for VCG is 93.5 and 50 percent. False negative ratio (FNR=FN/(FN+TP)) and false positive ratio (FPR=FP/(FP+TN)) for ECG is 40% and 30% and for VCG is 30% and 14% respectively.

Previous studies also showed that VCG has higher sensitivity and accuracy than ECG for other diseases. Hurd *et al.* (1981) showed 82% and 34% sensitivity for VCG and ECG on patients suffering from MI. Also Eriksson *et al.* (1991) studied patients with left and right bundle branch block in order to diagnose MI. They found that sensitivity of VCG in patients with right and left bundle branch block is 71% and 78% respectively.

3   Synthesized VCG

As explained before, in the case that recording of real VCG is not possible; the synthesizing of VCG from ECG could have contribution to improved analysis of electrical activities of heart and detection of certain electrocardiographic abnormalities. One of the first works for producing synthesized VCG from ECG was produced by Dower using the following transformation matrix:

$$
\begin{pmatrix} VCG_X(n) \\ VCG_Y(n) \\ VCG_Z(n) \end{pmatrix} = \begin{pmatrix} -0.172 & -0.073 & 0.122 & 0.231 & 0.239 & 0.193 & 0.156 & -0.009 \\ 0.057 & -0.019 & -1.06 & -0.022 & 0.040 & 0.048 & -0.227 & 0.886 \\ -0.228 & -0.310 & -0.245 & -0.063 & 0.054 & 0.108 & 0.021 & 0.102 \end{pmatrix} \begin{pmatrix} V_1(n) \\ V_1(n) \\ V_1(n) \\ V_1(n) \\ V_1(n) \\ V_1(n) \\ II(n) \\ II(n) \end{pmatrix}. \quad (4)
$$

where $[VCG_X(n), VCG_Y(n), VCG_Z(n)]^T$ shows the value of VCG vector in the point time n, and $[V_1(n), V_2(n),....,V_6(n), I(n), II(n)]^T$ shows the corresponding value of ECG leads. In SVD method, we don't have any explicit transformation matrix. After calculating singular values of ECGs, the eigenvectors corresponding to 3 biggest singular values is chosen as transformation matrix. In LSV method statistical least square fitting of an affine function is proposed. Each VCG lead is proposed as a linear combination of ECG leads and the transformation matrix is obtained based on applying LS method. The final transformation matrix in this method would be as follows:

$$
\begin{pmatrix} VCG_X(n) \\ VCG_Y(n) \\ VCG_Z(n) \end{pmatrix} = \begin{pmatrix} -0.226 & 0.027 & 0.065 & 0.131 & 0.203 & 0.220 & 0.370 & -0.154 \\ 0.088 & -0.088 & -0.003 & -0.042 & 0.047 & 0.067 & -0.131 & -0.717 \\ -0.319 & -0.198 & -0.167 & -0.099 & -0.009 & 0.060 & 0.184 & -0.114 \end{pmatrix} \begin{pmatrix} V_1(n) \\ V_1(n) \\ V_1(n) \\ V_1(n) \\ V_1(n) \\ V_1(n) \\ II(n) \\ II(n) \end{pmatrix}. \quad (5)
$$

In the following, the synthesized and real VCGs are compared using the above methods in terms of visual representation, correlation and mutual information. Figure 2 shows a view of loops developed by above mentioned techniques. The results of correlation between real VCG and synthesized VCGs for various methods are also concluded in Table 4. We also calculated mutual information as another metric to evaluate the similarity between synthesized VCGs and real VCG. The results are depicted in Figure 3. According to the results we can conclude that LSV method has the best results. We also evaluated these synthesized VCG signals by comparing the extracted features from VCG for an ischemic patient (Table 5). The correlation between these 22 features (that we name it feature signal) extracted from real VCG and synthesized VCG obtained by LSV, SVD and Dower methods are 0.7205, 0.5079 and 0.5762 respectively. We also calculated the correlation between feature signals of healthy and ischemic patients for each method. It's clear that best method must have the lowest correlation in order to be able to distinguish between healthy and ischemic patients as more as possible.This correlation measure for real VCG, LSV, SVD and Dower methods are 0.0631, 0.1881, 0.2931 and 0.1307 respectively.

Figure 4 compares the sagittal, frontal and horizontal loops of synthesized VCGs with real VCG for an ischemic patient. The highest correlation between real VCG and synthesized VCG obtained by LSV, SVD and Dower methods are 0.7105, 0.6649 and 0.6058 respectively. According to the mentioned simulation results it can be concluded that in most cases LSV method outperforms the others.

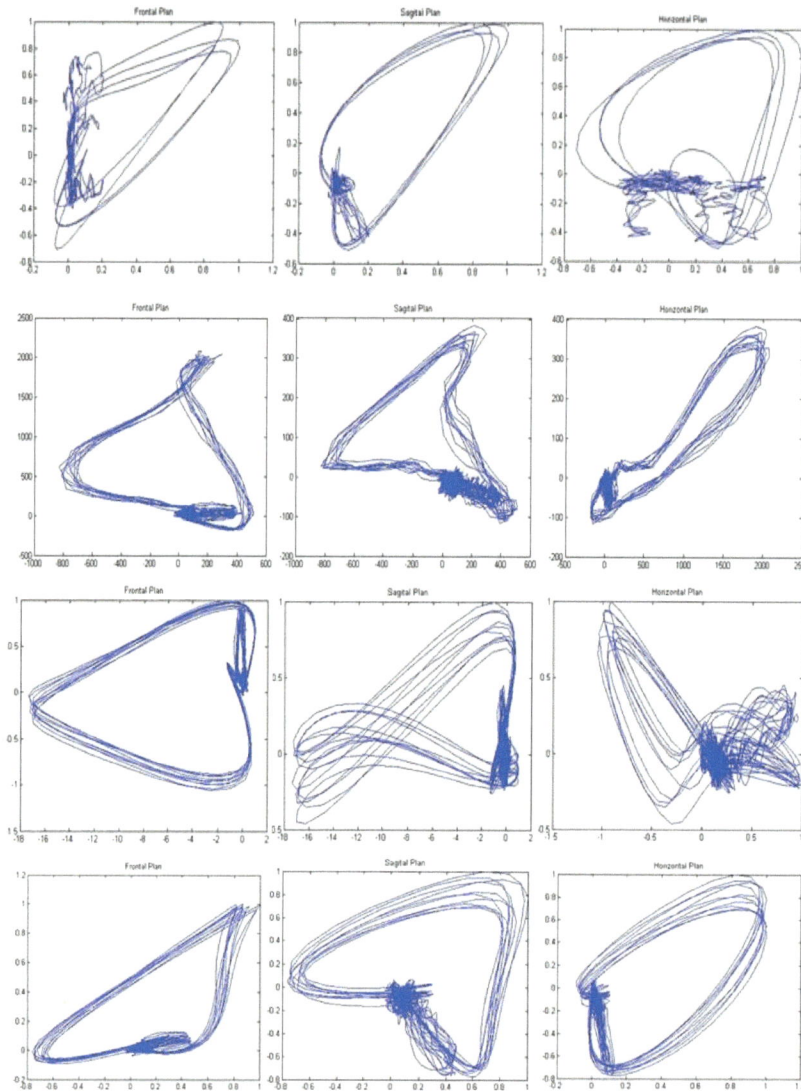

Figure 2: From top to down: (Frontal, sagittal and horizontal plans of) real VCG and synthesized VCG obtained by LSV, SVD and Dower method.

Method	Leads	Correlation
VCG & Dower	X,X_D	0.0280
	X,Y_D	0.0197
	X,Z_D	0.0055
	Y,X_D	0.0676
	Y,Y_D	0.0068
	Y,Z_D	0.0131
	Z,X_D	0.0345
	Z,Y_D	0.0370
	Z,Z_D	0.0181
VCG & SVD	X,X_S	0.0188
	X,Y_S	0.0306
	X,Z_S	0.0415
	Y,X_S	0.0166
	Y,Y_S	0.0537
	Y,Z_S	0.0820
	Z,X_S	0.0388
	Z,Y_S	0.0326
	Z,Z_S	0.0352
VCG & LSV	X,X_L	0.0331
	X,Y_L	0.0243
	X,Z_L	0.0331
	Y,X_L	0.0794
	Y,Y_L	0.0141
	Y,Z_L	0.0203
	Z,X_L	0.0090
	Z,Y_L	0.0316
	Z,Z_L	0.0142

Table 4: The correlation measures between real VCG and synthesized VCGs.

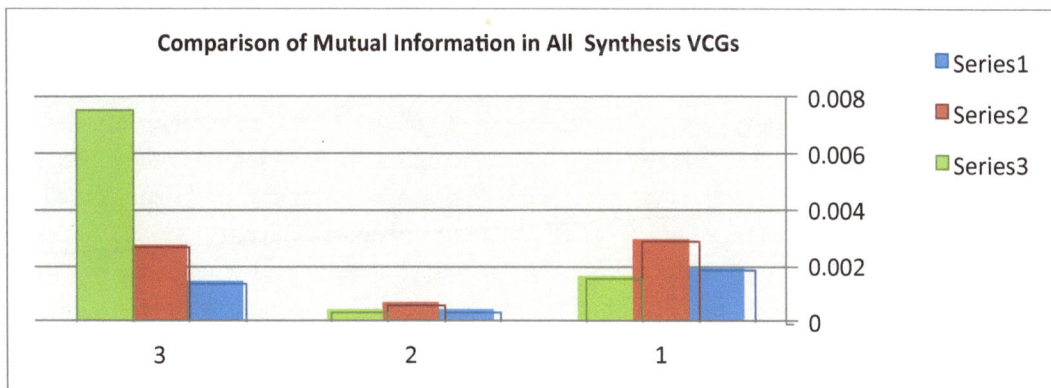

Figure 3: Comparison between mutual information of real VCG and synthesized VCG. 1, 2, 3 are respectively for SVD, Dower and LSV methods and Series1, 2, 3 respectively shows the results of X,Y,Z directions.

Feature	VCG (real)	VCG (Dower)	VCG (SVD)	VCG (LSV)
$VCG_{azimuth}$	1.49	-1.29	-1.41	-1.04
$VCG_{elevation}$	0.69	0.768	-1.51	0.070
QRS_{AF}	70.87	47.43	63.05	44.59
QRS_{AS}	-22.78	-88.67	-36.87	-20.26
QRS_{AH}	-53.83	11.52	-12.76	-70.29
T_{AF}	86.26	-47.49	-70.77	26.48
T_{AS}	-4.14	-17.84	-58.45	-8.15
T_{AH}	41.14	74.93	1.70	-86.17
$QRS\_T_{ratio\ AF}$	0.82	-0.99	-0.89	1.68
$QRS\_T_{ratio\ AS}$	5.52	2.48	0.63	2.48
$QRS\_T_{ratio\ AH}$	-1.30	-0.24	-7.50	0.81
Max QRS_T_{AF}	1.87	101.36	154.45	43.80
Max QRS_T_{AS}	29.13	88.73	37.87	12.24
Max QRS_T_{AH}	75.43	35.41	33.27	18.30
MA	75.43	101.36	154.45	43.80
RMMV	2.26	2.21	2.07	2.31
DEA	4.07	4.55	4.07	4.36
$T_{Loop\ Length}$	136	151	151	151
$QRS_{Loop\ Length}$	60	50	50	50
$T_{Loop\ area}$	$-2.16e^{-0.004}$	$-1.29e^{-0.004}$	$-8.56e^{-0.005}$	$-2.65e^{-0.005}$
$QRS_{Loop\ area}$	$-5.33e^{-0.004}$	$-1.77e^{-0.004}$	$-2.44e^{-0.005}$	$-8.50e^{-0.005}$
$QRS\_T_{ratio\ area}$	2.46	1.37	3.50	3.20

Table 5: Comparison between the values of extracted features from real VCG and synthesized VCGs.

4   Posterior ECG: Extracting V7, V8, V9 Leads of ECG Signal from VCG Using Partial Linear Transformation

In special situations like ambulatory care and emergency condition using VCG recording that is less elec-trodes is much easier and more useful. However, most cardiologists are accustomed to the 12-lead ECG even though some of the leads are either nearly aligned with or derived from the others and consequently contain redundant information. The ability to transform from orthogonal 3-lead VCG to 12-lead ECG enables the use of fewer leads for computer visualization, signal analysis and wireless transmission of signals. This can also improve mobility, albeit limited, to the patients.Furthermore, in special cardiac cas-es like AF and posterior MI the cardiologist needs some information from posterior side of the patient heart, that it can be achieved by using right-posterior ECG method (17-lead ECG). In this section VCG signals are used as a tool for providing total information from all sides of the heart (especially posterior side). However because for cardiologists is much easier to work with ECG signals for detecting some cardiac diseases, in this study new methods based on partial linear transformation is introduced to convert VCG signals to 15 channel ECG. In this trend for each part of VCG and ECG signals like P, QRS or ST segments, new conversion coefficients are obtained.

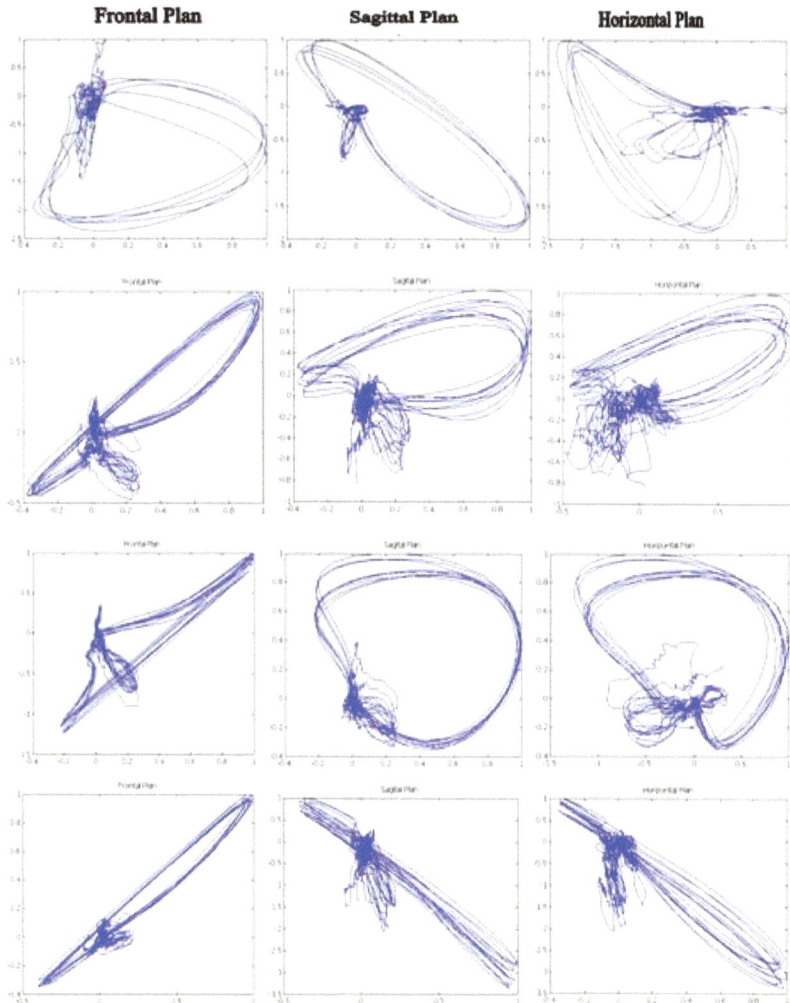

Figure 4: From top to down: (Frontal, sagittal and horizontal plans of) real VCG and synthesized VCG obtained by LSV, SVD and Dower method for an ischemic patient.

In this method we got the ECG data of each patient or case by applying this partial conversion on real VCG data.Converting VCG to ECG signals leads to reach posterior information of heart. So, just with 3 leads (Frank leads) and one VCG test of the patient and using this partial linear transformation the information about all sides of the heart will be prepared. ECG test is a fashionable diagnosing tool for cardiologist for the primary exam. So, by converting VCG to ECG, the data would be more understandable and useful for cardiologist, and also the information about posterior side of the heart (V7, V8, V9) would be prepared.

4.1 Existed Transformation Functions between ECG and VCG

Pioneering studies on lead transformation by Dower has down. This conversion made happen for the first time the possibility to derive the 12-lead ECG from the Frank leads. Dower used geometric transformation principles to obtain a matrix based on Frank's torso model, widely referred to as the Dower transformation matrix. In Dower transformation this matrix is multiplied to VCG samples for getting ECG signal from that, as showed below:

$$S = D \times V \tag{6}$$

where

$$D = \begin{bmatrix} -0.515 & 0.157 & -0.917 \\ 0.044 & 0.164 & -1.387 \\ 0.882 & 0.098 & -1.277 \\ 1.213 & 0.127 & -0.601 \\ 1.125 & 0.127 & -0.086 \\ 0.831 & 0.076 & 0.230 \\ 0.632 & -0.235 & 0.059 \\ 0.235 & 1.066 & -0.132 \end{bmatrix} \tag{7}$$

$$S(n) = [V_1(n)\ V_2(n)\ V_3(n)\ V_4(n)\ V_5(n)\ V_6(n)\ I(n)\ II(n)]^T \tag{8}$$

$$V(n) = [X(n)\ Y(n)\ Z(n)]^T \tag{9}$$

S contains the voltages of the corresponding leads, n denotes sample index and D is called the Dower-transformation matrix. From $S = D \times V$ it follows that the VCG leads can be synthesized by the 12-leads. The other method to derive ECG data from VCG, was developed transformation matrixes using statistical LS fitting of an affine function. Every derived lead is a linear combination of the known leads values plus a constant. The affine transformation structure provides a convenient means to automatically compensate for some of these constant biases so that the resulting empirical transformation scan would be more consistent and accurate.

Linear regression model assumes that every derived lead (the individual 8-lead value and posterior leads V_1, V_2,..., V_6, I, II, V_7, V_8, V_9) is denoted as a row vector with length of n (e.g., ECG(.) = [ECG(1), ECG(2) ,..., ECG(n)]) and the ECG matrix Z = $[V_1(.)^T, V_2(.)^T,..., V_6(.)^T, I(.)^T, II(.)^T, V_7(.)^T, V_8(.)^T, V_9(.)^T]^T$, can be obtained from a linear combination of the 3 Frank VCG values (the 3 leads are denoted as X = $[VCG_X(.)^T, VCG_Y(.)^T, VCG_Z(.)^T]^T$) as follows:

$$Z = AX + e \tag{10}$$

where A is 11×3 transformation matrix and eis the error. Thus, from knowing the input lead values, the corresponding coefficient vectors can be used to derive each of the 11 leads from VCG.

4.2 Partial Linear Transformation

In this investigation we compare the overall accuracies of the partial linear transformation and some generalized linear estimation methods with affine transformation method for correctly deriving the 15-lead ECG from the known 3-lead Frank XYZ, for healthy cases.We have used 50 healthy cases in this study. The sampling rate was 500 Hz, and the samples were typically gathered for 16-second duration and the recorder device was Cardiax recorder. The 15-lead ECG and VCG signals were used in the following investigation:

First of all it must be attended that because of changing of duration of P-QRS-ST segments of VCG and ECG signal for each case related with heart rate changing, the algorithm of transformation must be resistance against the R-R interval changing. Therefore, instead of applying partial linear transformation for P-QRS-ST segments separately, we can use some generalized least square methods like iterative generalized least square (IGLS) and non-linear recursive extended least square (NL-RELS). Using these generalized transformations the process would be on-line so the error of changing R-R interval would be compensated.

For applying partial linear transformation for P-QRS-ST segments separately, at first step ECG and VCG signals for each case must be synchronized. So, by using differential threshold method we could find the R peak of each signal and synchronize the ECG and VCG signals for each case. This process must be taken because in recording VCG signal, the position of the case is changed from the position in ECG recording. Cardiax recorder has the ability to give some information about duration of the P, QRS and ST segments of the ECG and VCG signals of each special case. So, we get duration of these segments in milliseconds, more ever we knew that the sampling frequency is 500 HZ. By employing this data we can get exactly each segment of our signals has how many samples using the following equation (for an example):

$$QRS\ segment = 40\ ms$$

$$\Longrightarrow \quad \frac{1000(ms)}{500(ms)} = \frac{40(ms)}{X\ sample} \tag{11}$$

$$Sampling\ rate = 500\ HZ$$

By this equation X would be calculated. So, after making ECG and VCG synchronized it would be possible to extract each segment of both signals. After that we use the least square fitting method to find partial coefficients for each segment of ECG & VCG signals. Final formula would be like this:

$$ECG(t) = aVCG_x(t) + bVCG_y(t) + cVCG_z(t) + d \tag{12}$$

$$ECG(t) = \begin{bmatrix} VCG_x(t) & VCG_y(t) & VCG_z(t) & 1 \end{bmatrix} \begin{bmatrix} a \\ b \\ c \\ d \end{bmatrix} \tag{13}$$

$$\begin{bmatrix} a \\ b \\ c \\ d \end{bmatrix} = (U^T U)^{-1} U^1 Y \tag{14}$$

where

$$U = \begin{bmatrix} VCG_x(1) & VCG_y(1) & VCG_z(1) & 1 \\ \vdots & \vdots & \vdots & \vdots \\ VCG_x(n) & VCG_y(n) & VCG_z(n) & 1 \end{bmatrix} \tag{15}$$

$$Y = \begin{bmatrix} ECG(1) \\ \vdots \\ ECG(n) \end{bmatrix} \qquad (16)$$

4 coefficients (a-b-c-d) are provided for each P-QRS-ST segment of the signal. In right-posterior method of electrocardiography, two electrodes locate on the right side of the heart and three electrodes locate at the back of the heart horizontally. In this way, we would have real information about posterior side of the heart too. By changing the position of the patient (lay down on right side of the body) the VCG test is given. Now, we have both signals and we could find local coefficients for each segment of our signals.

For testing this method we calculated the coefficients for 5,10,20,30,40,50 healthy cases and observed that when the number of our cases increased from 15 persons the coefficients are approximately constant, so we got that this method is trustable. In this study we did our process with age and gender separation too, to observe the effect of them in this transformation function. In addition, some generalized LS methods (Rao *et al.*, 1999; Plackett, 1950; Strutz, 2010) like IGLS and NL-RELS is used to improve the estimation process or compensate some issues such as the effect of changing R-R intervals by their on-line process.

4.3   IGLS Method

IGLS stands for iterative generalized least square method. In this method the point is finding the dynamic noise of the signal to improve the performance of estimator in the presence of non- additive white Gaussian noise (AWGN). To perform this method we do these steps (V_t is AWGN and $d_1,...,d_l$ show the dynamic of noise):

1.   Initialization: $d_i = 0$ for $i = 1,...,l$, $\hat{V}(i) = 0$ for $i = -l,..., -1$

2.   Define

$$ECG'(t) = ECG(t) + d_1 ECG(t-1) + \cdots + d_l ECG(t-l). \qquad (17)$$

$$VCG_x'(t) = VCG_x(t) + d_1 VCG_x(t-1) + \cdots + d_l VCG_x(t-l). \qquad (18)$$

$$VCG_y'(t) = VCG_y(t) + d_1 VCG_y(t-1) + \cdots + d_l VCG_y(t-l). \qquad (19)$$

$$VCG_z'(t) = VCG_z(t) + d_1 VCG_z(t-1) + \cdots + d_l VCG_z(t-l). \qquad (20)$$

3.   Form matrix U and Y

$$U = \begin{bmatrix} VCG_x'(1) & VCG_y'(1) & VCG_z'(t) & 1 \\ \vdots & \vdots & \vdots & \vdots \\ VCG_x'(n) & VCG_y'(n) & VCG_z'(n) & n \end{bmatrix}. \qquad (21)$$

$$U = \begin{bmatrix} ECG'(1) \\ \vdots \\ ECG'(n) \end{bmatrix}. \qquad (22)$$

4. Parameters estimation

$$\hat{I} = \begin{bmatrix} \hat{a} \\ \hat{b} \\ \hat{c} \\ \hat{d} \end{bmatrix} = (U^T U)^{-1} U^T Y. \tag{23}$$

5. Calculating the dynamic of noise in order to fine the error between original ECG and converted one as below:

$$\hat{Y} = \begin{bmatrix} \hat{Y}(1) \\ \vdots \\ \hat{Y}(n) \end{bmatrix} = U\hat{I}. \tag{24}$$

$$\hat{V} = \begin{bmatrix} \hat{V}(1) \\ \vdots \\ \hat{V}(n) \end{bmatrix} = Y - \hat{Y}. \tag{25}$$

$$\hat{V}(t) = \begin{bmatrix} -\hat{V}(t-1) & \cdots & -\hat{V}(t-l) \end{bmatrix} \begin{bmatrix} d_1 \\ \vdots \\ d_l \end{bmatrix}. \tag{26}$$

$$U_d = \begin{bmatrix} \hat{V}(1-1) & \hat{V}(1-2) & \cdots & \hat{V}(1-l) \\ \vdots & \vdots & \vdots & \vdots \\ \hat{V}(n-1) & \hat{V}(n-2) & \cdots & \hat{V}(n-l) \end{bmatrix}. \tag{27}$$

$$D = \begin{bmatrix} d_1 \\ \vdots \\ d_l \end{bmatrix} = \left(U_d^T U_d \right)^{-1} U_d \hat{V}. \tag{28}$$

After step 5, we must return to step 1 with new dynamic of noise obtained and after several iterations a, b, c, d coefficients would be extracted in step 4. We tested the degree of dynamic of noise in this study up to $l=5$ and found $l=3$ is the best choice.

4.4 NL-RELS Method

The other suggested method to compensate changing of R-R intervals in our cases is using NL-RELS method that can be used for on-line processing of data. In this paper we define the recursive formula as follows:

$$ECG(t) = \begin{bmatrix} \|VCG(t)\| & ECG(t-1) & 1 & \hat{V}(t-1) \end{bmatrix} \begin{bmatrix} a \\ b \\ c \\ d \end{bmatrix}. \tag{29}$$

where

$$\|VCG(t)\| = \sqrt{VCG_x^2(t) + VCG_y^2(t) + VCG_z^2(t)}. \tag{30}$$

To implement this method we have got 5 basic steps as follows:

1. Initialization:

$$\hat{V}(i) = 0 \text{ for } i = ...,-2,-1, t = 1, P_0 = K \begin{bmatrix} 1 & 0 & 0 & 0 \\ 0 & 1 & 0 & 0 \\ 0 & 0 & 1 & 0 \\ 0 & 0 & 0 & 1 \end{bmatrix} \text{where } K \text{ is a constant.}$$

2. Calculate the initial values of parameters using LS method:

$$\hat{I}_0 = \begin{bmatrix} \hat{a}(0) \\ \hat{b}(0) \\ \hat{c}(0) \\ \hat{d}(0) \end{bmatrix} = \left(U^T U \right)^{-1} U^T Y. \tag{31}$$

$$U = \begin{bmatrix} \|VCG(1)\| & ECG(1-1) & 1 & \hat{V}(1-1) \\ \vdots & \vdots & \vdots & \vdots \\ \|VCG(n)\| & ECG(n-1) & n & \hat{V}(n-1) \end{bmatrix}. \tag{32}$$

$$Y = \begin{bmatrix} ECG(1) \\ \vdots \\ ECG(n) \end{bmatrix}. \tag{33}$$

$$u_t^T = \begin{bmatrix} \|VCG(t)\| & ECG(t-1) & 1 & \hat{V}(t-1) \end{bmatrix}. \tag{34}$$

$$P_t = P_{t-1} - \frac{P_{t-1} \cdot u_t \cdot u_t^T \cdot P_{t-1}}{1 + u_t^T \cdot P_{t-1} \cdot u_t}. \tag{35}$$

$$\hat{I}_t = \begin{bmatrix} \hat{a}(t) \\ \hat{b}(t) \\ \hat{c}(t) \\ \hat{d}(t) \end{bmatrix} = \hat{I}_{t-1} + P_t \cdot u_t \left(ECG(t) - u_t^T \cdot \hat{I}_{t-1} \right). \tag{36}$$

3. Compute the error of computation and return to step three for making u_{t+1}^T. The formula of error $\hat{V}(t)$ would be like this:

$$\hat{V}(t) = ECG(t) - u_t^T \hat{I}_t. \tag{37}$$

This method processes our data in on-line format so we can say that the R-R interval changing of one person (case study) would be compensated. To receive the perfect result, initialization must be started from small values to reach the proper value.

4.5 Weighted Least Square (WLS) Method

The other method can be used to improve the results is WLS estimation. This method is used when we want to emphasize in special parts of the ECG and VCG segments or extract special parts of the signals. For instance, when cardiologist needed middle information of P, QRS or ST segments of signals the weighted function highlights the middle parts of signal segments. In this study the weighted matrix with emphasizing in middle rows and columns was used. The schedule would be like this: The weighted matrix was multiplied to VCG signals before converting to ECG. The mathematical formula is:

$$ECG(t) = \begin{bmatrix} VCG_x(t) & VCG_y(t) & VCG_z(t) & 1 \end{bmatrix} \begin{bmatrix} a \\ b \\ c \\ d \end{bmatrix}. \tag{38}$$

$$\begin{bmatrix} a \\ b \\ c \\ d \end{bmatrix} = \left(U^T W U \right)^{-1} U^T W Y. \tag{39}$$

$$U = \begin{bmatrix} VCG_x(1) & VCG_y(1) & VCG_z(t) & 1 \\ \vdots & \vdots & \vdots & \vdots \\ VCG_x(n) & VCG_y(n) & VCG_z(n) & n \end{bmatrix}. \tag{40}$$

$$Y = \begin{bmatrix} ECG(1) \\ \vdots \\ ECG(n) \end{bmatrix} \tag{41}$$

$$W = \begin{bmatrix} .1 & 0 & 0 & \cdots & 0 & 0 & 0 \\ 0 & .1 & 0 & \cdots & 0 & 0 & 0 \\ \vdots & \vdots & \vdots & \vdots & \vdots & \vdots & \vdots \\ 0 & 0 & 0 & .9 & 0 & \cdots & 0 \\ 0 & 0 & \cdots & 0 & .9 & \cdots & 0 \\ \vdots & \vdots & \vdots & \vdots & \vdots & \vdots & \vdots \\ 0 & 0 & 0 & \cdots & 0 & 0 & .1 \end{bmatrix}. \text{ (diagonal matrix)} \tag{42}$$

At last for comparing our suggested methods with affine transformation, we use affine matrix to convert the VCG signals to ECG ones and then calculate some statistical parameters for comparing the precision of our methods and existed one.

4.6 Evaluation of Various Partial Linear Transformation Methods

For evaluating different conversion methods used in this study first of all the transformation coefficients (a, b, c, d) are compared with each other in Table 6 and Table 7 for leads II and V$_9$.

Lead II QRS segment	Partial linear method	Dower method	Affine method	IGLS method	NL-RELS method	WLS method
a	0.50	0.23	0.01	0.4	1.90	0.48
b	-0.02	1.06	0.03	0.12	0.20	0.06
c	-0.03	-0.13	-0.01	-0.02	-0.03	-0.03
d	27.12		73.62	30.24	35.70	25.06

Table 6: Comparison between VCG and ECG signals for partial linear, Dower,affine, IGLS,NL-RELS and WLS methods for lead II.

For lead V_9		P	QRS	ST
Partial linear method	a	-0.0359	0.3415	0.2997
	b	0.0290	0.0949	0.1259
	c	-0.1390	-0.1261	-0.1660
	d	11.0267	24.247	-16.5325
Affine method	a	0.0061	0.0061	0.0061
	b	0.0157	0.0157	0.0157
	c	-0.0299	-0.0299	-0.0299
	d	33.2653	33.2653	33.2653
IGLS method	a	-0.0359	0.3365	0.2998
	b	0.0289	0.0928	0.1264
	c	-0.1390	-0.1261	-0.1660
	d	11.0327	26.619	-16.5478
methodRELS	a	-0.0540	0.4326	0.2760
	b	-0.2478	0.1246	0.1197
	c	-0.1390	-0.1279	-0.1530
	d	11.032	26.8021	-15.2308
WLS method	a	-0.073	0.2917	0.3867
	b	0.0478	-0.0883	0.0213
	c	-0.1997	0.1266	-0.1936
	d	5.152	19.407	-40.7115

Table 7: Comparison between VCG and ECG signals for partial linear, dower, affine, IGLS,NL-RELS and WLS methods for posterior lead V_9

R^2 is a statistic parameter that is used to quantify the extent to which a transform captures the trends in the relationship between the inputs (3 VCG leads) and each of the measured data. An R^2 statistic of 100% indicates that the transform is able to correctly reproduce the actual measured data (lead value) every single time. An R^2 statistic is given by:

$$R^2 = \left\{ 1 - \frac{\sum_k \left[\text{derived(samle k)} - \text{measured(sample k)} \right]^2}{\sum_k \left[\text{measured(sample k)} \right]^2} \right\} \times 100 \qquad (43)$$

R^2 is used to evaluate how close the outputs are calculated from the model relative to the actual measured lead values. When we compared statistical parameter (R^2) and correlation coefficients (C.C) of the conversion in partial linear method and generalized ones with affine transforms, we observed that our recommended method was much more reliable and accurate than affine and dower transforms. So for healthy cases, the partial linear transformation presented here yields improved accuracy (R^2 values) over affine transform (see following Tables for statistical details for all 15 leads).

In Table 8 there is comparison between the partial linear transformation method and the other ones that was used in this study to extract 12 lead ECG from VCG without segregation age and gender using statistical parameters like R2 and correlation coefficient. In Table 9 there is a comparison between partial linear method and generalized ones. In Table 10 partial linear transformation method is applied with segregation age and gender. In Table 11 statistical parameters like R2 and correlation coefficient is showed for posterior leads V7, V8, V9 and for all transformation methods. In Table 12 partial linear transformation method is applied with segregation of age and gender for posterior leads and QRS segments.

lead	R^2 Partial linear method	R^2 Dower method	R^2 Affine method	C.C Partial linear method	C.C Dower method	C.C Affine method
I	60.70	20.90	37.08	0.79	0.67	0.80
II	68.64	34.66	57.45	0.79	0.68	0.43
V_1	68.44	56.11	59.38	0.84	0.43	0.64
V_2	75.17	35.51	67.30	0.69	0.54	0.22
V_3	58.51	35.60	53.61	0.76	0.31	0.40
V_4	78.10	17.25	78.15	0.70	0.10	0.79
V_5	75.36	74.36	74.75	0.77	0.16	0.50
V_6	43.08	23.28	33.36	0.77	0.35	0.72

Table 8: Comparison between partial linear transformation method and the other existed ones to extract 12 lead ECG from VCG.

lead	R^2 partiallinear method	R^2 IGLS method	R^2 NL-RELS method	R^2 WLS method	C.C partiallinear method	C.C IGLS method	C.C NL-RELS method	C.C WLS method
I	60.70	59.04	21.08	43.07	0.79	0.79	0.48	0.66
II	68.64	67.13	24.12	46.95	0.79	0.79	0.50	0.71
V_1	68.44	67.96	30.73	50.03	0.84	0.84	0.52	0.76
V_2	75.17	74.61	32.10	56.34	0.69	0.68	0.39	0.62
V_3	58.51	57.23	21.96	35.91	0.76	0.76	0.43	0.67
V_4	78.10	78.01	36.14	64.13	0.70	0.70	0.57	0.69
V_5	75.36	73.95	31.23	61.06	0.77	0.76	0.55	0.66
V_6	43.08	42.68	20.04	26.41	0.77	0.75	0.68	0.69

Table 9: Comparison between partial linear transformation and generalized partial methods.

lead	R^2 Partial linear method for all data	R^2 For men	R^2 For women	R^2 Under age 60	R^2 Above age 60	C.C Partial linear method for all data)	C.C For men	C.C For women	C.C Under age 60	C.C Above age 60
I	60.70	38.25	32.86	45.57	69.83	0.79	0.78	0.56	0.68	0.70
II	68.64	49.91	40.44	50.21	70.65	0.79	0.79	0.61	0.67	0.75
V_1	68.44	49.88	38.52	53.13	68.95	0.84	0.80	0.65	0.74	0.79
V_2	57.17	59.07	44.62	60.21	77.80	0.69	0.60	0.49	0.62	0.69
V_3	58.80	39.03	36.64	52.41	60.32	0.76	0.59	0.57	0.70	0.74
V_4	78.10	59.56	58.83	51.41	78.73	0.77	0.51	0.55	0.69	0.70
V_5	75.36	67.12	49.77	69.60	73.99	0.77	0.60	0.56	0.58	0.65
V_6	43.08	37.08	22.90	36.13	49.14	0.77	0.70	0.68	0.70	0.73

Table 10: Partial linear transformation method with segregation age and gender.

Methods		P	R^2 QRS	ST	P	(C.C) QRS	ST
partial linear method	V_7	72.53	43.81	90.40	0.5640	0.8879	0.9025
	V_8	45.01	58.16	83.01	0.1499	0.9057	0.8630
	V_9	88.49	62.05	87.41	0.2574	0.9210	0.8058
WLS method	V_7	69.52	33.06	86.98	0.5210	0.8837	0.8832
	V_8	43.36	39.14	79.60	0.1197	0.8308	0.8247
	V_9	86.93	48.55	87.16	0.2770	0.8868	0.8058
IGLS method	V_7	70.06	43.80	88.84	0.5633	0.8773	0.9011
	V_8	42.97	55.05	81.94	0.1398	0.8986	0.8599
	V_9	85.09	61.60	87.40	0.2574	0.9208	0.8059
NL-RELS method	V_7	59.04	35.66	79.40	0.0871	0.7145	0.7602
	V_8	26.73	33.04	64.24	0.0906	0.7127	0.6411
	V_9	60.97	43.52	69.37	0.2232	0.8721	0.6003
Affine method	V_7	63.46	29.04	79.16	0.4365	0.3211	0.5205
	V_8	42.25	39.96	75.01	0.1341	0.2882	0.6713
	V_9	87.74	41.08	73.95	0.0497	0.0720	0.6450

Table 11: Statistical parameters R2 and correlation coefficient for posterior leads V7, V8, V9 and for all transformation methods.

lead	R^2 Partial linear method for all data	R^2 For men	R^2 For women	R^2 Under age 60	R^2 Above age 60	C.C Partial linear method for all data	C.C For men	C.C For women	C.C Under age 60	C.C Above age 60
V_7	43.81	31.12	29.75	23.61	43.88	0.88	0.88	0.54	0.69	0.80
V_8	58.16	39.05	33.07	44.90	60.04	0.90	0.89	0.63	0.83	0.77
V_9	62.05	42.82	37.01	47.35	72.65	0.92	0.93	0.67	0.80	0.82

Table 12: Partial linear transformation method with segregation of age and gender for posterior leads and QRS segments.

Regarding the results of comparison between all transformation methods and segregation of age and gender we can obviously say that:

1. Partial linear transformation method has more efficiency and accuracy than other introduced ones in this study. In other words it can be said that the priority of accuracy of all methods are like this:
   a. Partial linear transformation method
   b. IGLS method
   c. NL-RELS method
   d. WLS method
   e. Affine method
   f. Dower method

2. Segregation of gender dos not have a positive effect on efficiency and accuracy of transformations.

3. Segregation of age with threshold in 60 showed that for people above 60 the result is much better because there is less cardiac arrhythmia for them than people under 60.

These results show that for healthy subjects, our method (partial linear transformation) presented here, which maps 3-lead VCG to 15-lead ECG, is more accurately than the generalized ones and affine and dower methods, but it must be noticed that the recursive partial linear methods acts in on-line format so they results are weaker than off-line way in original partial linear transformation. In figures below (Figures 5-8) the similarity of real ECG and extracted one from VCG is showed for all transformation method for lead II and lead V9.

This comparison is applied between 7 persons and 1 segment from each one of their real ECG and extracted one is showed continuously. Red line introduces the real ECG and green line introduces the extracted one from VCG. In graphs below horizontal vector shows number of samples and vertical one shows the amplitude of each sample.

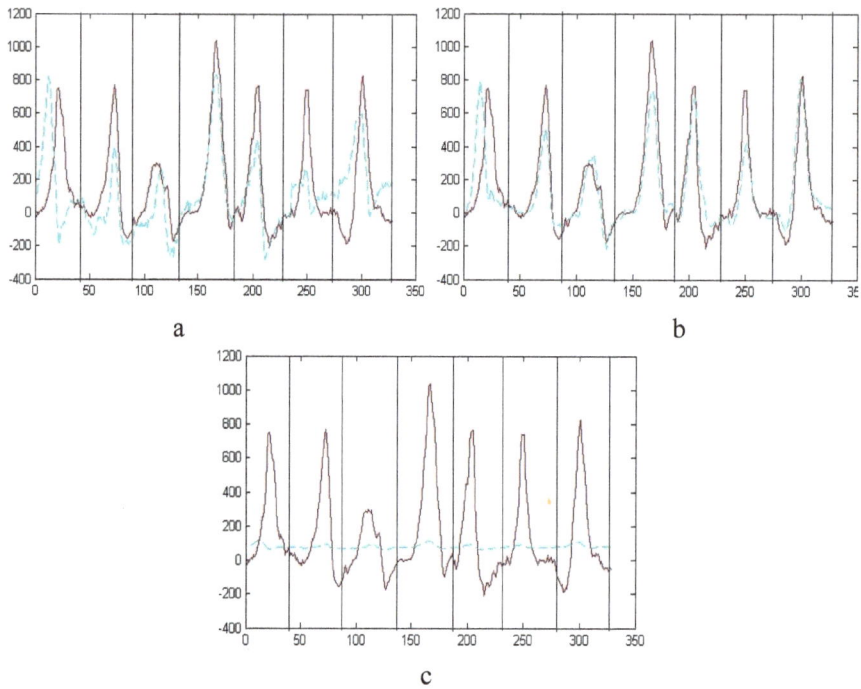

Figure 5: Extracted QRS segment from VCG signal (lead II) for 7 test samples using various methods. a) QRS segments in partial linear method, b) QRS segments in Dower method, c) QRS segments in Affine method,

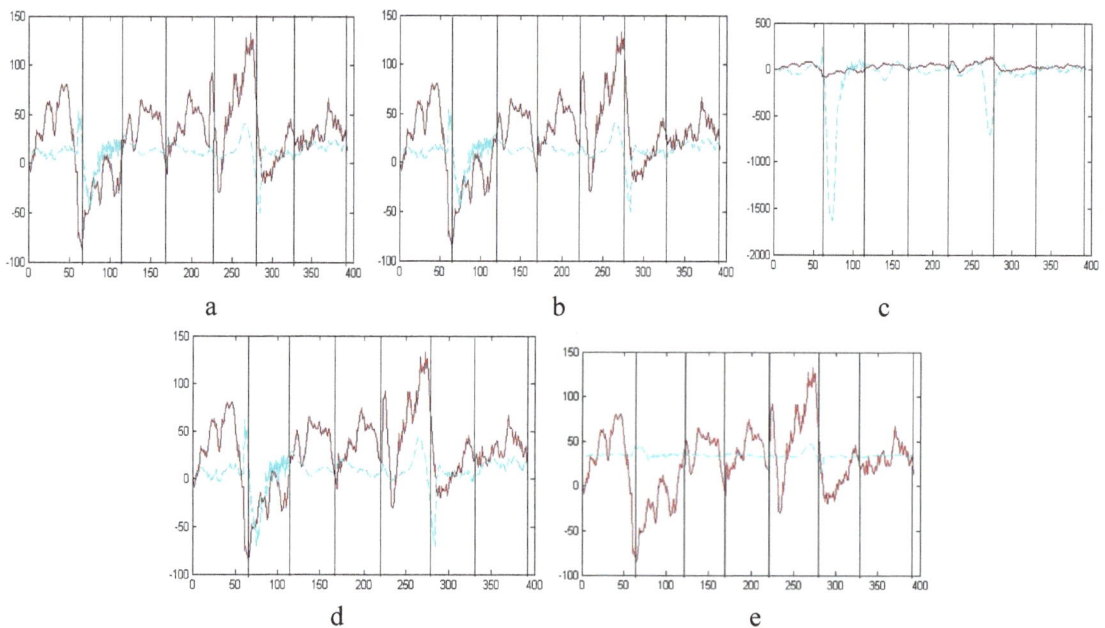

Figure 6: Extracted P segment from VCG signal (lead V_9) for 7 test samples using various methods. a) P segments in partial linear method, b) P segments in IGLS method, c) P segments in NL-RELS method, d) P segments in WLS partial linear method, e) P segments in affine method

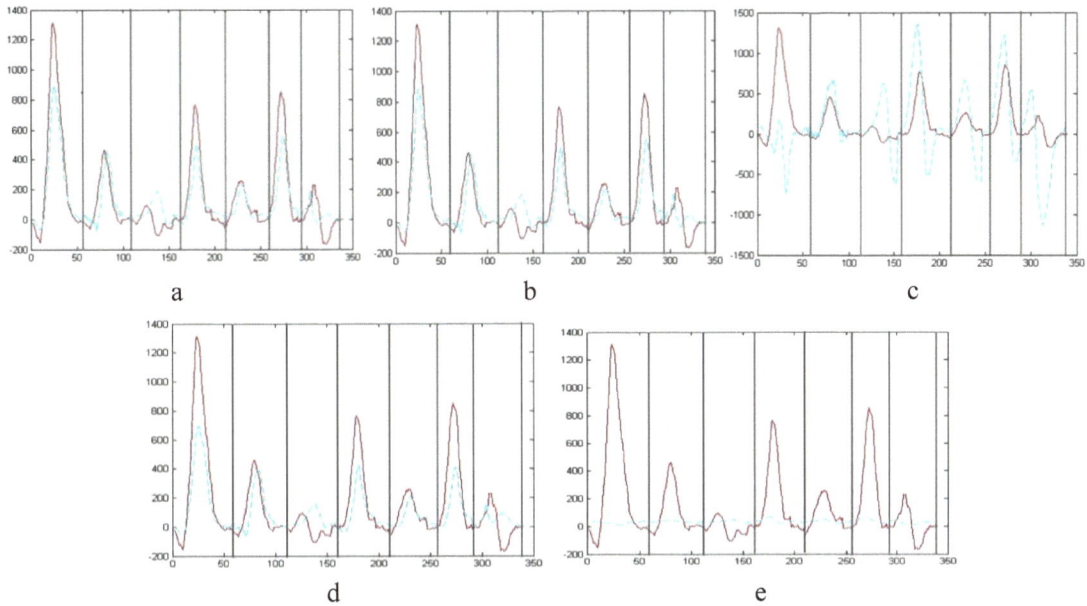

Figure 7: Extracted QRS segment from VCG signal (lead V_9) for 7 test samples using various methods. a) QRS segments in partial linear method, b) QRS segments in IGLS method c) QRS segments in NL-RELS method, d) QRS segments in WLS partial linear method Lead, e) QRS segments in affine method

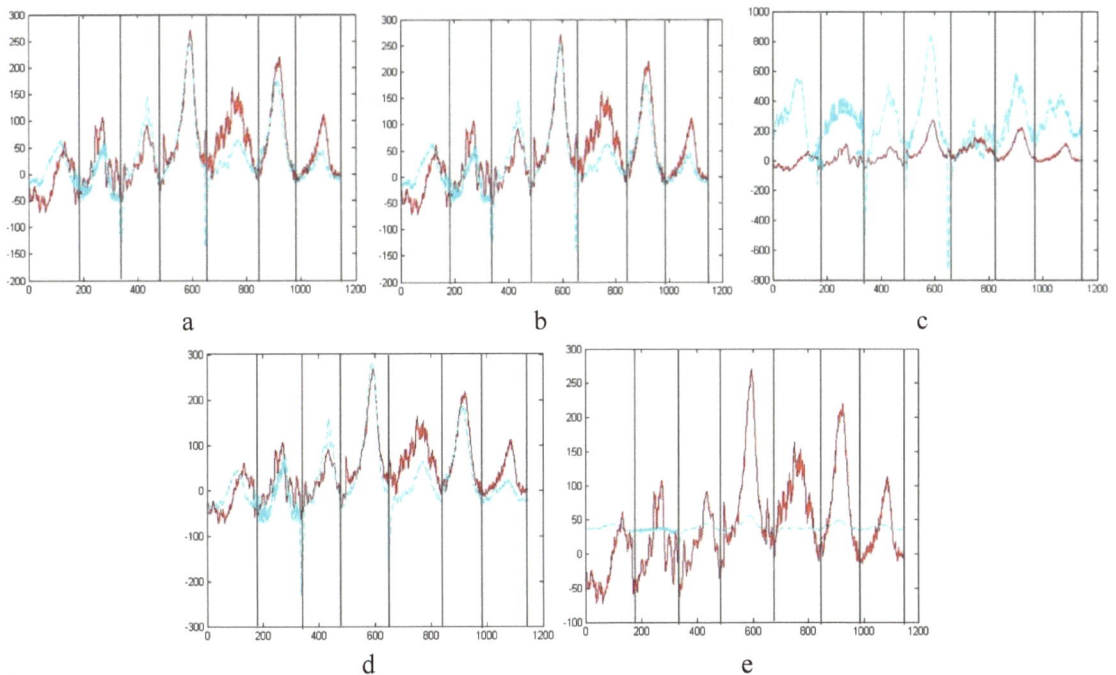

Figure 8: Extracted ST segment from VCG signal (lead V_9) for 7 test samples using various methods. a) ST segments in partial linear method, b) ST segments in IGLS method c)ST segments in NL-RELS method, d) ST segments in WLS partial linear method Lead, e) ST segments in affine method

As graphs showed we can see that the most similarity between real ECG and extracted one for both leads II and V9 is in partial linear method. After that figures of IGLS and WLS methods follow the real ECG and at last figures from NL-RELS, Affine and Dower methods have the least similarity to real ECG signal.

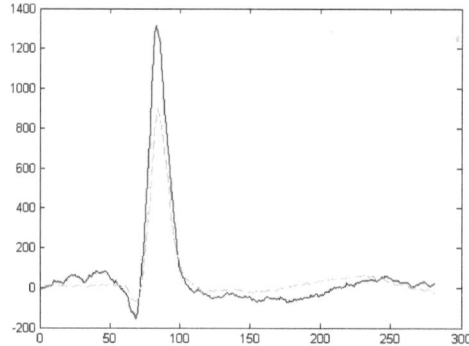

Figure 9: Comparison of real ECG and extracted one from VCG for all segments (P+QRS+ST) in partial linear transformation method.

In Figure 9, real ECG signal and extracted one for all segments (P, GRS, ST) and for just one case is showed that presents the similarity of 2 ECG signals in partial linear transformation method. Regarding the obtained results in this study, ECG signals that derived from VCG signals by using our methods (partial linear transformation, IGLS, RELS and weighted LS) had more similarity with general ECG leads than ones derived by using affine transformation. As a result by finding a reasonable and more accurate method for converting ECG and VCG signals to each other it would be possible to reach the information from all sides of the heart specially the posterior side of the heart (i.e., V_7, V_8, V_9 in original ECG) from VCG using partial linear transformation function. So, in some cardiac diseases like posterior MI and AF that they need information from posterior side of the heart walls to be detected, this method will be really useful and beneficial. Furthermore using partial linear transformation method makes it possible to take signal in VCG format only with 3 leads in emergency situation like in ambulance and transfer them to medical center. In medical center data can be transformed to ECG signals and be used by medical team. So capacity of data is decreased for telemedicine and taking signal is speed up.

At last it can be said that by providing total information from all sides of heart walls for cardiologist just from 3-lead VCG, it could be really helpful for them to have a better recognition of patient diseases, the time of diagnosing process would be decreased dramatically and sending and receiving ECG & VCG signals in telemedicine would be much easier.

References

Bishop CM. (1995). Neural Networks for Pattern Recognition, Oxford: Oxford University Press.

Comon P (1994). Independent Component Analysis: a new concept? Signal Processing, 36(3), 287–314.

Eriksson P, Andersen K, Swedberg K, Dellborg M. (1997). Vectorcardiographic monitoring of patients with acute myocardial infarction and chronic bundle branch block. Eur Heart J., 18(8), 1288–95.

Frank E. (1954). A direct experimentalstudy of threesystems of spatial vectorcardiography. Am HeartAssoc 101-113.

Frank E. (1956). An accurate, clinicallypractical system for spatial vectorcardiography. Am HeartAssoc, 737-749.

Hurd HP, Starling MR, Crawford MH, Dlabal PW, O'Rourke RA. (1981). Comparative accuracy of electrocardiographic and vectorcardiographic criteria for inferior myocardial infarction. Circulation. 63(5), 1025–9.

Jolliffe IT (2002). Principal Component Analysis, Springer (second edition).

Karsikasthe M (2011). New methods for vectorcardiographic signal processing. University of Oulu, PhD Thesis.

Rao CR, Toutenburg, Fieger A, Heumann C, Nittner T and Scheid S (1999). Linear Models: Least Squares and Alternatives. Springer Series in Statistics.

Strutz T (2010). Data Fitting and Uncertainty (A practical introduction to weighted least squares and beyond). Vieweg+Teubner. ISBN 978-3-8348-1022-9.

Cardiovascular Disease in Patients with Liver Cirrhosis

Margarida Antunes
Intensive Care Unit
Hospital Curry Cabral, Lisboa, Portugal

Susan Marum
Intensive Care Unit
Hospital Curry Cabral, Lisboa, Portugal

Paulo Marcelino
Intensive Care Unit
Hospital Curry Cabral, Lisboa, Portugal

1   Introduction

Cardiovascular diseases (CVD), mainly regarded as coronary artery disease and stroke, are the leading cause of mortality in western countries. Its incidence in patients with liver cirrhosis (LC) is still confounding but specific cardiovascular pathology in these patients is now well established. These include cirrhotic cardiomyopathy, hepatopulmonary syndrome and porto-pulmonary hypertension.

Nonetheless, cardiovascular complications in the patient with LC are a major cause of perioperative mortality and graft loss even in donor liver transplant recipients [1-4]. For these reasons, research has focused on this pathology, studying the potential reversibility of these cardiovascular alterations, early diagnosis and effective treatment. Although the specific cardiovascular conditions of LC are known for almost 60 years [5], its true prevalence remains unknown, perhaps because it was not observed in all patients with LC, but only in those with more advanced disease. Only recently the distinctive characteristics of ethanol-induced cardiomyopathy and LC-induced cardiomyopathy were recognized, and regular and careful previous cardiological evaluation usually fails its detection [6].

Apart from these facts, the hemodynamic profile of patients with LC is distinctive and deserves our best understanding. This may compromise patients in stressful situations, such as sepsis and after major surgery, including liver transplantation (LT).

2   Overview of Cardiovascular Disease in Liver Cirrhosis

Patients with LC present a higher mortality when compared to the general population [7,8]. For an adequate and accurate approach for this theme, it should be considered that the aetiology of LC is quite diverse, although in an end-stage condition there can be more unifying syndromes [9]. So, the natural history of each disease that evolves into LC must be taken into account: post-necrotic (viral), biliary tract diseases, liver steatosis, genetic conditions, alcohol consumption or even the presence of two or more risk factors.

Co-morbidities are important in this risk stratification and it includes the presence of CVD. Several authors studied the incidence of CVD in patients with LC. Kalaitzakis *et al* [10] studied this issue in a European population and found that although the incidence of coronary artery disease (CAD) was higher in patients with liver cirrhosis, it was independently related to the presence of diabetes, alcoholic aetiology and age . The same fact is reported for the risk of stroke in LC, although the incidence of intracranial bleeding is higher in these patients [11, 12], due to the inherent coagulopathy. It means that the actual incidence of CVD in patients with LC appears not to differ from general population although one finds it difficult to consider LC as a protective factor for CVD.

Patients with advanced LC have frequently lower levels of serum cholesterol and higher levels of serum triglycerides. However, it does not contribute to a hypothetical lower incidence of CVD in this group of patients. Nonetheless, known risk factors for the development of CVD in the general population are the most relevant, such as obesity, hypertension, hypercholesterolemia and diabetes. A distinctive incidence of CVD was observed in patients with LC due to specific conditions, such as non-alcoholic fatty liver disease and primary biliary cirrhosis [13-18]. In the first condition there is a plurimetabolic syndrome with severe fatty liver disease that can evolve into LC; the second condition regards a biliary system disease that, as a rule, is accompanied by hypercholesterolemia.

Heavy alcohol consumption is frequently present in patients with LC. The protective role of alcohol intake regarding CVD is to be established. In a nationwide study covering the years 1950 to 2002, Kerr *et al.* [19] found that a protective effect was noted for beer and wine consumption and a deleterious effect for stronger beverages. But it was also pointed that the incidence of CVD increased 1% per year and per litre of alcohol consumed, regardless of origin. This study may unveil other bias in this type of analysis, such as culture of drinking, genetic background and type of diet (Mediterranean versus non-Mediterranean). Another study by Kokolis *et al.* [20] verified that in a population which presented with chest pain, alcohol consumption was related with lower incidence of angiographically determined CAD, but related to systolic dysfunction. Based on these facts, it is not possible to determine that alcohol consumption protects from CVD, neither the right amount of consumption; it is not possible to distinguish the frontier between a healthy consumption and the development of other side effects, namely on the cardiac muscle.

There are muscular changes induced by alcohol consumption, called alcoholic myopathy [21]. It is characterized by atrophy of Type I muscle fibres (anaerobic, white glycolic), while Type II are relatively protected (aerobic, red oxidative). The clinical effect is reduced muscle mass, cramps, myalgia and difficulty in gait. It seems to affect more often chronic alcoholics than patients with pure alcoholic LC (incidence from 40-60% for the first group; 15-20% for the second). These changes also include the formation of acetaldehyde adducts, membrane changes and increases in cholesterol hyperoxides, inducing a radical-mediated damage to membrane. Although myopathy related to LC may be different, these patients are at increased risk for development of acute myopathy and rabdomyolisis [22, 23], as well as, more benign clinical entities such as muscle cramps [24]. Myocardial changes due to alcohol intake are also well known, and are mainly characterized by a pattern of dilated cardiomyopathy, undistinguished from other aetiologies. However, little data is available on myocardial changes due solely to LC. The course of progressive damage to the cardiovascular system can be silent and precipitate after stress manoeuvres, making both diagnosis and treatment, in most cases, late and difficult. This particular issue will be presented ahead as cirrhotic cardiomyopathy.

3   Electrophysiological Alterations in Liver Cirrhosis

In a study by Bernardi *et al.* [25] the incidence of prolonged corrected QT interval (QTc) was observed in 46.8% of patients. The factors associated with it were the CTP class and the serum norepinephrine levels. Other electrophysiological changes have been described in patients with cirrhosis such as rhythm disturbances, ventricular desynchrony and chronotropic incompetence. The rhythm disturbances more frequently reported are atrial fibrillation, atrial flutter and extrasystoles. These may be due to changes in the permeability of the cell plasma membrane [26]. The QTc interval is an indicator of ventricular depolarization and repolarization. Therefore, QTc prolongation is due to changes in myocardial repolarization and can lead to ventricular arrhythmias such as *Torsade de Pointes*, ventricular tachycardia, ventricular fibrillation and even sudden death [27]. The QT prolongation is more common when the etiology of cirrhosis is alcoholic than viral (83.3% vs 20%) [28]. Liver transplantation can improve the QTc interval of patients who have it prolonged [29]. Table 1 presents a list of common drugs that can prolong the QT interval.

Risk of *torsades de points* (strong evidence of QT prolongation when used as directed in label)	Amiodarone; Astemizol; Azithromycin; Chloroquine; Chlorpromazine; Cisapride; Citalopram; Clarithromycin; Disopyramide; domperidone; droperidol; erythromycin; escitalopram; flecainide; haloperidol; levomethadyl; mezoridasine; methadone; moxifloxacine; pentamidine; probucol; procainamide; quinidine; servoflurane; sotalol; thioridazine.
Potential risk (substantial evidence, but insufficient evidence as the effect if used as directed in the label)	Amantadine; atazanavir; chloral hydrate; clozapine; dolasetron; dronedarone; famotidine; fingolimod; foscarnet; phenytoin; gemifloxacin; ganisetron; indapamide; isradipine; levofloxacin; lithium; mirtazapine; nircadipine; octreotide; ofloxacin; olanzapine; ondasetron; oxytocin; quetiapine; risperidone; sunitinib; tacrolimus; tamoxifen; vardenafil; venlafaxine; voriconazol.
Conditional risk (evidence existing but only under certain conditions (over-dosage, drug interactions)	Amisulpiride; amitripyptiline; ciprofloxacin; diphenydramine; fluconazol; fluoxetin; imipramide; itraconazol; ketoconazol; paroxetin; ritonavir; sertraline; trazodone; trimethoprim/sulfamethoxazol;

Table 1: Common drugs that can prolong the QT interval

It has been suggested that an enhanced sympathetic activity can be responsible for this electrophysiological abnormality. Of notice, it was recently found that beta-blockers can induce higher mortality in patients with LC and refractory ascites [30]. This medication is part of the treatment for variceal bleeding as it decreases the porto-systemic pressure gradient. There is no plausible explanation for this fact, but it can be attributed to the influence of this class of drugs on the QT interval. Also, beta-blockers are nowadays a standard therapy for patients with heart failure. To understand this point one must look to the distinguishing hemodynamic profile of heart failure and LC.

4   Hemodynamic Alterations in Liver Cirrhosis

The main characteristics of the hemodynamic profile of heart failure patients are low cardiac output (CO), high peripheral vascular resistance (PVR) and signs of vascular congestion (high central venous pressure, high pulmonary capillary wedge pressure, dilated inferior vena cava without respiratory variation) [31].

In patients with heart failure the density of the beta receptors on the surface of the cardiomyocytes is low due to the internalization of the beta receptors secondary to the excess sympathetic activity; in this situation, the response to adrenergic stimuli can be affected. In patients, the use of beta-blockers can expose the internalized adrenergic receptors in a process that requires several weeks and that can initially worsen the symptoms; but with time, the higher density of these receptors on the surface of the cardiomyocytes can enhance the inotropic response to adrenergic stimuli and thus improve the systolic performance of the left ventricle.

The main cardiovascular disorders of the LC are portal hypertension and a permanent state of hyperdynamic circulation. The increased blood flow in the splanchnic bed exacerbates the portal hypertension and consequently increases the incidence of esophageal varices, variceal bleeding and ascites. Peripheral vasodilation also contributes to the pathophysiology of ascites, resulting in a decreased effective circulating volume, which is sensed by the kidney as hypovolemia, leading to salt and water retention.

In this state of hyperdynamic circulation of LC, heart rate (HR), CO and Left Ventricular Ejection Fraction (LVEF) are increased, and PVR, mean arterial pressure (MAP) and blood vessel contraction are decreased. The pathophysiology is multifactorial. It has been reported that arterial vasodilation activates the sympathetic nervous system and the renin-angiotensin-aldosterone system, resulting in a tachycardic response. Blood volume is decreased at a central level (heart, lungs and great vessels) and increased in the periphery (mainly the splanchnic circulation) . With the evolution of the illness, there are other precipitating factors of clinical worsening such as autonomic dysfunction and desensitization of myocardial beta-adrenergic receptors [32, 33] - conditioning hypo-responsiveness to treatment with vasoactive drugs - or nitration of cardiac proteins [34].

In an experimental model with rats with induced portal hypertension, a reduction in myocardial contractility and beta-adrenergic response was observed and the authors associated these findings with a possible altered excitation-contraction coupling, decreased sarcolemma L-type calcium channel density and reduced calcium in the sarcoplasmic reticulum [35]. In recent reports, an inadequate adrenergic stimulus due to the presence of a relative suprarenal insufficiency has been noticed. This inadequacy of the adrenergic system can lie on the basis of the incompetent response to stressful situations, ranging from exercise to severe medical conditions like sepsis or major surgery. Thus, it may not be possible to further increase the cardiac output or further decrease the peripheral systemic vascular resistance, the known adaptive phenomena to stress situations. If beta-blockers are added to the medication, this inadequate response can also be further compromised.

5   Cirrhotic Cardiomyopathy

For many years cirrhotic cardiomyopathy was thought to be due to alcoholic heart muscle disease. However, "cirrhotic cardiomyopathy" (CCM) is the term used to describe a group of features indicative of abnormal cardiac performance in cirrhotic patients which seems to be an independent entity, different from ethanol-induced cardiomyopathy [36].

Only scattered clinical studies have specifically studied the features of the CCM, which would justify that there are no diagnostic criteria widely accepted between experts. The working definition was proposed in the World Congress of Gastroenterology in Montreal (Canada) in 2005 and is detailed in Table 2. The main characteristics of this condition are depicted in Table 3.

CCM is defined as a chronic cardiac dysfunction in patients with LC characterized by a blunted response to stress, with systolic and/or diastolic dysfunction, electrophysiological changes and without known history of heart disease. There is little information about the epidemiology of such entity since its diagnosis is difficult due to near normal cardiac function at rest. Most of the patients are diagnosed during an episode of cirrhosis decompensation, probably having been assymptomatic during the first stages of the disease [37]. If CCM is not diagnosed in time or is treated improperly, it can lead to cardiac failure [38]. There have been reported rates up to 50% of pulmonary edema and 27% of haemodynamically significant arrhythmias in the perioperative period of orthotropic liver transplant (OLT) [39]. Fouad *et al.* in a study of 197 post-OLT patients found a prevalence close to 50% of cardiac decompensation, which was the main cause of death in these patients [40].

The pathogenesis of CCM is likely to be attributed to the increase of intra-abdominal pressure in cirrhotic patients, particularly those with ascites, resulting in an increased intrathoracic pressure and consequent myocardial dysfunction. However, as the CCM has been described in patients without ascites, it appears that other factors, not mechanical, could cause progressive cardiac deterioration. Within these factors, nitric oxide, TNFα, bile acids, endotoxin and beta-adrenergic receptor dysfunction have been proposed.

Systolic dysfunction	• Blunted increase in cardiac output with stress • Resting LVEF <55%
Diastolic dysfunction	• E/A ratio <1 • Prolonged DT (>200 msec) • Prolonged IVRT (>80 msec)
Supportive criteria	• Electrophysiological abnormalities • Altered chronotropic response • Electromechanical desynchrony • Prolonged QTc • Enlarged LA • Increased cardiac mass • Increased BNP/proBNP • Increased troponin I

Table 2: The working definition of cirrhotic cardiomyopathy (Montreal, 2005)

Altered function of β-adrenergic receptor: Several studies have demonstrated a reduced receptor density in cirrhotic patients and animal models.
Enhanced muscarinic tone that could contribute to the negative inotropic effect on the myocardium.
Altered membrane fluidity, these changes have a profound effect on the β-adrenoceptor function that includes impairing the receptor-ligand interaction; affects the function of membrane-bound ion channels (Ca^{++} and K^+) (3)
NO, carbon monoxide and endocannabinoids exerts a negative effect on cardiac contractility.

Table 3: Pathophysiological characteristics of cirrhotic cardiomyopathy

The histopathology of the CCM is nonspecific. The autopsy findings are increased ventricular volumes and mass, hypertrophy of cardiomyocytes, interstitial and intracellular edema and signs of cellular injury. The left ventricle (LV) is thickened and less compliant. These findings are more evident in patients with ascites [41], and they are more frequent in the LV that in the right ventricle [42].

Ventricular systolic function has been the most studied feature of CCM, which is normal at rest but, in situations of physical stress (surgery, infection, bleeding and exercise), psychological or pharmacological stress (dobutamine, sodium load) is affected [43]. In CCM the ejective period is shortened and pre-ejective time is lengthened [44].

Diastolic dysfunction is due to a defect in ventricular compliance that alters its physiological filling, which usually precedes systolic dysfunction in ischemic heart disease. However, this has not yet been demonstrated in cirrhotic patients. Some authors suggest that diastolic dysfunction is present in all cases of CCM and that the echocardiographic findings of a pathological E/A ratio may be sufficient for diagnosis [45] (se Figure 1). However, it has been described in most cirrhotic patients without cardiomyopathy, so its individual use for diagnosis is not enough.

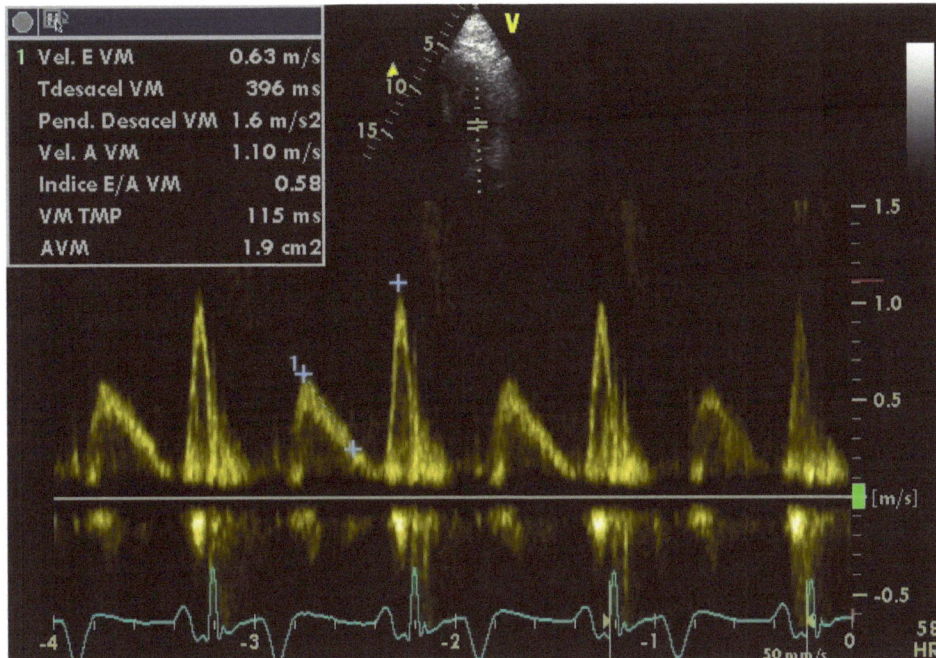

Figure 1: Diastolic dysfunction in a cirrhotic patient diagnosed during pre-transplantation echocardiographic study (E/A ratio <0.8, DTE >240.

Diastolic dysfunction in CCM may also be due to left ventricular hypertrophy, fibrosis or interstitial edema. If diastolic dysfunction is present, it will be more deteriorated after OLT, especially in the first 3 months [45]. It appears to be more common in patients with ascites and paracentesis improves diastolic and systolic functions [46]. Left ventricular hypertrophy (LVH) leads to an increased myocardial stiffness and, therefore, changes in contractility, relaxation and conductivity. In patients with LC, LVH is thought to be an adaptive phenomenon to the chronic overload of blood volume by retaining sodium and water. Therefore, in CCM we find a heart with increased ventricular mass, rigid, less compliant and proarrhythmogenic. Chronotropic incompetence is associated with increased risk of perioperative complications, greater incidence of arrhythmia and myocardial infarction. The failure to achieve 82% of predicted heart rate after dobutamine echocardiography was associated with an increased risk of death of almost 4 times in the first months after liver transplantation (22% versus 6%) [47]. We cannot however conclude that chronotropic incompetence is an independent predictor of mortality in patients with cirrhosis.

Limited studies suggested that, in an earlier stage of CCM, mechanical desynchrony preceded LV dysfunction - in fact, mechanical desynchrony is one of the diagnostic criteria in the working definition of CCM. Recently, Aljaroudi *et al.* [48] performed a study with 178 patients with LC who underwent stress-gated Tc-99m sestamibi myocardial perfusion imaging and found no differences in desynchrony indexes between survivors and non-survivors, and then concluded that in patients with LC there is insufficient evidence of a higher incidence of LV desynchrony.

The Transjugular Porto-systemic Shunt (TIPS) produces an acute increase in preload by shifting traffic from the portal vein circulation to the systemic circulation, leading to a worsening of the hyperdynamic state by increasing CO, bi-atrial end-diastolic volume and a decrease in SVR. It is estimated that 1% of cirrhotic patients without cardiac history developed heart failure after TIPS [49]. With TIPS, the central filling pressure increases more than 2 times and the stroke volume index increases up to 20% immediately [50]. Within two years, both CO and SVR tend to normalize, also occurring mild LV hypertrophy. These consequences are responsible for an increased probability of death in patients with CCM immediately after TIPS [51]. Another trigger for CCM is LT. In the perioperative period of LT, CCM is the third leading cause of death after rejection and infection [52]. 47% of patients have radiographic acute pulmonary edema immediately after OLT [53] and 3% developed new dilated cardiomyopathy in the first 6 months [54].

Several studies support the correlation between CCM and elevated laboratory parameters such as atrial natriuretic peptide (ANP), brain natriuretic peptide (BNP), pro-BNP and troponin I, which could be used in screening. It seems that ANP is less specific, since its alteration is related to atrial distension or distortion that can sometimes exist alongside effective hypovolemia [55]. Several studies have shown that when pro-BNP and BNP are elevated, these are related to the severity of cirrhosis, myocardial dysfunction, myocardial hypertrophy and QT prolongation [56, 57]. B-type natriuretic peptide (BNP) concentrations are higher in cirrhosis possibly due to the hyperdynamic state and cirrhotic cardiomyopathy. Pimenta et al. [58], in a study that included 83 patients hospitalized with decompensated cirrhosis, observed that BNP levels in cirrhosis reflects cardiac systolic function and is an independent predictor of medium-term survival in advanced cirrhosis. Median BNP levels were 130.3 (65.2 – 363.3) pg/ml, BNP levels above the median were associated with an increased occurrence of death within 6 months of discharge (p=0.023).

Troponin I is a key parameter for the diagnosis of myocardial ischemia and has also proved to be useful for diagnosis of other entities such as sepsis-induced myocardial dysfunction, hypertrophic cardiomyopathy and LC. Pateron et al. [59] showed that in patients with LC who had elevated serum troponin I, it correlated with lower left ventricular stroke volume and mass index.

Risk assessment with ECG, coronary angiography and myocardial perfusion scintigraphy has failed to predict a perioperative CCM. Late gadolinium enhancement (LGE) in cardiac magnetic resonance (CMR) was traditionally considered to be associated with cardiac fibrosis in ischemic heart disease, but it is also described in infiltrative cardiomyopathies, myocarditis and sepsis [60, 61]. Lössnitzer et al. [62] performed CMR in 20 patients with end-liver disease listed for liver transplantation and found hyperdynamic state and LGE in all of them, suggesting a common mechanism originating from cirrhosis. The pattern of LGE was patchy, similar to myocarditis [63], so it cannot be ruled a possible partial reversibility of LGE. A greater extent of LGE was found in patients with ethanol-induced cardiomyopathy. The authors suggested that CMR should be the gold standard for diagnosis of CCM [64].

The most common form to study the LV systolic function is by using the LVEF calculus measured by two-dimensional echocardiography and Simpson's modified biplane method. However, this approach has serious limitations because LVEF is preload and afterload-dependent. For the analysis of diastolic function, E / A ratio has been analysed in most reported studies of CCM, concluding that a ratio ≤1 is associated with increased mortality risk. The E / A ≤ 1 is present in 50-70% of patients with end-stage liver disease, being more evident with the progression of the disease (MELD ≥ 20), and lowest in patients with ascites [65]. However, E/A ratio is also preload dependent [66], which doesn't allow the diagnosis of a pseudo normal pattern (grade II diastolic dysfunction) and thus leads to underestimation of the real incidence of diastolic dysfunction in patients with LC.

For these reasons, recent studies using new echocardiographic technologies such as Doppler Tissue Imaging (DTI) are promising, since it lacks the limitations above cited and, therefore, becomes an attractive diagnostic tool [67]. Kazantov *et al.* [68], in a pioneer study using DTI, studied LV systolic and diastolic function at rest in 44 cirrhotic patients without previous known heart disease, and simultaneously analysed tissue velocities and strain rate in various segments of the LV in the same cineloop. They noted that all patients had systolic dysfunction and 54% had diastolic dysfunction (25% impaired diastolic relaxation pattern, 27% pseudo normal filling pattern and 2% restrictive filling pattern) at rest. These findings suggest that the current characterization of CCM is doubtful, further studies are needed in this field and that advanced methods such as echocardiography with DTI and Speckle Tracking may become the gold standard for diagnosis of CCM. Accumulating evidence also suggest that dobutamine stress echo test cannot be recommended routinely for the diagnosis of CCM, being reserved for patients with severe ischemic heart disease before transplantation [69].

Unfortunately there is no specific treatment for CCM [70]. Few treatments have been proposed to date and many of them are just experimental. The clinical management of patients with CCM will be, therefore, with supportive measures, treating heart failure as if it they were not cirrhotic patients. Accumulating evidence also suggests the use of cardioprotective therapy - beta-blockers, statins, angiotensin-converting enzyme inhibitors or anti-aldosterone agents could have a very important role [71-74].

Albumin dialysis using the Molecular Adsorbent Recirculating System (MARS) has been shown to improve hemodynamic status of patients with end-liver disease decreasing the levels of nitric oxide, TNFα and intrahepatic vasoconstriction. These effects disappeared four days after cessation of MARS. (75, 76). However, it has not shown improved survival in patients treated. LT is one of the treatments proposed for the CCM, but the high incidence of perioperative complications in these patients makes this option be reconsidered.

6   Porto-pulmonary Hypertension (PPH)

PPH is defined by criteria obtained by right heart catheterization in patients with portal hypertension (PoH): elevated mean pulmonary artery pressure (>25 mmHg at rest or > 30 mmHg with exercise), increased pulmonary vascular resistance (> 240 dynes s/cm^5), normal pulmonary artery occlusion pressure (<15 mmHg). Its prevalence varies according to the population studied being that in patients with end-stage liver disease it can range from 3.5 to 16.1% [77, 78].

PoH either precedes or is diagnosed concurrently with PPH, supporting the hypothesis that the pathogenesis of PPH may be related to vasoactive substances not metabolized or produced by the cirrhotic liver that are found in the pulmonary circulation. It is thought that these mediators possibly induce vasoconstriction or direct toxic damage to the pulmonary arteries, since high concentrations of mediators such as serotonin, interleukin-1, endothelin-1, glucagon, secretin and thromboxane A2 have been found in plasma of patients with PoH [79, 80].

Early stage of PPH is generally asymptomatic or patients may have symptoms of the underlying liver disease. With advancing disease exertional dyspnea is the most frequent presenting symptom of PPH (81%); other symptoms, such as syncope, chest pain, and fatigue, are seen in a third of the patients. Most importantly, this specific entity is quite important, due to the fact that is a contraindication for liver transplantation. The pre-transplant screening of signs of right heart overload using echocardiography is therefore mandatory.

7   Hepato-pulmonary Syndrome (HPS)

The HPS is characterized by a defect in arterial oxygenation induced by pulmonary vascular dilation and pulmonary arterial-venous shunting in the setting of liver disease. It has been reported to be present in 4 to 29% of patients with liver disease [81-83] and from 15 to 30% in patients waiting for LT.

HPS can affect all ages and occasionally occur in non-cirrhotic patients with portal hypertension (PoH) and may also been reported in mild liver disease. The exact mechanism of pathogenesis is unclear but it can be the result of alteration in the production or clearance of chemical mediators causing intrapulmonary vascular vasodilatation and arteriovenous shunting through the lungs with a ventilation-perfusion mismatch. Hypoxia occurs as a result of inability of oxygen to diffuse through the markedly dilated lung capillaries. The capillaries are known to dilate to 15–500 μm (n = 8–15 μm) in HPS. There is a pulmonary vascular dilation, intrapulmonary shunts and low pulmonary vascular resistance, which seems to be due to the effect of multiple vasoactive substances; some studies point to increase NO levels in cirrhotic patients. According to the alveolar-capillary disequilibrium hypothesis, pulmonary vascular dilation and intrapulmonary shunts in patients with liver cirrhosis are the leading contributors to hypoxemia in advanced liver disease. The low pulmonary vascular resistance leads to a reduction in the intrapulmonary transit time, subsequently a decreased oxygen diffusion across the dilated pulmonary vessels. Another pattern of intrapulmonary vascular dilation is characterized by localized dilation of parts of the pulmonary vasculature and is associated with large arteriovenous shunting, with poor response to oxygen supplementation (84). This syndrome is characterized by the presence of liver disease, pulmonary vascular vasodilatation, associated with significant arteriovenous shunting (AVS) and hypoxemia; capillary vasodilatation is most pronounced at the lung bases, explaining orthodeoxia and platypnea associated with HPS. VQ mismatch appears to be a major event in the pathogenesis of hypoxemia in HPS as a result of extensive pulmonary vasodilatation, a decrease in V/Q ratio in alveolar-capillary units and resultant low PO_2 and O_2 content of blood leaving the lungs; defect in oxygenation, Due to pulmonary capillaries dilatation oxygen encounters difficulty in diffusing into the center of the larger capillaries. Increased cardiac output and the associated reduced transition time of blood through the pulmonary vascular bed also impair diffusion, leading to a diffusion–perfusion defect or alveolar capillary oxygen disequilibrium.

Clinical presentation is characterized by dyspnea of insidious onset associated with cyanosis in 90% of all cases, platypnea and orthodeoxia. The presence of clubbing has the highest positive predictive value (75%) and dyspnea the highest negative predictive value (100%) for HPS. Spider nevi are a common clinical feature of patients with HPS with significant relationship between cutaneous spider angiomata and systemic and pulmonary vasodilatation suggesting that spider nevi may represent a cutaneous marker for intrapulmonary vascular dilatation.

Two types of HPS have been described: Type I is associated with vascular dilation at the precapillary level close to the normal gas exchange units of the lung and Type II with focal larger dilations amounting to AVS distant from the gas exchange units. Supplementary oxygen improves Type I HPS PaO_2 but not Type 2 HPS [84].

The HPS is associated with an increased risk of death - the median survival time in cirrhotic patients has been reported as 10,6 months compared to 40,8 months in cirrhotic patients without HPS. The leading cause of death is hemorrhagic shock due to gastrointestinal bleeding. Survival is worse with base-line PaO_2 < 50 mmHg irrespective of the decision to perform LT [85, 86]. The diagnosis relies on imaging techniques and arterial gas analysis. The cut-off values for PaO_2 are controversial. Schenk and colleagues suggested that arterial hypoxemia defined as a PaO_2<70 mmHg or below the age-related threshold predicted the presence of HPS with high probability in the absence of intrinsic cardiopulmonary diseases. A chest radiograph (CXR) and pulmonary function tests must be used to help exclude other causes of hypoxia such as pulmonary atelectasis, ascites, chronic obstructive pulmonary disease, hepatic hydrothorax. A definitive diagnosis of HPS can be made by demonstration of pulmonary vasodilation associated with functional arteriovenous shunting. Imaging studies that can identify such shunts include contrast echocardiography and perfusion scintigraphy with 99mTc, which are usually carried out following analysis of arterial gases to identify elevated alveolar-arterial differences in O_2 or hypoxemia.

Most patients being cared for in hospital setting have undergone a conventional CXR, which is not only useful in the diagnosis of HPS but is crucial for excluding other causes of hypoxemia. A CXR in HPS shows bibasilar nodular or reticulonodular opacities in 5–13.8% of patients with chronic liver disease and 46–100% of patients with HPS. High-resolution computed tomography (CT) is useful in excluding pulmonary fibrosis or emphysema as the cause of these opacities.

Liver transplantation is the only definitive treatment for HPS with at least 85% of patients experiencing significant improvement or complete resolution of hypoxemia following surgery; however these patients have a higher post-transplant mortality rate related to pulmonary hypertension, cerebral embolic hemorrhages and prolonged mechanical ventilation. [84] Several therapeutic trials in HPS have shown poor results such as somatostatin analogues, cyclooxygenase inhibitors, and immunosuppressive agents such as corticosteroids and cyclophosphamide. [87]. Some reports have shown improvement in gas exchange with the use of TIPS in HPS [88]. Martínez-Pallí G et al. [89] in another study concluded that TIPS neither improved nor worsened pulmonary gas exchange in patients with portal hypertension and the data does not support the use of TIPS as a specific treatment for HPS.

8   Non Alcoholic Fatty Liver Disease (NAFLD)

NAFLD is defined as the presence of hepatic steatosis in the absence of other cause for secondary hepatic fat accumulation. It is known that it can progress to cirrhosis and is thought to be a major cause of cryptogenic cirrhosis [90]. The prevalence of NAFLD in the US is 20-30%, with a greatest incidence in the fifth decade of life [91]. It is associated with other metabolic disorders such as diabetes, dyslipidemia, hypertension and obesity and is, thus, a known risk factor for cardiovascular disease [92]. However, recent studies have also shown that patients with NAFLD but with no hypertension, diabetes or previous heart condition, have cardiac function abnormalities, such as echocardiographic features of early LV diastolic dysfunction and impaired LV energy metabolism [93-95].

Rijzewijk et al. [96] has conducted a study on diabetic type 2 patients where it was found that on those with a higher degree of liver steatosis, there was an impaired myocardial perfusion and lower high-energy phosphates content on P-magnetic resonance spectroscopy but similar values of LV function and morphology on MRI. Abnormalities, such as echocardiographic features of early LV diastolic dysfunction and impaired LV energy.

Another recent study by Bonapace et al [97] has made a similar evaluation and it is proposed that the systemic release of inflammatory mediators from the steatotic liver may lead to the abnormality of cardiac function, whether possibly through subclinical myocardial infarction or ectopic deposition of fat in different organs, including the myocardium [98]. Nevertheless, recent data are conflicting, suggesting a complex relationship between these entities. Further studies are necessary to enlighten the mechanisms through which NAFLD leads to diastolic cardiac dysfunction [99, 100].

References

1. Raval, Z., Harinstein, M.E., Skaro, A.I., Erdogan, A., DeWolf, A.M., Shah, S.J., Fix, O.K., Kay, N., Abecassis, M.I., Gheorghiade, M., Flaherty, J.D. (2011) Cardiovascular Risk assessment of the Liver Transplant Candidate. J Am Coll Cardiol., 58(3):223-31.

2. Johnston, S.D., Morris, J.K., Cramb, R., Gunson, B.K., Neuberger, J. (2002) Perioperative considerations in Patients with Cirrhotic Cardiomyopathy. Transplantation, 73(6):901-6.

3. Desai, S., Hong, J.C., Saab, S. (2010) Cardiovascular Risk Factors following Orthotopic Liver Transplantation: predisposing factors, incidence and management. Liver Int., 30(7):948-57.

4. Mackram, F., Eleid, R., Hurst, T., Vargas, H., Rakela, J., Mulligan, D., Appleton, C. (2010) Short-Term Cardiac and Noncardiac Mortality Following Liver Transplantation. Journal of Transplantation, Article ID 910165.

5. Kowalski, H.J., Abelmann, W.H. (1953) The cardiac output at rest in Laennec's cirrhosis. J Clin Invest, 32:1025-1033.

6. Alqahtani, S.A., Fouad, T.R., Lee, S.S. (2008) Cirrhotic cardiomyopathy. Semin Liver Dis, 28(1):5-69.

7. Fouad, T.R., Abdel-Razek, W.M., Burak, K.W., Bain, V.G., Lee, S.S. (2009) Prediction of cardiac complications after liver transplantation. Transplantation, 87(5):763-770.

8. Fleming, K.M., Aithal, G.P., Card, T.R., West, J. (2012) All-cause mortality in people with cirrhosis compared with the general population: a population-based cohort study. Liver Int., 32(1):79-84.

9. Jepsen, P., Vilstrup, H., Andersen, P.K., Lash, T.L., Sørensen, H.T. (2008) Comorbidity and survival of Danish cirrhosis patients: a nationwide population-based cohort study. Hepatology, 48(1):214-20.

10. Kalaitzakis, E., Rosengren, A., Skommevik, T., Björnsson, E. (2010) Coronary artery disease in patients with liver cirrhosis. Dig Dis Sci., 55(2):467-75.

11. Grønbaek, H., Johnsen, S.P., Jepsen, P., Gislum, M., Vilstrup, H., Tage-Jensen, U., Sørensen, H.T. (2008) Liver cirrhosis, other liver diseases, and risk of hospitalisation for intracerebral haemorrhage: a Danish population-based case-control study. BMC Gastroenterol., 8:16.

12. Huang, H.H., Lin, H.H., Shih, Y.L., Chen, P.J., Chang, W.K., Chu, H.C., Chao, Y.C., Hsieh, T.Y. (2008) Spontaneous intracranial hemorrhage in cirrhotic patients. Clin Neurol Neurosurg., 110(3):253-8.

13. Solaymani-Dodaran, M., Aithal, G.P., Card, T., West, J. (2008) Risk of cardiovascular and cerebrovascular events in primary biliary cirrhosis: a population-based cohort study. Am J Gastroenterol., 103(11):2784-8.

14. Kadayifci, A., Tan, V., Ursell, P.C., Merriman, R.B., Bass (2008) Clinical and pathologic risk factors for atherosclerosis in cirrhosis: a comparison between NASH-related cirrhosis and cirrhosis due to other aetiologies. NMJ Hepatol, 49(4):595-9.

15. Caldwell, S., Argo, C. (2010) The natural history of non-alcoholic fatty liver disease. Dig Dis., 28(1):162-8.

16. Chen, Y.H., Chen, K.Y., Lin, H.C. (2011) Non-alcoholic cirrhosis and the risk of stroke: a 5-year follow-up study. Liver Int., 31(3):354-60.

17. Wong, V.W., Wong, G.L., Yip, G.W., Lo, A.O., Limquiaco, J., Chu, W.C., Chim, A.M., Yu, C.M., Yu, J., Chan, F.K., Sung, J.J., Chan, H.L. (2011) Coronary artery disease and cardiovascular outcomes in patients with non-alcoholic fatty liver disease. Gut, 60(12):1721-7.

18. Arslan, U., Türkoğlu, S., Balcioğlu, S., Tavil, Y., Karakan, T., Cengel, A. (2007) Association between nonalcoholic fatty liver disease and coronary artery disease. Coron Artery Dis, 18(6):433-6.

19. Kerr, W.C., Karriker-Jaffe, K., Subbaraman, M., Ye, Y. (2011) Per capita alcohol consumption and ischemic heart disease mortality in a panel of US states from 1950 to 2002. Addiction, 106(2):313-22.

20. Kokolis, S., Marmur, J.D., Clark, L.T., Kassotis, J., Kokolis, R., Cavusoglu, E., Lapin, R., Breitbart, S., Lazar, J.M. (2006) Effects of alcoholism on coronary artery disease and left ventricular dysfunction in male veterans. J Invasive Cardiol., 18(7):304-7.

21. Lee, O.J., Yoon, J.H., Lee, E.J., Kim, H.J., Kim, T.H. (2006) Acute myopathy associated with liver cirrhosis. World J Gastroenterol, 12(14):2254-8.

22. Dopazo, C., Bilbao, I., Lázaro, J.L., Sapisochin, G., Caralt, M., Blanco, L., Castells, L., Charco, R. (2009) Severe rhabdomyolysis and acute renal failure secondary to concomitant use of simvastatin with rapamycin plus tacrolimus in liver transplant patient. Transplant Proc, 41(3):1021-4.

23. Jones, J.C., Coombes, J.S., Macdonald, G.A. (2012) Exercise capacity and muscle strength in patients with cirrhosis. Liver Transpl, 18(2):146-51.

24. Chatrath, H., Liangpunsakul, S., Ghabril, M., Otte, J., Chalasani, N., Vuppalanchi, R. Prevalence and morbidity associated with muscle cramps in patients with cirrhosis.

25. Bernardi, M., Maggioli, C., Dibra, V., Zaccherini, G. (2012) QT interval prolongation in liver cirrhosis: innocent bystander or serious threat? Expert Rev Gastroenterol Hepatol., 6(1):57-66.

26. Zambruni, A., Trevisani, F., Caraceni, P., Bernardi, M. (2006) Cardiac electrophysiological abnormalities in patients with cirrhosis. J Hepatol, 44:994-1002.

27. Mandell, M.S., Lindenfeld, J., Tsou, M.Y., Zimmerman, M. (2008) Cardiac evaluation of liver transplant candidates. World J Gastroenterol, 14:3445-3451.

28. Sun, F.R., Wang, B.Y., Tong, J., et al. (2011) Relationship between model for end-stage liver disease and left ventricular function in patients with end-stage liver disease. Hepatobiliary Pancreat Dis Int, 10:50-54.

29. Bal, J.S., Thuluvath, P.J. (2003) Prolongation of QTc interval: relationship with aetiology and severity of liver disease, mortality and liver transplantation. Liver Int, 23:243-248.

30. Sersté, T., Melot, C., Francoz, C., Durand, F., Rautou, P.E., Valla, D., Moreau, R., Lebrec, D. (2010) Deleterious effects of beta-blockers on survival in patients with cirrhosis and refractory ascites. Hepatology., 52(3):1017-22.

31. Iwakiri, Y., Groszmann, R. (2006) The hyperdynamic circulation of chronic liver diseases: from the patient to the molecule. Hepatology, 43:S121-31.

32. Lee, S.S., Marty, J., Mantz, J., et al. (1990) Desensitization of myocardial beta-adrenergic receptors in cirrhotic rats. Hepatology, 12:481-485.

33. Ma, Z., Meddings, J.B., Lee, S. (1994) Membrane physical properties determine cardiac beta-adrenergic receptor function in cirrhotic rats. Am J Physiol, 267:G87-93.

34. Manny, A.R., Ippolito, S., Ollosson, R., Moore, K.P. (2006) Nitration of cardiac proteins is associated with abnormal cardiac chronotropic responses in rats with biliary cirrhosis. Hepatology, 43:847-856.

35. Zavecz, J.H., Battarbee, H.D., Bueno, O.F., et al. (2000) Cardiac excitation-contraction coupling in the portal hypertensive rat. Am J Physiology-Gastrointestinal and Liver Phys, 279:G28-29.

36. Gaskari, S.A., Honar, H., Lee, S.S. (2006) Therapy insight: Cirrhotic cardiomyopathy. Nat Clin Pract Gastroenterol Hepatol, 3:329-337.

37. Zardi, E., Abbate, A., Zardi, D.M., Dobrina, A., Margiotta, D., Van Tassel, B.W., Afeltra, A., Sanyal, A.J. (2010) Cirrhotic Cardiomyopathy. Journal of the American College of Cardiology Vol. 56, No. 7.

38. Donovan, C.L., Marcovitz, P.A., Punch, J.D., et al. (1996) Two-dimensional and dobutamine stress echocardiography in the preoperative assessment of patients with end-stage liver disease prior to orthotopic liver transplantation. Transplantation, 61(8):1180-1188.

39. Lee, F., Glenn, T.K., Lee, S.S. (2007) Cardiac dysfunction in cirrhosis. Best Pract Res Clin Gastroenterol, 21:125-140.

40. Pozzi, M., Redaelli, E., Ratti, L., et al. (2005) Time-course of diastolic dysfunction in different stages of chronic HCV related liver diseases. Minerva Gastroenterol Dietol, 51:179-186.

41. Alexander, J., Mishra, P., Desai, N., et al. (2007) Cirrhotic cardiomyopathy: Indian scenario. J Gastroenterol Hepatol, 22:395-399.

42. Milani, A., Zaccaria, R., Bombardieri, G., et al. (2007) Cirrhotic cardiomyopathy. Dig Liver Dis, 39:507-515.

43. Wong, F., Girgrah, N., Graba, J., Allidina, Y., Liu, P., Blendis, L. (2001) The cardiac response to exercise in cirrhosis. Gut, 49:268-275.

44. Torregrosa, M., Aguade, S., Dos, L., et al. (2005) Cardiac alterations in cirrhosis: reversibility after liver transplantation. J Hepatol, 42:68-74.

45. Pozzi, M., Carugo, S., Boari, G., et al. (1997) Evidence of functional and structural cardiac abnormalities in cirrhotic patients with and without ascites. Hepatology, 26:1131-37.

46. Umphrey, L.G., Hurst, R.T., Eleid, M.F., et al. (2008) Preoperative dobutamine stress echocardiographic findings and subsequent short-term adverse cardiac events after orthotopic liver transplantation. Liver Transpl, 14:886-892.

47. Harinstein, M.E., Flaherty, J.D., Ansari, A.H., et al. (2008) Predictive value of dobutamine stress echocardiography for coronary artery disease detection in liver transplant candidates. Am J Transplant, 1523-1528.

48. Aljaroudi, W., Aggarwal, H., Igbal, F., Heo, J., Iskandrian, A.E. (2011) Left ventricular desynchrony in patients with LC. J Nucl Cardiol, 18(3):451-455.

49. Gazzera, C., Roghi, D., Valle, F., et al. (2009) Fifteen years' experience with transjugular intrahepatic portosystemic shunt (TIPS) using bare stents: retrospective review of clinical and technical aspects. Radiol Med, 114:83-94.

50. Kovacs, A., Schepke, M., Heller, J., et al. (2010) Short-term effects of transjugular intrahepatic shunt on cardiac function assessed by cardiac MRI: preliminary results. Cardiovasc Intervent Radiol, 33(2):290-6.

51. Braverman, C., Steiner, M.A., Picus, D., White, H. (1995) High-output congestive heart failure following transjugular intrahepatic portal-systemic shunting. Chest, 107(5):1467-1469.

52. Therapondos, G., Flapan, A.D., Plevris, J.N., Hayes, P.C. (2005) Cardiac morbidity and mortality related to orthotopic liver transplantation. Liver Transpl, 10:1441-1453.

53. Snowden, C.P., Hughes, T., Rose, J., Roberts, D.R. (2000) Pulmonary edema in patients after liver transplantation. Liver Transpl, 6:466-470.

54. Dec, G.W., Kondo, N., Farrell, M.L., et al. (1995) Cardiovascular complications following liver transplantation. Clin Transplant, 9:463-471.

55. Rector Jr, W.G., Adair, O., Hossack, K.F., Rainquet, S. (1990) Atrial volume in cirrhosis: relationship to blood volume and plasma concentrations of atrial natriuretic factor. Gastroenterology, 99:776-770.

56. Wong, F., Siu, S., Liu, P., Blendis, L.M. (2001) Brain natriuretic peptide: is it a predictor of cardiomyopathy in cirrhosis? Clin Sci, 101:621-628.

57. Henriksen, J.H., Gotze, J.P., Fuglsang, S., et al. (2003) Increased circulating pro-brain natriuretic peptide (proBNP) and brain natriuretic peptide (BNP) in patients with cirrhosis: relation to cardiovascular dysfunction and severity of disease. Gut, 52:1511-1517.

58. Pimenta, J., Paulo, C., Gomes, A., Silva, S., Rocha-Gonçalves, F., Bettencourt, P. (2010) B-type natriuretic peptide is related to cardiac function and prognosis in hospitalized patients with decompnesated cirrhosis. Liver International, Vol. 30, pp. 1059 – 1066.

59. *Pateron, D., Beune, P., Laperche, T., et al. (1999) Elevated circulating cardiac troponin I in patients with cirrhosis. Hepatology, 29:640-643.*

60. *Bernal, V., Pascual, I., Esquivias, P., García-Gil, A., Fernández, C., Mateo, J.M., González, M., Simón, M.A. (2009) Cardiac hemodynamic profiles and pro-B-type natriuretic Peptide in cirrhotic patients undergoing liver transplantation. Transplant Proc., 41(3):985-6.*

61. *Ruiz-Bailén, M., Romero-Bermejo, F.J., Rucabado-Aguilar, L., et al. (2010) Myocardial dysfunction in the critically ill patient: is it really reversible? Int J Cardiol, 145(3):615-6.*

62. *Lossnitzer, D., Steen, H., Zahn, A., Lehrke, S., Weiss, C., Weiss, K.H., Giannitsis, E., Stremmel, W., Sauer, P., Katus, H.A., Gotthardt, D.N. (2010) Myocardial late gadolinium enhancement cardiovascular magnetic resonance in patients with cirrhosis. J Cardiovasc Magn Reson, 13;12:47.*

63. *Friedrich, M.G. (2008) Tissue characterization of acute myocardial infarction and myocarditis by cardiac magnetic resonance. JACC Cardiovasc Imaging, 1(5):652-662.*

64. *Goitein, O., Matetzky, S., Beinart, R., et al. (2009) Acute myocarditis: Non-invasive evaluation with cardiac MRI and transthoracic echocardiography. AJR Am J Roentgenol, 192(1):254-258.*

65. *Valeriano, V., Funaro, S., Lionetti, R., et al. (2000) Modification of cardiac function in cirrhotic patients with and without ascites. Am J Gastroenterol, 95:3200-3205.*

66. *Abeles, R.D., Shawcross, D.L., Auzinger, G. (2007) E/A ratio alone cannot reliably diagnose diastolic dysfunction in the assessment before and after TIPS. Gut, 56:1642.*

67. *Andersen, U.B., Moller, S., Bendtsen, F., Henriksen, J.H. (2003) Cardiac output determined by echocardiography in patients with cirrhosis: comparison with the indicator dilution technique. Eur J Gastroenterol Hepatol, 15:503-7.*

68. *Kazantov, K., Holland-Fischer, P., Andersen, N.H., et al. (2011) Resting myocardial dysfunction in cirrhosis quantified by tissue Doppler imaging. Liver Int, 31(4):534-40.*

69. *Moller, S., Henriksen, J.H. (2010) Cirrhotic cardiomyopathy. J Hepatol, 53:179-190.*

70. *Gaskari, S.A., Honar, H., Lee, S.S. (2006) Therapy insight: Cirrhotic cardiomyopathy. Nat Clin Pract Gastroenterol Hepatol, 3:329-337.*

71. *Brilla, C.G., Matsubara, L., Weber, K.T. (1993) Antifibrotic effects of spironolactone in preventing myocardial fibrosis in systemic arterial hypertension. Am J Cardiol, 71:12A-6.*

72. *Bos, R., Mougenot, N., Findji, L., et al. (2005) Inhibition of catecholamine-induced cardiac fibrosis by an aldosterone antagonist. J Cardiovasc Pharmacol, 45:8-13.*

73. *Zambruni, A., Trevisani, F., Di Micoli, A., et al. (2008) Effect of chronic beta-blockade on QT interval in patients with liver cirrhosis. J Hepatol, 48:415-421.*

74. *Abraldes, J.G., Albillos, A., Bañares, R., et al. (2009) Simvastatin lowers portal pressure in patients with cirrhosis and portal hypertension: A randomized controlled trial. Gastroenterology, 136:1651-8.*

75. *Catalina, M.V., Barrio, J., Anaya, F., et al. (2003) Hepatic and systemic haemodynamic changes after MARS in patients with acute on chronic liver failure. Liver Int, 23(Suppl 3):39-43.*

76. *Sen, S., Mookerjee, R.P., Cheshire, L.M., et al. (2005) Albumin dialysis reduces portal pressure acutely in patients with severe alcoholic hepatitis. J Hepatol, 43:142-148.*

77. *Benjaminov, F.S., Prentice, M., Sniderman, K.W., et al. (2003) Portopulmonary hypertension in decompensated cirrhosis with refractory ascites. Gut, 52:1355.*

78. *Castro, M., Krowka, M.J., Schroeder, D.R., et al. (1996) Frequency and clinical implications of increased pulmonary artery pressures in liver transplant patients. Mayo Clin Proc, 71:543.*

79. *Khan, A.N., Al-Jahdali, H., Abdullah, K., Irion, K.L., Sabih, Q., Gouda, A. (2011) Pulmonary vascular complications of chronic liver disease: Pathophysiology, imaging, and treatment. Annals of Thoracic Medicine, 6:57 – 65.*

80. Robalino, B.D., Moodie, D.S. (1991) Association between primary pulmonary hypertension and portal hypertension: analysis of its pathophysiology and clinical, laboratory and hemodynamic manifestations. J Am Coll Cardiol, 17: 492 – 498.

81. Hoeper, M.M., Krowka, M.J., Strassburg, C.P. (2004) Portopulmonary hypertension and hepatopulmonary syndrome. Lancet, 363.

82. Martinez, G.P., Barbera, J.A., Visa, J., et al. (2001) Hepatopulmonary syndrome in candidates for liver transplantation. J Hepatol, 34:651-657.

83. Huffmyer, J.L., Nemergut, E.C. (2007) Respiratory dysfunction and pulmonary disease in cirrhosis and other hepatic disorders. Respir Care, 52:1030-1036.

84. Cortese, D.A., Krowka, M.J. (1994) Hepatopulmonary syndrome - Current concepts in diagnostic and therapeutic considerations. Chest, 105: 1528 – 1537.

85. Krowka, M.J., Cortese, D.A. (1990) Hepatopulmonary syndrome: an evolving perspective in the era of liver transplantation. Hepatology, 11: 54 - 58.

86. Swanson, K.L., Wiesner, R.H., Krowka, M.J. (2005) Natural history of hepatopulmonary syndrome: Impact of liver transplantation. Hepatology, 41: 1122 – 1129.

87. Al-Hamoudi, W. K. (2010) Cardiovascular changes in cirrhosis: pathogenesis and clinical implications. The Saudi J Gastroenterol, 16:145 – 153.

88. Krowka, M.J., Dickson, E.R., Cortese, D.A. (1993) Hepatopulmonary syndrome - Clinical observations and lack of therapeutic response to somatostatin analogue. Chest, 104: 515 – 521.

89. Selim, K.M., Akriviadis, E.A., Zuckerman, E., Chen, D., Reynolds, T.B. (1998) Transjugular intrahepatic portosystemic shunt: A successful treatment for hepatopulmonary syndrome. J Am Coll Gastrenterol, 93: 455 – 458.

90. Martínez-Pallí, G., Drake, B.B., García-Pagán, J., Barberà, J., Arguedas, M.R., Rodriguez-Roisin, R., Bosch, J., Fallon, M.B. (2005) Effect of transjugular intrahepatic portosystemic shunt on pulmonary gas exchange in patients with portal hypertension and hepatopulmonary syndrome. World J Gastroenterol, 11 6858 – 6862.

91. Caldwell, S.H., Crespo, D.M. (2004) The spectrum expanded: cryptogenic cirrhosis and the natural history of non-alcoholic fatty liver disease. J Hepatol, 40:578-84.

92. Bayard, M., Holt, J., Boroughs, E. (2006) Nonalcoholic fatty liver disease. Am Fam Physician, 73(11):1961–1968.

93. Targher, G., Day, C.P., Bonora, E. (2010) Risk of cardiovascular disease in patients with nonalcoholic fatty liver disease. N Engl J Med, 363:1341–1350.

94. Goland, S., Shimoni, S., Zornitzki, T., et al. (2006) Cardiac abnormalities as a new manifestation of nonalcoholic fatty liver disease: echocardiographic and tissue Doppler imaging assessment. J Clin Gastroenterol, 40:949–955.

95. Fotbolcu, H., Yakar, T., Duman, D., et al. (2010) Impairment of the left ventricular systolic and diastolic function in patients with non-alcoholic fatty liver disease. Cardiol J, 17:457–463.

96. Perseghin, G., Lattuada, G., De Cobelli, F., et al. (2008) Increased mediastinal fat and impaired left ventricular energy metabolism in young men with newly found fatty liver. Hepatology, 47:51–58.

97. Rijzewijk, L.J., Jonker, J.T., van der Meer, R.W., et al. (2010) Effects of hepatic triglyceride content on myocardial metabolism in type 2 diabetes. J Am Coll Cardiol, 56:225–233.

98. Stefan, N., Kantartzis, K., Häring, H.U. (2008) Causes and metabolic consequences of fatty liver. Endocr Rev, 29:939–960.

99. Bonapace, S., Perseghin, G., Molon, G., Canali, G., Bertolini, L., Zoppini, G., Barbieri, E., Targher, G. (2012) Nonalcoholic fatty liver disease is associated with left ventricular diastolic dysfunction in patients with type 2 diabetes. Diabetes Care, 35(2):389-95.

100. Ray, K. (2013) NAFLD: Getting to the heart of NAFLD. Nat Rev Gastroenterol Hepatol, doi:10.1038/nrgastro.2012.243.

www.ingramcontent.com/pod-product-compliance
Lightning Source LLC
Chambersburg PA
CBHW050819220326
41598CB00006B/256